CHRONIC OBSTRUCTIVE PULMONARY DISEASE

LUNG BIOLOGY IN HEALTH AND DISEASE

Executive Editor: **Claude Lenfant**

Director, National Heart, Lung, and Blood Institute
National Institutes of Health
Bethesda, Maryland

CHRONIC OBSTRUCTIVE PULMONARY DISEASE

A BEHAVIORAL PERSPECTIVE

Edited by

A. John McSweeny

Medical College of Ohio
Toledo, Ohio

Igor Grant

University of California, San Diego
San Diego Veterans Administration Medical Center
La Jolla, California

MARCEL DEKKER, INC.   New York • Basel

Library of Congress Cataloging-in-Publication Data

Chronic obstructive pulmonary disease.

  (Lung biology in health and disease ; v. 36)
  Includes bibliographies and indexes.
  1. Lungs--Diseases, Obstructive--Psychological
aspects. I. McSweeny, A. John. II. Grant, Igor,
    . III. Series. [DNLM: 1. Behavior Therapy.
2. Behavioral Medicine. 3. Lung Diseases, Obstructive
--prevention & control. 4. Lung Diseases, Obstructive
--psychology. 5. Lung Diseases, Obstructive--therapy.
W1 LU62 v. 36 / WF 600 C5517]
RC776.03C476   1988   616.2'4   88-11807
ISBN 0-8247-7693-3</p>

MARCEL DEKKER, INC.
270 Madison Avenue, New York, New York 10016

Current printing (last digit):
10 9 8 7 6 5 4 3 2 1

Printed in the United States of America

INTRODUCTION

When a cure is impossible, it is the duty of the physician to bring contentment, comfort or even happiness to his patients to lighten their afflictions. But this does not mean necessarily that he should limit living to prolong life.

W. T. Longcope, M.D. (1932)

Perhaps no disease entity deserves such an admonition as much as chronic obstructive pulmonary disease (COPD). Indeed, COPD is a debilitating, lingering disease that affects physical performance and causes neuropsychological impairment. Many of the patients, if not bedridden, have considerably impeded activity as well as emotional distress and a diminished quality of life. It is now well established that the hallmarks of the disease, shortness of breath, hypoxia, and hypercardia, have definite psychological effects.

In the United States alone, approximately 10 million people have COPD, and a sizable number of them have reached the lingering state. Moreover, we know that most of these patients can benefit from effective palliative treatment and from psychological support. Thus, not to follow Dr. Longcope's admonition would be truly irresponsible. It therefore remains very puzzling that, as stated by Dr. Parker (Chapter 11), "chronic obstructive pulmonary disease is a condition that has been largely ignored by the behavioral science community."

The treatment of COPD is no longer the responsibility of the pulmonary disease specialist alone—it utilizes a team approach that includes the chest clinician, the nurse, the behavioral scientist, and the psychiatrist. Such a team is in fact represented by the contributors to this volume, which is edited by a psychologist, A. John McSweeny, and a psychiatrist, Igor Grant. It offers a new perspective that many will do well to adopt. The first chapter is titled "COPD: A Brief Introduction for Behavioral Scientists." All the other chapters can be viewed as "behavioral science: a comprehensive introduction to pulmonary disease specialists!"

iii

Dr. Longcope, who taught such distinguished physicians as Alvan Barach, would be happy to see this beautiful contribution to the series of monographs Lung Biology in Health and Disease, for now we have the tools to "bring contentment, comfort or even happiness" to COPD patients.

Claude Lenfant, M.D.
Bethesda, Maryland

PREFACE

This volume represents the culmination of the editors' 10 years of interest and efforts in a topic that was initially somewhat unique for behavioral scientists: respiratory disease. Until the 1980s only a handful of empirical studies existed concerning behavioral aspects of chronic obstructive pulmonary disease (COPD). Pulmonologists A. J. Block and Thomas Petty, psychiatrist Donald Dudley, and their colleagues provided the few exceptions to the general state of affairs. Fortunately this situation has changed. Spurred by developments in behavioral medicine as well as by the theoretical writings of field leaders such as George Engel, behavioral scientists, physicians, and other investigators have produced a new source of information that has immediate and/or potential application for the management and prevention of COPD.

We have attempted to bring together chapters that represent the current state of the art in behavioral science as applied to the problem of COPD. In doing so, we have covered a series of topics that will interest both pulmonologists and behavioral scientists as well as other physicians and health-care workers. Some of the chapters, of course, will be of greater interest than others to particular readers. It is our belief, however, that most readers will find all of the chapters informative and useful.

The first chapter, by pulmonologist David Cugell, provides an introduction to COPD. This chapter will be especially useful for behavioral scientists who are not familiar with COPD but should also serve as a good review for all readers. Chapter 2, by Berry and Block, represents a collaborative effort by a psychologist and a pulmonologist to cover an area with important biomedical and behavioral implications in COPD, that of sleep disorders. The authors note that the sleep disorders common in COPD patients are influenced by behavioral patterns and have an influence on cognitive and emotional functioning. In many ways, the active multidisciplinary efforts in the area of sleep research illustrate the advantages of investigating a human problem from both biomedical and behavioral perspectives.

Chapter 3, by neuropsychologist George Prigatano and psychiatrist Igor Grant, covers the neurobehavioral effects of COPD. Their review indicates that the chronic hypoxemia associated with COPD does have an impact on brain function and, consequently, on the cognitive functions which depend on the integrity of the brain. This basic finding may not surprise many clinicians, but Prigatano and Grant reveal that the relationship between COPD and different brain functions is complex. Some brain functions appear to be relatively impervious to variations in oxygen supply, while others are more sensitive. Thus, the new knowledge about COPD, brain function, and cognitive function provides an expanded understanding of the workings of the brain as well as the systems that sustain it with oxygen.

Chapter 4, by psychologist A. John McSweeny, is also concerned with the relationship of COPD to behavior. This chapter deals with the emotional, experiential, and social aspects of COPD. McSweeny notes that these aspects are closely related to brain function, as discussed by Prigatano and Grant, although one's social environment and premorbid personality also play important roles. Chapter 4 ends on an optimistic note with suggestions for researchers as well as for pulmonary clinicians on maximizing the quality of life of COPD patients.

Chapters 5 through 10 deal with the management and prevention of COPD. In Chapter 5, Thomas Petty, who has edited previous volumes in this series, reviews the current state of the art in the medical management of COPD. Like Chapter 1, by Cugell, this chapter serves as an excellent introduction or review, depending on the experience of the reader.

Chapters 6, 7, and 8 provide examples of the application of behavioral science in the management and prevention of COPD; all are written by psychologists. In Chapter 6, Robert Heaton assesses the impact of oxygen therapy on neuropsychological functioning and quality of life. His review indicates that the results are perhaps not as dramatic as we might hope in the short term but does offer some cautious optimism about the longer-term benefits of oxygen therapy on cognitive-behavioral functioning.

In Chapter 7, Robert Kaplan and Catherine Atkins report alternative methods of increasing exercise among COPD patients. Their research will have practical import to rehabilitation programs designed to achieve maximum physical performance with COPD patients. Judith Flaxman, in Chapter 8, reviews behavioral and other approaches to dealing with the major etiological agent in the development of COPD—cigarette smoking. Flaxman notes that physicians can and should give some fairly simple advice in the context of their office practices concerning smoking cessation.

In Chapter 9, Donald Dudley, a pioneer in behavioral research as applied to respiratory disorders, and Judith Sitzman, a nurse-clinician colleague, provide information on the psychosocial management of COPD patients as well as the treatment of psychiatric problems seen in COPD patients. Their chapter includes a review of psychotropic medications that may have application in COPD, information that physicians should find especially useful.

In Chapter 10, Marcia Kopacz, a nurse-clinician with considerable experience with COPD patients, discusses the management of COPD patients from a nursing point of view. The material she presents has applicability to all health professionals but is particularly well suited to the broad responsibilities that nurses have in the care of COPD patients.

In the last chapter, psychologist and National Institutes of Health officer Sydney Parker provides a summary and review of the topic of the book. Parker's chapter ties the contents of the first 10 chapters together from a historical perspective and suggests future directions that behavioral and biomedical researchers might consider.

In conclusion, we believe that this book represents an example of the fruits of the biopsychosocial model and the prediction that follows from it: that the addition of a behavioral perspective strengthens the science and practice of medicine.

A. John McSweeny
Igor Grant

CONTENTS

CONTRIBUTORS

Catherine J. Atkins, Ph.D. Division of Family Medicine, University of California, San Diego, California

David T. R. Berry, Ph.D. Assistant Professor, Department of Psychology, University of Kentucky, Lexington, Kentucky

A. Jay Block, M.D. Professor and Chief, Pulmonary Division, Department of Medicine, University of Florida, Gainesville, Florida

David W. Cugell, M.D. Bazley Professor of Pulmonary Diseases, Department of Medicine, Northwestern University Medical School, Chicago, Illinois

Donald L. Dudley, M.D. Medical Director, Washington Institute of Neurosciences, and Clinical Professor, Department of Neurological Surgery, University of Washington, Seattle, Washington

Judith Flaxman, Ph.D. Illinois School of Professional Psychology, Chicago, Illinois

Igor Grant, M.D. Professor and Acting Chairman, Department of Psychiatry, University of California, San Diego, and Assistant Chief of Psychiatry, San Diego Veterans Administration Medical Center, La Jolla, California

Robert K. Heaton, Ph.D. Professor and Co-Director, UCSD/SDSU Joint Doctoral Program in Clinical Psychology, Department of Psychiatry, University of California, San Diego, California

Robert M. Kaplan, Ph.D. Professor of Psychology and Director, Center for Behavioral and Community Health Studies, San Diego State University, and

Professor of Community and Family Medicine, University of California, San Diego, California

Marcia A. Kopacz, R.N., M.S.N.* Clinical Nurse Specialist, Division of Pulmonary and Critical Care Medicine, Henry Ford Hospital, Detroit, Michigan

A. John McSweeny, Ph.D. Associate Professor, Department of Psychiatry, Medical College of Ohio, Toledo, Ohio

Sydney R. Parker, Ph.D. Chief, Prevention, Education, and Research Training Branch, Division of Lung Diseases, National Heart, Lung, and Blood Institute, National Institutes of Health, Bethesda, Maryland

Thomas L. Petty, M.D. Professor of Medicine, and Director, Webb-Waring Lung Institute, University of Colorado Health Sciences Center, Denver, Colorado

George P. Prigatano, Ph.D. Chairman, Section of Neuropsychology, Department of Neurology, Barrow Neurological Institute, St. Joseph's Hospital and Medical Center, Phoenix, Arizona

Judith Sitzman, D.N.Sc., R.N. Adjunct Professor, Institute of Health Professions, Massachusetts General Hospital, Boston, Massachusetts, and Psychotherapist, Comprehensive Psychiatric Centers, Santa Rosa, California

---

Present affiliation:
*Quality Assurance Consultant, Department of Utilization Management, Oakland General Hospital, Madison Heights, Michigan

1

COPD: A Brief Introduction for Behavioral Scientists

DAVID W. CUGELL

Northwestern University Medical School
Chicago, Illinois

What is chronic obstructive pulmonary disease (COPD): why use such a cumbersome term, and what does it mean? Is this some type of mystical obscurantism, a concession to the "lumpers" at the expense of the "splitters" or a term that is precise and accurately descriptive? As with most things in life, it depends upon one's point of view. An obvious shortcoming of this term is the lack of either a causative or pathologic definition. Nevertheless, the term *chronic obstructive pulmonary disease* has been in widespread use for the past 25 years, is firmly entrenched in our medical literature, and has achieved a general consensus of meaning. In the 1950s an increasing prevalence of "chronic bronchitis" was observed among middle-aged male urban dwellers in Great Britain, whereas similar patients in the United States were labeled as having "emphysema." Several commissions examined this apparent discrepancy. Eventually, new terms, endorsed by professional groups on both sides of the Atlantic, emerged, and they have achieved general usage (Ciba, 1959; ATS, 1962). The single common feature linking all of the diseases included by this designation, and its convenient abbreviation COPD, is expiratory airflow obstruction.

Table 1. Lung Disease Associated with
Chronic Airflow Obstruction

Upper airway obstructive disease

    Laryngeal lesions

    Tumors

    Tracheomalacia

Lower airway obstructive diseases

    Asthma

    Chronic bronchitis

    Emphysema

    Small airway obstruction, bronchiolitis

Other chronic airway diseases

    Cystic fibrosis

    Bronchiectasis

Table 1 lists the diseases associated with some degree of airflow obstruction, and therefore eligible for inclusion in the broad designation COPD. All of these diseases have some unique or characteristic feature that permits differentiating one from another despite the universality of airflow obstruction.

In an effort to be more specific about COPD, the terms *bronchitis* and *emphysema* will be used. These terms have the advantage of describing the basic lung pathology and identifying specific abnormalities. Most patients with COPD that is not due to asthma or some unusual cause will have some pathologic changes of both bronchitis and emphysema. Since many of the symptoms that characterize these two diseases are similar, separation of one from the other on the basis of clinical manifestations is usually not possible; and use of the combined term *bronchitis-emphysema,* although cumbersome, is highly appropriate. Asthma, another lower airway obstructive lung disease, differs in many ways from the bronchitis-emphysema complex. A major distinction is that asthma is an intermittent malady. For most patients, effective treatment enables them to pursue a normal or near-normal existence. During the symptom-free interval the typical asthmatic patient not only feels well but also functions in a normal manner. The onset of asthma generally occurs at a younger age than bronchitis-emphysema, although there are many exceptions. When asthma appears in childhood, it tends to disappear in late adolescence. When asthma first appears in the fourth or fifth decade of life, effective treatment is more difficult and symptoms tend to progress. The typical complaints of the asthma patient—dyspnea, wheeze, cough, and chest tightness—are the direct result of airway narrowing and its associated partial airflow obstruction. Because the decrease in airway diameter is produced by spasmodic contraction of smooth muscle within the airways, and can be completely reversed either spontaneously or with medication, this intermittent airway constriction is known as *bronchospasm.*

Many of the same clinical manifestations experienced by asthmatic patients, such as intermittent increases in dyspnea, cough, and wheezing, also occur in patients with COPD. The major mechanisms for this transient increase in symptoms are increased airway secretions and bronchospasm with their attendant aggravation of airflow obstruction. Despite these similarities, COPD patients differ substantially from patients with typical asthmas. They seldom exhibit the heightened responses to plant or animal products; they do not revert to normal between episodes; and they tend to be much more refractory to the same drugs that relieve bronchospasm in most asthmatic patients.

The tracheobronchial tree (Fig. 1) is commonly divided into an upper and lower portion, although there is no universal agreement on where the separation occurs. The larynx and the tracheal bifurcation are two frequently used sites. Pathologic change and functional impairment in patients with asthma, bronchitis, and emphysema usually occur in airways several generations distal to the trachea and main stem bronchi. Therefore, we are concerned to only a limited degree with upper airway diseases. Another partition of the tracheobronchial tree that is functionally useful but lacks anatomical definition is a division of the airways into those that are outside and those within the thorax. Airways within the thorax are subject to the mechanical forces associated with breathing and coughing on both their internal and external surfaces whereas extrathoracic airways are subject to those same forces on only their internal or lumenal surface. A vigorous cough may produce a transient increase of intrathoracic pressure of 100 to 200 cm H_2O. Pressures of that magnitude could easily cause lung damage if dissipated across the airway wall. However, when those pressures result from vigorous expiratory maneuvers the pressure is applied to both the pleural and luminal surfaces so that no damage results. In asthma, bronchitis, and emphysema the major sites of obstruction are in airways from the second or third down to the eighth or ninth of the 25 or so generations of airways. The term *small airways* refers

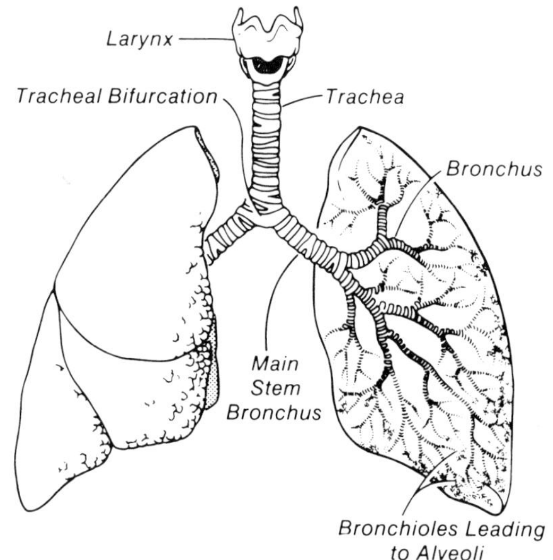

Figure 1 Normal anatomy of the lung, airways, and their subdivisions. Each of the main bronchi branch 16 to 26 times before terminating in alveolar structures. Accompanying the bronchi as they subdivide progressively are corresponding branches of the pulmonary artery that eventually become a capillary network in the alveoli where gas exchange occurs. The right lung is subdivided into three lobes—upper, middle, and lower— whereas on the left side there are only two distinct lobes.

to more distal portions (approximately tenth to twenty-fifth generations of the tracheobronchial tree) where airways are 2 mm in diameter or less (Fig. 1).

Although all of the diseases in Table 1 qualify as members of the COPD group, this term is commonly restricted to describing patients with either bronchitis, emphysema, or some combination thereof. The effects of and adaptations to these two specific forms of obstructive lung disease are the subject of this volume.

I. Chronic Bronchitis and Emphysema

A. Pathogenesis

Most patients with bronchitis and emphysema are male. In a large, multicenter cooperative study of advanced COPD conducted in the United States and Canada, 160 patients were male and only 43 were female (NOTT, 1980). Once the disease becomes established, its progress is generally similar in both sexes. Because the onset is insidious the age at which the disease first develops is difficult to determine. Significant symptoms and functional defects are usually present by the fourth decade although patients may deny any disability but readily admit to a chronic cough. Additional symptoms and disability may develop over the course of several years, but it can take 20 years or more. The ultimate cause for these diseases is unknown, but they are almost universally associated with heavy cigarette consumption, and frequently with recurrent bronchial infections. The common clinical unit of cigarette use is the pack-year(20 cigarettes per day for 1 year). Virtually all patients with these disorders have a cigarette consumption of at least 20 pack-years, and the majority have consumed two to three times that amount. The association between excessive cigarette use and subsequent bronchitis-emphysema is sufficiently great that in some studies a history of heavy cigarette use is considered essential; without it the diagnosis is not complete. Despite this extremely high degree of association, a very few patients—identical in every respect to all other patients—with bronchitis-emphysema have not been smokers. Also, not all heavy smokers develop bronchitis or emphysema. These apparent inconsistencies merely reflect variations in host response to a common injury.

Another strong association is the frequent occurrence of respiratory tract infections. Patients often report that whenever they develop a head cold it "goes down to my chest," and some patients report several antecedent episodes of pneumonia. Healthy people have a bacteria-free tracheobronchial tree; secretions removed from below the larynx are invariably sterile. In a patient with established bronchitis-emphysema the secretions frequently con-

tain microorganisms, but it is often difficult to differentiate between those
that have taken up chronic residence and intermittent "invaders" that are responsible for an increase in symptoms plus a change in the quantity and character of the sputum. *Hemophilus influenzae, Streptococcus pneumoniae,
Mycoplasma pneumoniae,* and rhinovirus, often in combination, are the most
frequent respiratory pathogens (Gump et al., 1976). Intermittent bronchial
infections with these and other pathogens probably contribute to the development of bronchitis-emphysema. Additional contributory factors are high
levels of air pollution, both in the community and at the work place; childhood asthma and respiratory infections; and recurrent pulmonary infections
among family members. All of these factors are associated with bronchitis
and emphysema, to a greater or lesser degree, but are not specific causes. The
strongest and most undeniable association is with tobacco.

Patients subjected to equal respiratory insults such as cigarette smoke,
air pollutants, and infections may either escape unscathed, develop bronchitis,
or develop emphysema. These different responses result not from minor dis-
similarities in exposure but from inherent differences between patients.
Robin and O'Neill (1963) designated some patients with obstructive lung
disease as "fighters," and others as "nonfighters." Fighters, primarily patients
with the lung tissue changes of emphysema, attempt to preserve the integrity
of their arterial blood gas composition no matter what the "cost" in breathing
effort. The result is a marked increase in the work of breathing, excessive dyspnea, but preservation of arterial blood gas composition. On the other hand,
patients with mucus hypersecretion and lower airway infection (signs of
chronic bronchitis) are content to accept a reduced level of alveolar ventilation
with concomitant abnormalities in blood gas content, and thus the designation
"nonfighter."

Other terms that have been even more widely used to describe the two
major categories of chronic obstructive pulmonary disease patients are "pink
puffer" and "blue bloater" (Dornhorst, 1955). The former term is equivalent
to the "fighter": the emphysematous patient who maintains normal arterial
blood gases, appears to be puffing all the time, and has severe dyspnea. The
"blue bloater" designation is equivalent to the "nonfighter," the bronchitic
patient with a low arterial oxygen tension and a cyanotic appearance (hence
the terms "blue") plus edema that creates the "bloated" appearance.

Recent studies provide some explanation for the divergent pathways
that patients follow in the course of developing obstructive lung disease. In
a study of the relatives of patients with bronchitis Mountain and co-workers
(1978) found that the healthy relatives of patients with abnormal arterial

blood gases (blue bloaters) were peculiarly resistant or had reduced sensitivity to the increase in ventilation normally provoked by the inhalation of carbon-dioxide-enriched or oxygen-deficient atmospheres. A similar insensitivity has been observed by some among endurance athletes and their nonathletic siblings (Saunders et al., 1976). It may be that the development of bronchitis in one patient and emphysema in another is in large measure determined by the premorbid sensitivity to respiratory stimuli. Perhaps those of us who happen to be born with a relative insensitivity to respiratory stimuli may be destined to develop the bronchitic form of obstructive lung disease whereas those of us with a heightened or normal response to the same stimuli will develop emphysema, should we be so misfortunate to develop obstructive lung disease at all.

B. Typical Clinical Presentation

The usual patient is a male, in his 60s or a bit older, with shortness of breath on activity and cough as the major complaints. There will likely be a long history of regular cigarette use; many years of cough, particularly in the morning; sputum production; and the gradual appearance and progression of breathing difficulty. Dyspnea is first noted during vigorous activity, and may subsequently appear in conjunction with changes in atmospheric conditions, upper respiratory infections, and during less strenuous maneuvers such as stair climbing, carrying small bundles, or bending over to tie one's shoes. Wheezing, especially in conjunction with respiratory infections, physical activity, or climatic changes, is often present. Some patients have daily sputum production, others have a nonproductive cough, and in some a productive cough is present in the early stages of their disease and subsequently the sputum production disappears. Smoking cessation is generally associated with a decrease in cough and sputum production, but with minimal improvement in effort dyspnea.

In the early and intermediate phases of the disease there will be few if any visible signs of disease, unless the patient is observed during some physical activity when respiratory distress far out of proportion to the degree of exertion may be obvious. Few abnormalities can be detected during physical examination of the patient at this early stage. The intensity of breath sounds heard through the stethoscope may be somewhat diminished. Wheezing and coarse, rattling sounds or rhonchi may be audible, especially during forced expiratory maneuvers. The chest x-ray film is usually normal. The expiratory airflow obstruction measured by simple lung function tests confirms the diagnosis.

As the disease becomes further advanced and symptoms increase in both

number and severity, clinical distinctions between obstructive lung disease due
to chronic bronchitis and due to emphysema may appear, although the majority of patients will have both types of tissue damage and a clear difference may
not be apparent. In the patient with predominant bronchitis there is usually
a more prominent history of cough, sputum production, and recurrent pulmonary infections. Symptoms generally begin at an earlier age than in patients
in whom the dominant tissue change is emphysema. The bronchitis patient
eventually develops cyanosis: a bluish pallor to the skin secondary to inadequate saturation of hemoglobin with oxygen. Wheezes, rhonchi, and coarse
crackles are audible upon auscultation of the chest. Right ventricular cardiac
failure with its attendant signs of an enlarged liver, swollen ankles, and increased abdominal girth due to fluid accumulation may occur in the late stages.
Radiologic examination of the chest usually demonstrates normal-appearing
lungs and some cardiac enlargement. Lung function tests show severe airflow
obstruction, marked increase in airway resistance, normal total lung capacity,
a gross mismatch in the distribution of air and blood within the lung, and significant arterial blood gas abnormalities with both an oxygen deficit and carbon dioxide excess. At this advanced stage of the disease—with cyanosis due
to a blood oxygen deficit and peripheral edema due to heart failure—"blue
bloater" becomes an apt designation.

Other patients with moderate to severe obstructive lung disease may
have little or no bronchitis, but do have severe anatomical emphysema. They
tend to be in their sixth or seventh decade and dyspnea is the major clinical
complaint. Cough and sputum production are often inconsequential at this
phase of the disease. Dyspnea can be so overwhelming and so disabling that
it takes hours for the patient to complete such simple tasks as shaving or
dressing. Additional complaints may include chest pain, episodes of near
panic due to air hunger, and weight loss. The latter is a grave prognostic sign.
The chest tends to enlarge and assumes a barrel shape. There is often a
marked disparity between the large thorax and the very thin abdomen and
extremities. One mechanism that is normally used to help achieve additional
ventilation, either in connection with vigorous physical activity in healthy
people or for simple tasks in patients with obstructive lung disease, is contraction of the neck muscles. These muscle bundles run from various locations on the base of the skull to the first rib, scapula, and clavicle. Chest
expansion is facilitated when they contract, and this may be obvious in patients following very limited activity. As a consequence of the frequent use
of these neck muscles patients will either maintain or sometimes increase
their collar size despite a considerable reduction in other body dimensions
(Fig. 2).

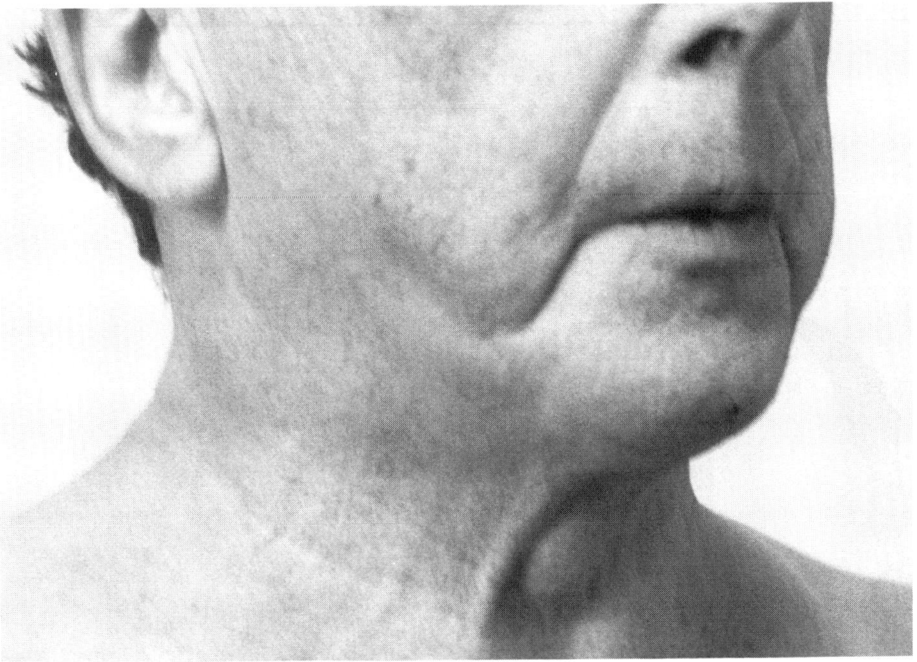

Figure 2 Pursed lip breathing in a patient with severe COPD. Because of hypertrophy of the neck muscles, the neck appears full although the patient has lost considerable weight.

The breath sounds become very distant or difficult to hear and the heart tones become faint. Patients have obvious respiratory distress and adopt a breathing pattern that consists of an inspiratory gasp and a prolonged expiratory phase. Some patients utilize a pursed lip expiratory maneuver (Fig. 2). This form of expiration has long been noted in patients with COPD. The increased intrathoracic pressures generated by exaggerated breathing efforts can produce excessive airway compression, with narrowing and increased airflow resistance, all of which make it much more difficult to breathe. Expiring with pursed lips results in a slight increase in pressure inside the airway, thereby decreasing its tendency to collapse during exaggerated breathing. Because some patients benefit from pursed lip breathing it has been recommended for use by all patients with COPD. However, unless it is adopted spontaneously, patients are unlikely to derive any benefit from the conscious use of the

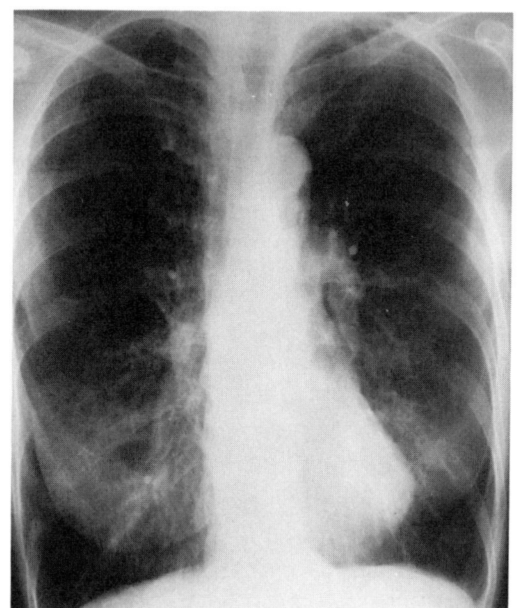

(a)

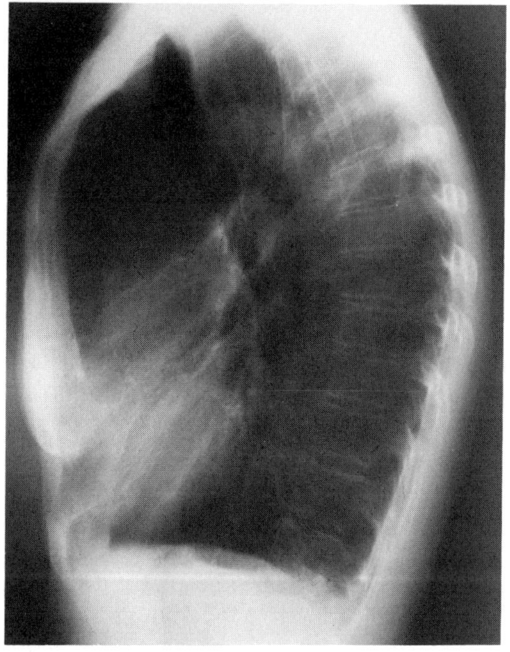

(b)

maneuver. Patients with advanced disease sometimes experience some relief from their dyspnea by leaning forward on their elbows if seated, or placing their outstretched arms and hands on a table edge when standing.

The chest x-ray film at this stage of the disease confirms the barrel-shaped thorax, a diaphragm that is flattened and in a lowered position, hyperinflated lung fields, and a small cardiac silhouette (Fig. 3). Occasionally, blebs or bullae (air-containing spaces that replace normal lung tissue) are seen on the chest film. Lung function tests show the same severe degree of airflow obstruction found in patients with bronchitis, but there is also a generous enlargement of the total lung capacity, a marked increase in residual volume, changes in other lung volume compartments, but with preservation of or only minor changes in arterial blood gas composition.

C. Pathology

In the clinical description of a "typical patient," few distinctions were made between those clinical manifestations attributable to bronchitis, which is characterized by inflammation, and emphysema, which is characterized by tissue destruction and loss of alveolar architecture. Although distinct and unique morphologic changes occur in both the airways and the lung parenchyma (tissue), they often coexist to a variable degree.

The walls of central bronchi consist of outer columnar epithelial cells, with cilia protruding from many of them (Fig. 4). Interspersed between the columnar cells are goblet cells, which are the source of some of the mucus that lines the respiratory tract. These and other epithelial cells are anchored to a basement membrane that separates them from a submucosal region containing supporting structures, muscle tissue, and additional mucous glands. The submucosa rests on plates or rings of cartilage. Patients with chronic bronchitis have excessive respiratory tract mucus and enlarged mucous glands. This is commonly expressed in a semiquantitative manner as the Reid index:

Figure 3 Posterioanterior (a) and left lateral (b) view of the thorax of a patient with far-advanced COPD, primarily emphysema. Note the low position and flattened contour of the diaphragms; sparse vascular markings, particularly in the upper lung zones; small cardiac silhouette; increased anterior-posterior diameter of the thorax best seen on the lateral view; and a large air space occupying the region between the sternum and the anterior surface of the heart seen only on lateral view.

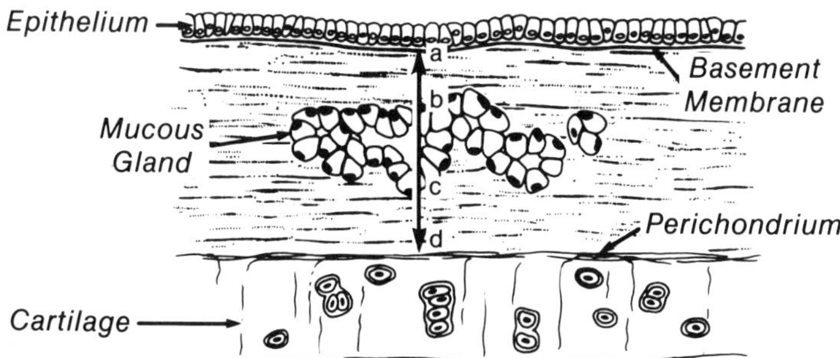

Figure 4 Schematic representation of the bronchial wall and underlying cartilage. The Reid index is the ratio of mucous gland width (b-c) to bronchial wall thickness measured from the basement membrane to the perichondrium (a-b). (Reproduced with permission from Thurlbeck, 1976.)

the ratio of the maximum thickness of the mucous gland to the bronchial wall (Fig. 4). Bronchial gland mucus is deposited in the airway lumen via small channels that can be seen with the unaided eye as pinpoint openings on the mucosal surface. The normal coordinated, rhythmic movement of the cilia is frequently depressed or virtually absent in patients with chronic bronchitis, thereby markedly depressing a major mechanism for disposing of impacted particulates (i.e., smoke, dust, and other particulate matter that enter the lungs). Bronchial epithelial cells observed in tissue culture show an abrupt cessation of ciliary movement when exposed to cigarette smoke and then a gradual recovery. Thus, the smoker may be plagued by not only excessive mucus production but also an impaired clearance mechanism. This results in plugging of smaller bronchi. Different changes have been observed in "small" airways: those that are 2 mm in diameter or less. In airways of those dimensions there are no mucous glands, no cilia, and no cartilage. Marked narrowing of the lumen of small airways due to mucosal thickening has been found in patients with chronic bronchitis, and in young asymptomatic smokers.

One of the "official" definitions of emphysema is ". . . a condition of the lung characterized by abnormal, permanent enlargement of the air spaces distal to the terminal bronchi accompanied by destruction of their walls" (Ciba, 1959). This definition includes a description of both tissue changes and the region of the lung where it occurs. These locations are defined as centrilobular, panlobular, and paraseptal. The functional unit to which these relate is the acinus. The progressive branching of the tracheobronchial tree ends with a terminal bronchiole, of which there are approximately 28,000 in human lungs (Thurlbeck, 1976). That portion of the lung distal to the terminal bronchial is the acinus, and it consists primarily of alveolar tissue, which is the gas-exchanging segment of the lung. The acinus, also known as a lobule, is visible to the unaided eye. Centrilobular emphysema is generally confined to the central portion of the lobule whereas in panlobular disease enlargement and destruction of the airspaces involve the entire acinus more or less uniformly. In paraseptal emphysema the peripheral portion of the acinus is primarily involved. Quantitative methods for expressing the degree or quantity of emphysema have been developed. They depend upon use of either a grid, point counting, light transmission, or comparable methods for scoring the presence or absence of tissue on a large slice of the lung. The more severe the disease, the greater the number and the larger the area of the "holes." The regions of the lung that are examined must be clearly specified because of the spotty distribution of emphysematous changes. From visual inspection of lung slices it is immediately obvious that anthracotic (carbon-containing, from tobacco and other smoke) pigment is most heavily deposited in those regions where lung tissue destruction is maximal. Despite this strong association, no cause and effect relationship has been demonstrated. It is not clear whether emphysema precedes the apparent increase in pigment or if the pigment serves as a nidus and "concentrates" agents or materials that are then capable of producing the tissue destruction.

A variety of changes in other lung structures, primarily blood vessels, occur in patients with obstructive lung disease, but these do not become significant until the COPD has become sufficiently severe to produce abnormal gas exchange, or cardiovascular complications, such as cor pulmonale and heart failure.

The normal aging process produces changes in lung structure that resemble the changes in patients with COPD. There is a progressive loss of elastic recoil, beginning between 20 and 30 years of age. This changes the balance of forces acting on the lungs so that the resting end-expiratory position tends to enlarge with age, and the alveolar dimensions increase. In many ways the alterations in structure and function that occur with aging resemble those that develop, although in an accelerated fashion, in patients with COPD. These include the frequent appearance of centrilobular emphysema and apical bullous disease in an elderly person in whom there have been no clinical signs of lung disease.

D. Clinical Variants

Bullous Disease

An occasional finding in patients with obstructive lung disease is the presence
of blebs or bullae. Both appear on the chest x-ray film as air-containing
spaces confined by an extremely thin tissue wall and an absence of normal
lung markings within the air-filled space. They are more common in the upper lung regions, frequently multiple, and generally circular in appearance.
A bleb is an air space that originates at the periphery of the lung due to a
separation of visceral pleura from lung parenchyma. A bulla is a more deeply
seated air-containing space with parenchyma on all sides. The radiologic appearance and clinical consequences of these lesions are similar and little purpose is served by attempting to differentiate one from another. Other air-
containing, circular abnormalities can be seen on chest x-ray films. Cavities
usually have thick walls and associated radiologic and clinical signs of current
or prior infection that readily differentiate them from blebs and bullae. Cysts
are rounded air space lesions, bronchial in origin, more central in location, and
also have thick walls.

Bullous disease, a term generally used to include blebs, bullae, or both,
has attracted considerable attention because in some patients these air-containing spaces enlarge and compress surrounding lung tissue. Surgical excision of
the offending bulla can produce dramatic benefit if the compressed lung is
capable of returning to near-normal function. When bullae are unilateral, uni-
locular, occupy more than one-third of the hemithorax, and are associated
with a loss of lung volume rather than airflow obstruction, the surgical results
are excellent. When there is severe airflow obstructive disease, the results are
uncertain. Among 15 patients followed for an average of 10.3 years, the
deterioration in expiratory airflow was similar to that observed in patients
with obstructive lung disease and no bullae (Gaensler et al., 1983). Selecting
patients who might benefit from surgical intervention can be extremely difficult. Serial radiographs that document progressive compression by expanding
bullae are extremely helpful. Computed tomographic lung scans may reveal
bullae that are not apparent on regular films. In addition to the customary
pulmonary function tests, special physiological measurements such as quantity of trapped gas in the lung, exercise studies, and measurements of regional
pulmonary perfusion using scintiscans are all useful in reaching a decision concerning surgery. Even patients with far advanced obstructive lung disease, in
whom any type of surgery would normally be contraindicated, may be candi-
dates because even a small increment in lung function can be very beneficial.

Complications of the bullous lesions themselves include periodic accumulation of fluid that can appear, subside, and recur in the absence of any obvious clinical infection. Bullae can also become infected and resemble a lung abscess, and they may rupture, creating a pneumothorax.

Genetic Factors

Normal human serum contains a protein, alpha-1-antiprotease, that is capable of inhibiting several types of proteolytic (protein-destroying) enzymes. One of these enzymes is elastase, and it is capable of digesting elastin, the major structural protein of the lung. A link between an absence of this protease inhibitor in the serum and pulmonary emphysema was first identified in 1963 and has subsequently provoked extensive studies of biochemical abnormalities and genetic factors that may contribute to the development of emphysema. Pulmonary infection and smoking greatly increase the population of monocytes, macrophages, and polymorphonuclear leukocytes in the lung, and all of these cells can release proteolytic materials. Enzyme inhibitors in the serum prevent proteolysis. Patients in whom there is a congenital absence of the alpha-1-protease inhibitor in the blood serum are at a very high risk of developing emphysema, particularly if they smoke. There are some clinical differences between patients who develop emphysema as a result of a serum enzyme deficiency, and the much greater number of patients with COPD and no measurable enzyme defect. Disease associated with the enzyme deficiency tends to start at the lung bases, occurs in men and women with approximately equal frequency, and first appears in the third to fourth decade of life; these features clearly distinguish it from the much more commonplace form of COPD. Not everyone with alpha-1-antiprotease deficiency develops emphysema. Patients who do not smoke and live in relatively unpolluted regions may be spared.

A large number of population surveys have been completed to determine the prevalence of obstructive lung disease. In general, the symptoms of bronchitis and airflow obstruction are two to three times higher among first-degree relatives of patients with definite COPD than among the population at large. Despite definite familial aggregation no specific genetic factors that might explain family clustering have been demonstrated conclusively.

Compensatory Emphysema

This refers to the radiologic appearance of an overdistended lung or portion thereof. This can occur in a patient following surgical resection, with compensatory overdistention of a portion of the remaining lung tissue. Unless the patient also has COPD the overdistention is not associated with expiratory airflow obstruction and has nothing in common with COPD. Compensatory emphysema does occur in an exaggerated form in infants and children in association with pneumonia, and is known as lobar emphysema. It can be sufficiently severe to displace the mediastinum and partially compress the remaining lung. The process is generally reversible, but may require surgical intervention. Two chronic diseases associated with long-standing lung infections—cystic fibrosis and bronchiectasis (Table 1)—may cause sufficient scarring and bronchial distortion to produce expiratory airflow obstruction. Their cause, course, and basic pathologic nature differ substantially from COPD, and should not be confused with this much more common clinical problem.

E. Laboratory Tests

The range of tests that can be used to evaluate patients with COPD can be comprehensive and include assessment of multiple organ systems, or they can be exceedingly simple and limited to a single quantitative measure of the most important functional disturbance: airflow obstruction.

Spirometry is commonly used in diagnostic work-ups. Such pulmonary function testing will generally demonstrate decreased expiratory airflow but a normal (or increased) vital capacity* (in restrictive lung disease, e.g., fibrosis, vital capacity is usually reduced). The most common and reliable flow measure is the forced expiratory volume (FEV) per unit time. $FEV_{1.0}$ measures the amount of air expelled during a forced vital capacity in 1 sec, and this will be reduced in COPD. Another commonly used test of airflow limitation is the midflow, also called the forced expiratory flow 25 to 75 (FEF 25-75%), which is calculated from the time required to exhale the midhalf of the vital capacity.

In its very early stages, when the patient has minimal symptoms that he considers more of a nuisance than a sign of disease, airflow obstruction and possible evidence of bronchospasm may be the only measurable abnormalities. These are most directly and simply assessed by measuring the forced expiratory volume in 1 sec before and after bronchodilator administration. A chest x-ray film should be obtained, primarily to exclude other pulmonary pathologic changes and to have as a baseline against which subsequent films can be compared. As the disease progresses and functional disturbances increase,

---

*Vital capacity is the volume of air expelled by maximum expiratory effort after a maximum inspiration.

many additional abnormalities can be detected by lung function testing.
Nevertheless, with some specific exceptions such as preoperative assessment
and disability evaluation, these additional studies are of minimal benefit to
the managing physician in his or her day-to-day care of the patient. At more
severe stages of the disease the most important additional laboratory test is
measurement of arterial blood gas content. Carbon dioxide retention, acid-
base imbalance, and hypoxemia may develop, either in combination or separately. If present, they have important therapeutic implications (see Chap 6).
Further laboratory testing is obviously indicated in the event that patients
develop complications, such as cor pulmonale, pulmonary infections, and
pneumothorax.

F. Complications

The major complication of importance is the onset of cardiac disease and
heart failure. When this occurs conventional treatment for heart failure
should be used, but it is unlikely to be very successful in the absence of aggressive treatment and some improvement in the underlying lung disease.
Associated with the complicating heart disease, or cor pulmonale, is a
reduction in blood oxygen, carbon dioxide retention, and an increase in
the concentration of red blood cells: polycythemia. Continuous supplemental oxygen is generally needed to restore cardiac compensation and reduce
the rate of red blood cell production. Cor pulmonale is associated with the
bronchitic form of COPD, and rarely develops, except as a terminal event, in
the "pink puffer," the patient with a loss of alveolar architecture and anatomical emphysema. Other events that occur in the course of COPD are
considered complications by some, but might just as well be considered manifestations of the underlying disease process. For example, bronchopulmonary
infections, respiratory failure, and rupture of a bleb or bulla have already been
noted in the "typical case" description.

II. Epilogue

Patients, their families, and their doctors all agree that COPD is a debilitating,
depressing, disabling, dismal malady. Apart from its multiple symptoms and
functional disturbances, some of which have been detailed above, COPD
also exerts a profound influence on the psychosocial aspects of life to a degree that is frequently not appreciated by those primarily concerned with the
patient's medical care. Careful medical management, as described in Chap 6,
plus a full understanding of the psychosocial implications of this disease—the

main subject of this text—will markedly enhance the quality of life for those who already have this disease. Prevention should be our ultimate objective. As of this writing, that can be best achieved by control of air pollution, primarily the personal type that results from cigarette smoking. Important as it may be to take care of our patients now, we should all look forward to the day when COPD no longer requires our attention.

References

American Thoracic Society (1962). Definitions and classification of chronic bronchitis, asthma, and pulmonary emphysema. *Am. Rev. Respir. Dis.* **85**:762-769.

Ciba Guest Symposium Report (1959). Terminology, definitions and classifications of chronic pulmonary emphysema and related conditions. *Thorax* **14**:286-299.

Dornhorst, A. C. (1955). Respiratory insufficiency. *Lancet* **1**:1185-1187.

Gaensler, E. A., Cugell, D., Knudson, R., and Fitzgerald, M. (1983). Surgical management of emphysema. *Clin. Chest Med.* **4**:443-463.

Gump, D. W., Phillips, D. A., Forsyth, B. R., McIntosh, K., Lamborn, K. R., and Stouch, W. H. (1976). Role of infection in chronic bronchitis. *Am. Rev. Respir. Dis.* **113**:465-474.

Mountain, R., Zwillich, C., and Weill, J. V. (1978). Hypoventilation in obstructive lung disease. The role of familial factors. *N. Engl. J. Med.* **298**: 521-525.

Nocturnal Oxygen Therapy Trial Group (1980). Continuous or nocturnal oxygen therapy in hypoxemic chronic obstructive lung disease: A clinical trial. *Ann. Intern. Med.* **93**:39-398.

Robin, E. D., and O'Neill, R. P. (1963). The fighter versus the nonfighter: Control of ventilation in chronic obstructive pulmonary disease. *Arch. Environ. Health* **7**:125-128.

Saunders, N. A., Leeder, S. R., and Rebuck, A. S. (1976). Ventilatory response to carbon dioxide in young athletes: A family study. *Am. Rev. Respir. Dis.* **113**:497-502.

Thurlbeck, W. B. (1976). *Chronic Airflow Obstruction in Lung Disease.* Philadelphia, W. B. Saunders.

2

Sleep-Disordered Breathing in Patients with COPD

DAVID T. R. BERRY

University of Kentucky
Lexington, Kentucky

A. JAY BLOCK

University of Florida
Gainesville, Florida

I. Introduction

Sleep-disordered breathing (SDB) involves respiratory dysfunction that occurs
during sleep. Although many patients with SDB have normal daytime respiratory parameters, the onset of sleep unmasks a nocturnal breathing disorder.
Overnight breathing disturbances have recently been linked to cardiopulmonary complications, daytime somnolence, and neuropsychological decline.
Significant physiological and behavioral sequelae are therefore attributable
to nighttime hypoxia.

Chronic obstructive pulmonary disease (COPD) patients are hypoxic on
a continuing basis, secondary to their pulmonary disorder. The physiological
and behavioral consequences of this chronic hypoxia are explored in other
chapters of this volume. However, it now appears that many COPD patients
suffer exacerbations of their chronic hypoxia during episodes of SDB. Given
the consequences of nocturnal breathing dysfunction in other patient groups,
it is likely that SDB aggravates the physiological and behavioral deficits seen
in COPD, resulting in a worsening of day-to-day functioning in affected patients.

This chapter will focus on SDB and its consequences in patients with chronic pulmonary disease. Initially, an overview of present knowledge of SDB and its sequelae in other patient groups will be presented, followed by a review of recent findings regarding SDB and associated deficits in COPD patients. Taken together, the two sections will provide the broad context of the SDB phenomenon as well as an outline of its characteristics and consequences in patients with chronic pulmonary disease.

II. Sleep-Disordered Breathing in Subjects with Normal Daytime Respiration

A. Definitions

Sleep-disordered breathing is a broad term subsuming a variety of respiratory disturbances that may occur during sleep. Some discussion of sleep-related physiological phenomena is necessary for an understanding of SDB. Sleep is now conceptualized as a time of complex neural events. During sleep, the brain moves cyclically through light sleep (stages 1 and 2), slow-wave sleep (stages 3 and 4), and rapid eye movement (REM) sleep. Each of these discrete stages is characterized by a distinct set of physiological events which are known to include alterations in control and expression of respiratory rhythms. The neural respiratory control mechanism tolerates different levels of hypoxia and hypercapnia in different sleep stages. For example, it appears that light sleep and REM sleep are the most likely periods for respiratory instabilities (i.e., apneas, hyponeas, and oxygen desaturations) to occur. Sleep-disordered breathing is thought to result from an interaction of central neural anomalies and structural abnormalities, which together result in a compromised airway (Sullivan et al., 1984).

Nocturnal breathing is, therefore, a multiply determined phenomenon. In the face of this complexity, clinical identification of pathologic aspects of nocturnal respiration has yet to reach a mature stage. Both qualitative and quantitative approaches have been utilized, but few, if any, validation studies of these criteria have been reported (George and Kryger, 1985). The most commonly reported SDB events include apneas, hypopneas, and oxygen desaturations, defined as follows:

Apnea: Pauses in respiration that last 10 sec or more (Guilleminault et al., 1978)

Hypopnea: Declines in respiratory amplitude accompanied by drops in oxygen saturation (Block et al., 1979b)

Oxygen desaturation: Drops in arterial oxygen saturation (Block et al., 1979b)

Characterization of these events has tended to emerge more from fortuitous availability of measurement technology than from a systematic exploration of normal and pathologic nocturnal respiration. It remains possible that future comprehensive research into the issue may result in identification of other pathologic respiratory events.

With these caveats aside, it must be acknowledged that measurement of apnea, hypopnea, and oxygen desaturations has proved clinically useful in indexing problematic levels of SDB, as well as in predicting significant daytime sequelae such as hypersomnolence and neuropsychological impairment. Additionally, the relative standardization of these events in diagnostic sleep studies has resulted in accumulation of much useful data on the SDB phenomenon. Until better validated criteria are introduced, it is important to measure comprehensively and report these events in research and clinical reports. Such comprehensive measurements will allow comparison with other reports, and build on the current database.

As alluded to above, measurements of apneas, hypopneas, and oxygen desaturations are frequently used to index the severity of SDB. One popular index is the apnea + hypopnea index (AHI). In calculating an AHI, the number of apneas and hypopneas observed are divided by the number of hours of sleep obtained. A patient with 10 apneas and 10 hypopneas in 5 hr of sleep would have an AHI of 4. This AHI, while not well validated, is widely used in comparing diagnostic or research studies in which different total sleep times are obtained.

Patients who experience multiple episodes of SDB associated with loud snoring and daytime hypersomnolence are diagnosed clinically with a sleep apnea syndrome (SAS) (ASDC, 1979). It has been proposed that an AHI greater than of equal to 5 is diagnostic of a sleep apnea syndrome (Guilleminault et al., 1978). However, it seems clear that use of such a cutoff score implicitly and improperly assumes a linear relationship between SDB and associated symptoms. That the relationship between SDB and daytime symptoms is a complex, probably multiply determined one is indicated by at least two reports. Orr et al. (1979) matched four SAS patients with four asymptomatic heavy-snoring males on absolute numbers of SDB events, but observed differences in daytime functioning. Although these subjects experienced similar numbers of SDB events, they presented grossly divergent daytime functioning, suggesting that numbers of SDB events are not the sole determinant of the disease. In a related report, Berry and co-workers (1984b) found that healthy older subjects were significantly more likely to display an AHI greater than 5 than were healthy younger subjects, indicating an interaction between age and level of SDB in subjects with normal daytime functioning. Taken together, these two reports indicate that the association between SDB and physiological and behavioral consequences is a multiply determined one, rather than a simple linear one as is implicitly assumed in utilization of a single diagnostic threshold.

B. Techniques for Monitoring Nocturnal Respiration

Diagnosis of sleep apnea syndrome and related nocturnal breathing disorders is accomplished by measurements obtained during overnight monitoring of various physiological parameters (polysomnography) in a sleep disorders laboratory. Typically, clinical sleep laboratories are run by neurologists, pulmonologists, or psychologists who have training and experience in the diagnosis and treatment of sleep disorders.

Interested readers are referred to Bornstein (1982) for a detailed description of techniques for monitoring respiration during sleep. In brief, a typical polysomnographic study includes measures of several aspects of nocturnal physiology, such as electrical activity of the brain and heart, airflow at mouth and nose, and arterial oxygen saturation. Neural electrical activity is recorded from surface-mounted electrodes attached to standardized positions on the scalp. Recorded electroencephalographic (EEG) signals are used to judge the stage of sleep throughout the night. Electrocardiographic (ECG) electrodes on the chest measure heart activity and document cardiac dysfunction during sleep. Respiration is recorded through thermistors at the mouth and nose, which measure temperature change and indicate whether airflow is attenuated or absent, as in hypopneas or apneas, respectively. Respiratory effort is measured through strain gauges that monitor muscular effort in breathing. An oximeter, mounted on the ear lobe, provides a continuous indication of arterial oxygen saturation and detects periods of oxygen desaturation.

All of these signals are routed to a polygraph, which transforms signals and records them on chart paper for a permanent record. Following completion of the study, each record is visually scored for EEG sleep stage, ECG abnormalities, and SDB events, which are scored from thermister, oximeter, and strain gauge signals. Although several systems exist for scoring SDB events, no reliability and validity studies have been offered in support of these criteria.

C. Physiological and Behavioral Deficits Associated with SDB

The gradual accumulation of data on SDB events has led to a better understanding of the physiological and behavioral sequelae of the disorder. These deficits associated with SDB may be loosely grouped into three categories: cardio-pulmonary abnormalities, sleep/wake cycle alterations, and intellectual deterioration. Of additional importance in a discussion of these sequelae is the concept of a continuum of SDB. This continuum of increasing SDB extends from groups such as young, healthy males and premenopausal women, who experience relatively little SDB (Block et al., 1980), through heavy-snoring, middle-aged men, who experience substantial amounts of SDB (Berry and Block, 1984), up to frank sleep apnea syndrome patients, who might experience up to hundreds of SDB events during a night's sleep (Guilleminault et al., 1978). However, this continuum of SDB is not the sole determinant of daytime symptoms in the disorder. As noted earlier, absolute level of SDB does not reliably predict presence or absence of daytime deficits. Other factors, such as age, or number of years suffering SDB events may mediate the daytime expression of the disorder (Block et al., 1979b). It seems then, that SDB may occur at low, apparently subclinical levels, or at significant (usually higher) symptomatic levels. It is important to distinguish these two levels in reviewing the literature, since they are not comparable.

Cardiopulmonary dysfunction represents an important area of deficit for the sleep-disordered breather. Very few reports examine possible cardiopulmonary changes in subclinical populations, although Berry et al. (1986b) note a significant correlation (r = 0.373; p < 0.05) between number of oxygen desaturations and systolic blood pressure in a group of heavy-snoring males. Several reports document cardiopulmonary changes in sleep apnea syndrome patients, including bradycardia (Zwillich et al., 1982), cardiac arrhythmias (Tilkian et al., 1978), and increased pulmonary and systemic hypertension (Buda et al., 1981). These reports indicate that cardiopulmonary deficits are a likely concomitant of symptomatic levels of SDB, while more limited evidence suggests a relationship between SDB and hypertension in subclinical populations. These cardiopulmonary sequelae undoubtedly have significant physiological and behavioral consequences in the affected patient, and treatment is clearly a priority in sleep apnea syndrome patients.

Alterations of the sleep/wake cycle are another frequent pathologic change in patients with SDB. The most commonly examined aspect of this area has been daytime hypersomnolence, a disorder with obvious behavioral consequences. Again, relatively few reports detail such data in subclinical subjects, although Berry et al. (1986b) note a significant correlation (r = 0.297; p < 0.05) between SDB and increasing subjective sleepiness (as measured by the Stanford Sleepiness Scale) in heavy-snoring males. Several reports document significantly shorter sleep latencies for daytime naps in patients with sleep apnea syndrome (Roth et al., 1980; Reynolds et al., 1982), while significant correlations between indices of SDB and nap latencies were reported by Carskadon et al. (1982). Thus, there is strong evidence linking SDB and daytime hypersomnolence in symptomatic sleep apnea syndrome patients, and more limited evidence linking the two in subclinical subjects.

A last area of deficit noted to accompany SDB involves intellectual deterioration. At least two reports describe such data in subclinical groups. Berry et al. (1984a) found significant relationships between SDB and deteriorating neuropsychological performance in heavy snoring males, as did Yesavage et al. (1985) in a heterogenous group of elderly subjects. In clinical sleep apnea syndrome patients, Findley et al. (1985) showed SAS patients to be impaired relative to controls on neuropsychological tests following treatment of the sleep apnea syndrome. Thus, there are strong and consistent relationships between nocturnal respiration and daytime cognitive status in both subclinical and clinical sleep apnea syndrome subjects.

This evidence indicates that SDB may well be a significant determinant of daytime physiological and behavioral parameters. Either directly, as in the case of hypersomnolence or intellectual declines, or indirectly, as in the case of cardiopulmonary dysfunction, SDB may have considerable impact on daytime functioning.

D. Associated Factors

Along with increased knowledge of the physiological and behavioral consomitants of SDB has come increased understanding of factors predisposing to nocturnal breathing dysfunction. Several variables have now been shown to correlate with SDB, including age, weight, hypertension, snoring, and male gender. Numerous reports have noted an association between age and SDB both in subclinical (Block et al., 1979; Bixler et al., 1982) and in clinical sleep apnea syndrome populations (Kreiger et al., 1983). Obesity also correlates with SDB in subclinical and clinical populations (Block et al., 1979; Kreiger et al., 1983) and high levels of SDB are reported in the morbidly obese (Harman et al., 1982). Kales et al. (1984) reported a significantly greater incidence of SDB in hypertensive patients than in matched controls. High levels of SDB are noted in heavy-snoring males (Berry and Block, 1984) and several studies have noted significantly more SDB in males than in premenopausal women (Block et al., 1979b; Smallwood et al., 1983). Interestingly, postmenopausal women display levels of SDB equivalent to those seen in males (Block et al., 1980).

These markers for SDB in subjects with normal daytime respirations, including age, weight, hypertension, snoring, and male gender, have implications for other populations as well. The relationship of these parameters to SDB in

other populations should be explored, as they may constitute risk factors for
SDB. Thus older, obese men who snore and have high blood pressure should
be carefully considered clinically for signs of nocturnal breathing dysfunction
(e.g., unexplained arrhythmias, hypersomnolence, and intellectual deterioration), and research into predictor factors in other populations should be pur-
sued as well.

E. Sleep-Disordered Breathing in COPD Patients

It is clear from the preceding discussion that SDB is associated with physiological and behavioral deficits in patients with normal daytime respiratory
parameters. It is now known that SDB frequently occurs in patients with
COPD. However, it appears that the mechanisms underlying SDB are perhaps
diverse in patients with chronic lung disease. Additionally, physiological and
behavioral deficits resulting from SDB may be altered in the presence of the
chronic lung disease. It is important to understand these mechanisms and
deficits in order to identify properly and treat SDB occurring in COPD
patients.

Mechanisms

Although severe oxygen desaturation during sleep in COPD patients was reported over 20 years ago (Trask and Cree, 1962), detailed investigations of
nocturnal respiration in these patients are relatively recent. It is now thought
that there are at least three mechanisms of SDB in COPD patients, including
sleep-related decline in baseline oxygen tension, classic apnea and hypopnea
events, and REM-related prolonged oxygen desaturations. Regarding baseline changes in oxygen saturation, sleep onset in normals is accompanied by
a modest decline in baseline oxygen saturation, thought to result from a loss
of wakefulness drive to respiration. Figure 1 illustrates the relationship between oxygen tension drops and oxygen saturation changes, which are mediated by the oxygen-hemoglobin dissociation curve. In normal subjects an 11
mm drop in oxygen tension results in a 2% change in oxygen saturation, a
typical fall in oxygen saturation during sleep in normal subjects. For COPD
patients however, a more severe change in oxygen saturation is observed. Because of their lung disease, COPD patients' baseline waking oxygen tension
is lower, and falls on the shoulder of the oxyhemoglobin dissociation curve.
In this region, a modest change of 15 mm in oxygen tension is accompanied
by a 9% drop in oxygen saturation. Thus, the loss of wakefulness drive to
respiration in COPD patients results in a relatively severe drop in oxygen

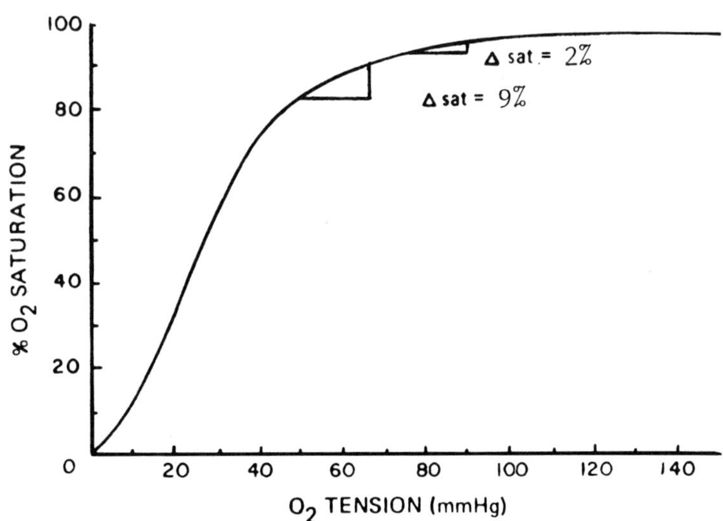

Figure 1 Oxyhemoglobin dissociation curve illustrating the difference in effect on saturation of a 11 mmHg drop on the flat portion vs. the steep portion of the curve. (Reproduced with permission from Block, A. J. (1985). Sleep apnea and related disorders. In *DM*. Edited by Cotsonas, N. J., Jr. et al. Copyright (©) 1985 by Year Book Medical Publishers, Inc., Chicago.)

saturation. A significant, chronic oxygen desaturation is therefore typically seen during sleep in COPD patients.

During light sleep, a second, more classic type of respiratory event is seen. Apneas, and more frequently hypopneas may be observed during stage 1 and 2 sleep in chronic lung disease patients. Most of these events are relatively brief, and only modest oxygen desaturation accompanies them. These events may be due to rhythmic cycling of breathing (periodic breathing), which is sometimes seen at sleep onset. Altered neural set points in changing sleep stage may underlie these events. That is, with different sleep stages, different levels of hypoxia and hypercapnia in blood gases are tolerated by the neural respiratory controller. Rapidly changing sleep stages (e.g., waking, stage 1, and stage 2) may result in unstable set points and hence disorganized breathing patterns.

Perhaps the most significant SDB of COPD patients occurs during REM sleep. Extremely low oxygen saturation values in the range of 50-60% may be observed for long periods of time. Analysis of recordings suggests that these profound desaturations are not due to simple apnea or hypopnea events, but may be the result of several factors. First, REM sleep results in alterations of neural respiratory set points such that greater hypoxia and hypercapnia are tolerated in REM state than in most other sleep stages. Additionally, arousal responses to hypoxia are blunted during REM stage. Thus loss of ventilatory and arousal responses to pathologic blood gas parameters may combine to allow development of relatively deep hypoxia during REM sleep. A second important factor involves a REM-related loss of tone in muscles subserving breathing. As a result of this decrease in muscle tone, ventilation/perfusion mismatches may develop, further exacerbating oxygen desaturation. Additionally, this loss of muscle tone increases upper airway resistance, and, further, the likelihood of shallow hypopnic breathing. Thus oxygen desaturation during REM sleep results from a combination of loss of ventilatory and arousal response to hypoxia and hypercapnia, ventilation/perfusion mismatches, and hypoventilation secondary to increased upper airway resistance. Given this evidence, it appears that mechanisms of SDB may be more complex in COPD patients than in subjects with normal daytime respiration (Block, 1985).

Frequency

The exact frequency of SDB in COPD patients is not yet known. However, a rapidly developing literature suggests that nocturnal respiratory disorder is relatively common in certain subgroups of COPD patients. Clinically, COPD patients may be divided into two types, blue bloaters (BB) and pink puffers (PP). Blue bloaters have been described as obese, hypoxic, hypercapnic (increased levels of arterial CO_2), and with a long history of chronic cough and cor pulmonale (right ventricular cardiac dysfunction). Also observed in these patients are polycythemia, enlarged hearts, and low ventilatory response to blood gas challenges. Pink puffers, in contrast, have relatively preserved blood gases, low body weight, hyperinflated lungs, small cardiac shadows, and few signs of cor pulmonale. It has not proved possible to classify reliably all COPD patients into these categories; however, some utility for this distinction may be found in relationship to SDB in these patients, as will be discussed below.

Table 1 presents data from several recent reports on SDB in COPD patients. Information on demographics, spirometrics, and SDB events is provided. Unfortunately, several reports that either failed to quantify, or presented idiosyncratic indices of SDB events were excluded because of lack of comparability. Even with this criterion imposed, however, a good deal of heterogeneity is observed.

Table 1 Characteristics of Sleep-Disordered Breathing in Patients with COPD

Reference	N M	N F	Age (yrs)	Weight (lbs)	FEV$_1$	FVC	% Experiencing Apnea	% Experiencing Hypopnea	% Experiencing Desaturation	Mean number of events Apnea	Mean number of events Hypopnea	Mean number of events Desaturation
Flick and Block (1977)	9	1	63	–	0.7	2.0	–	–	100 (10%)[a]	–	–	–
Wynne et al. (1979)	7	–	46	167	0.7	–	71	71	85 (4%)[a]	32[b]	32[b]	13.8
Littner et al. (1980)	9	–	59	190	0.42	–	–	–	67 (4%)[a]	–	–	–
Arand et al. (1981)	10	–	56-62	–	0.37[c]	–	–	–	70 (5%)[a]	–	–	–
Hudgel et al. (1983)	5	1	63	–	0.7	–	0	100	0	–	20	–
	7	–	62	–	1.3	–	0	100	100 (10%)[a]	–	14	–
Stradling and Lane (1983)	41	–	63	–	0.84	–	17[d]	95	–	–	–	–
Douglas et al. (1979)												
BB	5	5	57	–[e]	0.5	1.5	–	–	100	–	–	3.0
PP	1	1	66	–[e]	0.7	1.7	–	–	0 (10%)[a]	–	–	0.0

Demarco et al. (1981)	4	–	57	230	0.9	–	100%[b]	100%[b]	100	30.8[b]	30.8[b]	22.7
	6	–	55	145	1.3	–	100%[b]	100%[b]	100	19.2[b]	19.2[b]	3.5
									(4%)[a]			
Tirlapur and Mir (1982)												
BB	3	4	60	–	0.5	1.0	–	–	100	–	–	4.1
PP	3	2	66	–	0.8	1.8	–	–	40	–	–	2.0
									(10%)[a]			
Catterall et al. (1983a)												
BB	7	6	57	–	0.7	–	–	–	100	–	–	2.9
PP	5	2	61	–	0.8	2.0	–	–	38	–	–	0.9
(1983a)									(10%)[a]			
Catterall et al. (1983b)												
BB	2	4	56	–	0.7	1.5	14	100	100	–	–	4.5
(1983b)									(10%)[a]			

[a]Desaturation criteria.
[b]Apneas + hypopneas combined.
[c]FEV_1/FVC.
[d]20 sec apneas.
[e]None 20% over ideal weight.

Considering first demographic data (i.e., N. sex, age, weight), it is noted that results from over 150 COPD patients are presented. However, only 26 of these patients were female. The mean age of most samples clusters rather tightly around 55-65 years of age. Finally, the weights of patients are rarely reported. The restricted range of sampling and lack of reporting on key demographic variables in these reports is problematic. Recalling that demographic variables are important predictors of SDB in other populations, it is essential to measure and report these parameters in COPD patients. With this information in hand, it may prove possible to forecast with some confidence the probability of SDB in a given COPD patient.

Turning to spirometric data, the information in the table indicates that FEV_1 (liters of air expired in the first second of exhalation) is commonly reported. Mean values from FVC (total volume of air expired) are less frequently reported. Two reports provide only a ratio of FEV_1/FVC. While the data suggest reasonable comparability among these reports, perhaps more complete reporting of spirometric data would allow identification of previously unsuspected relationships between pulmonary function measurements and SDB.

The final section of the table deals with SDB events. Clearly, there are difficulties in interpreting these data. Most reports fail to report comprehensively on SDB events (i.e., apneas, hypopneas, and desaturations). Many criteria for events are relatively idiosyncratic. For example, definitions of apneas and hypopneas very somewhat. Particular heterogeneity is apparent in reports of oxygen desaturations, which are variously defined as 4%, 5%, and 10% drops in arterial oxygen saturation. An additional difficulty lies in the frequent failure to count and report the numbers of SDB events.

Given these limitations, interpretation of SDB data from the table will necessarily be largely qualitative. To facilitate interpretation, those reports detailing data from blue bloaters and pink puffers separately are presented following the reports that fail to make this distinction. Considering first data from general COPD populations, it is noted that apnea and hypopnea events are apparently common in these COPD patients. Desaturation is also frequent, although some variations in proportions of patients desaturating are noted. Based on this evidence, events are not unusual in the general COPD patient population. Turning next to reports distinguishing blue bloaters and pink puffers, provocative patterns appear. When the two subgroups of COPD patients are compared, BBs exhibit a higher prevalence of oxygen desaturation (100%), and a greater number of desaturations (3-23, varying with definition) than do PPs (mean of about 40% desaturation: zero to two events, depending on definition). These differences emerge despite some variance in desaturation definitions. Apnea/hypopnea events are not commonly reported although there is some suggestion that these events are more common in blue bloaters as well.

SDB events appear to be quite common in COPD patients. Available data indicate that these events may be more frequent and intense in the blue and bloated subgroup of COPD patients. These differences have been noted previously, and have led to the suggestion that nocturnal hypoxemia in blue bloaters leads to cor pulmonale and polycythemia (higher than normal concentrations of red blood cells) (Block et al., 1979a).

Physiological and Behavioral Consequences

Based on the data just reviewed, it is clear that SDB occurs with some regularity in COPD patients. Given the physiological and behavioral deficits secondary to SDB in other populations, it is logical to explore these parameters in COPD patients as well. We hope the promising results outlined below will stimulate further research in the area.

Physiological and behavioral changes secondary to SDB in chronic pulmonary patients may again be loosely grouped into cardiopulmonary complications, sleep/wake cycle alterations, and intellectual deficits. Block (1985) notes that systemic artery pressures in COPD patients typically remain within normal limits during sleep while pulmonary artery pressures increase progressively as sleep deepens toward REM stage. Thus, the highest pulmonary artery pressures are observed during REM stage. Pulmonary artery pressures recorded during sleep tend to correlate negatively with oxygen saturation in chronic pulmonary patients. It is thought that pulmonary vasoconstrictive response to local hypoxia in the lungs underlies this relationship. The clinical implications of this finding are that episodic oxygen desaturation during sleep may eventually lead to cor pulmonale (Block et al., 1979a). ECG abnormalities, including arrhythmias, conduction and repolarization deficits, as well as other abnormalities have been temporally related to episodic oxygen desaturations (Tirlapur and Mir, 1982). It may be that REM-related oxygen desaturations occurring during the period of maximum density of this sleep stage (early morning) account for the increased mortality of COPD patients during the 6-7 AM hour (Block, 1985). Clearly, cardiopulmonary abnormalities secondary to SDB events have important physiological and behavioral implications for the COPD patient.

Sleep/wake cycle alterations are also observed secondary to SDB in chronic pulmonary patients. COPD patients frequently complain of troubled sleep and EEG studies confirm frequent arousals and awakenings near the termination of SDB events. While these frequent arousals may function to protect the COPD patient from slipping into deeper hypoxia (through awakening and "resetting" of neural respiratory set points), they also result in disorganized sleep that rarely reaches deeper stages (i.e., slow wave sleep). Although subjective sleepiness is not a major complaint of many COPD patients, no objective measures of daytime sleepiness have yet been reported. It may be that a chronic but low-level sleepiness is present in these patients, masked by subjective readjustment of their frame of reference for assessing this sleepiness. This may prove an interesting question for further investigation. Thus sleep/wake cycle alterations secondary to SDB exert some physiological and behavioral effects on COPD patients, and hypersomnolence remains a possible sequela.

Intellectual deficits secondary to SDB have not yet been conclusively demonstrated in COPD patients. However, at least two pieces of information support this notion. First, it seems logical that the strong, consistent relationship between SDB and neuropsychological and performance observed in other populations will be replicated in COPD patients. Additionally, indirect evidence for this relationship exists in the Nocturnal Oxygen Therapy Trial (Heaton et al., 1983; see Chap. 6), which showed that oxygen delivered during sleep reversed some neuropsychological deficits observed in COPD. It would be of interest to determine whether hypoxia secondary to SDB had a stronger relationship to neuropsychological performance than did daytime PaO_2. Therefore, suggestions that nocturnal hypoxia results in some exacerbation of daytime neuropsychological deficits are presently likely, but unproven.

Thus, current research suggests physiological and behavioral deficits secondary to SDB in COPD. The strongest evidence involves cardiopulmonary deficits secondary to nocturnal breathing dysfunction, with weaker evidence supporting sleep/wake cycle alterations and intellectual deterioration. These promising preliminary findings should be followed up with more comprehensive investigations.

Treatment

Block (1985) has reviewed the current thinking regarding treatment of SDB in COPD patients. While treatment criteria are formalized for patients with chronic daytime hypoxia unresponsive to medical therapy, guidelines for the treatment of hypoxia occurring only at night are more speculative. In selected patients, positive pressure ventilators such as nasal continuous positive airway pressure (CPAP) devices may be useful. A more accepted approach involves low-flow oxygen therapy. Although early reports warned of the possibility of inducing hypercapnia or acidosis through such treatments, recent controlled studies indicate the safety and efficacy of this approach. Fletcher and Levin (1984), as well as Goldstein et al. (1984), report on the utility of oxygen treatment, and note no significant detrimental side effects. Low-flow oxygen is reported to prevent episodic pulmonary hypertension and cardiac arrhythmias, improve the quality of sleep, and relieve morning headache, all thought to result from reversal of nocturnal hypoxia secondary to SDB.

An alternative treatment approach involves drug therapy. Theoretically, a variety of agents with respiratory stimulant properties might be useful. However, surprisingly few reports have examined the issue. Medroxyprogesterone acetate, an oral form of progestational female sex hormone, may improve daytime blood gases in COPD patients. Those patients with the best response may also show improvement of nightime blood gas parameters (Skatrud et al., 1983). However, this effect is not consistent in the general COPD population (Dolly and Block, 1983b). Further research, evaluating both daytime and nighttime response to respiratory stimulant, seems in order.

Exacerbating Factors

Two recent reports indicate that certain commonly ingested substances exacerbate SDB in COPD patients. Dolly and Block (1983a) using a double-blind, controlled design, found that consumption of 1 ml alcohol/kg body weight prior to bedtime significantly increased the number of premature ventricular contractions recorded during sleep. Similarly, Block et al. (1984), again utilizing a double-blind controlled design, found that flurezepam, a commonly prescribed hypnotic, significantly increased the number of SDB events observed, and exacerbated their depth and duration. These reports suggest that COPD patients should restrict their alcohol consumption prior to bedtime, as well as avoid the use of hypnotics to induce sleep. Further research should explore the possibility of other substances that potentiate SDB in chronic pulmonary patients.

III. Summary and Conclusions

Sleep-disordered breathing has been linked to physiological and behavioral deficits in patients with normal daytime respiration. Recent work has shown that SDB occurs frequently in chronic pulmonary patients as well. The frequency and severity of SDB is particularly high in those patients with the blue and bloated type of the disease. Although still relatively undeveloped, research into the daytime concomitants of SDB in COPD patients suggests that cardiopulmonary deficits, sleep/wake cycle alterations, and intellectual deterioration may result from, or be exacerbated by, the nocturnal breathing disorder. Thus SDB may prove to be an important determinant of physiological and behavioral parameters in COPD patients. Treatment studies suggest that reversal of SDB may be accomplished by low-flow oxygen therapy, and possibly respiratory stimulants. Other work indicates that COPD patients should avoid alcohol and hypnotics prior to sleep, as they appear to increase sleep-disordered breathing. A plethora of important research questions in the area remain to be addressed, many with significant implications for the COPD patient.

References

Arand, D. L., McGinty, D. J., and Littner, M. R. (1981). Respiratory patterns associated with hemoglobin desaturation during sleep in COPD. *Chest* **80**:183-190.

Association of Sleep Disorders Centers (1979). Diagnostic classification of sleep arousal disorders. *Sleep* **2**:1-137.

Berry, D. T., Bauer, R. M., Webb, W. B., Block, A. J., and Switzer, D. A. (1984a). Nocturnal hypoxia and neuropsychological deficits. *INS Bull.* November, 5-6.

Berry, D. T., Webb, W. B., Block, A. J., Bauer, R. M., and Switzer, D. A. (1986a). Nocturnal hypoxia and neuropsychological variables. *J. Clin. Exp. Neuropsychol.* **8**:229-238.

Berry, D. T., Webb, W. B., and Block, A. J. (1984b). Sleep apnea syndrome: A critical review of the apnea index as a diagnostic criterion. *Chest* **86**: 529-531.

Berry, D. T., Webb, W. B., Block, A. J., and Switzer, D. A. (1986b). Sleep-disordered breathing and its concomitants in a subclinical population. *Sleep* **9**:478-483.

Berry, R., and Block, A. J. (1984). Positive airway pressure cures snoring and obstructive sleep apnea syndrome. *Chest* **85**:15-20.

Bixler, E., Kales, A., Soldatos, C., Vela-Bueno, A., Jacoby, J., and Scarone, V. (1982). Sleep apnea activity in a normal population. *Res. Commun. Chem. Pathol. Pharmacol.* **36**:141-152.

Block, A. J. (1985). Sleep apnea and related disorders. *DM*, May. Chicago, Year Book Med. Pub., Inc.

Block, A. J., Boysen, P., Wynne, J. W. (1979a). The origin of cor pulmonale: A hypothesis. *Chest* **75**:109.

Block, A. J., Boysen, P., Wynne, J., and Hunt. L. (1979b). Sleep apnea, hypopnea, and oxygen desaturation in a normal population. *N. Engl. J. Medicine* **30**:513-517.

Block, A. J., Wynne, P., and Boysen, P. (1980). Sleep-disordered breathing and nocturnal desaturation in post-menopausal women. *Am. J. Med.* **69**:75-79.

Block, A. J., Dolly, F. R., and Slayton, P. C. (1984). Does flurazepam ingestion affect breathing and oxygenation during sleep in patients with COPD? *Am. Rev. Respir. Dis.* **129**:230-233.

Bornstein, S. K. (1982). Respiratory monitoring during sleep: polysomnography. In *Sleeping and Waking Disorders: Indications and Techniques.* Edited by C. Guilleminault. Reading, MA, Addison-Wesley, pp. 183-212.

Boysen, P., Block, A. J., Wynne, J. W., Hunt, L. A., and Flick, M. R. (1976). Nocturnal pulmonary hypertension in patients with COPD. *Chest* **76**: 536-542.

Buda, A. J., Schroeder, J. S., and Guilleminault, C. (1981). Abnormalities of pulmonary artery wedge pressures in sleep-induced apnea. *Int. J. Cardiol.* **1**:67-74.

Calverley, P. M., Brezinova, V., Douglass, N., Catterall, J. R., and Flenley, D. C. (1982). The effect of oxygenation on sleep quality in COPD. *Am. Rev. Respir. Dis.* **126**:206-210.

Carskadon, M., Brown, E., and Dement, W. C. (1982). Sleep fragmentation in the elderly. *Neurobiol. Aging* **3**:321-327.

Catterall, J. R., Douglass, N. J., Calverley, P. M., Shapiro, C. M., Brezinova, V., Brash, H. M., and Flenley, D. C.(1983a). Transient hypoxia during sleep in COPD is not a sleep apnea syndrome. *Am. Rev. Respir. Dis.* **128**:24-29.

Catterall, J. R., Douglass, N. J., Calverly, P. M., Shapiro, C. M., and Flenly, D. C. (1983b). Arterial oxygenation during sleep in patients with right to left cardiac or intrapulmonary shunts. *Thorax* **38**:344-348.

Cherniak, N. A. (1980). The control of breathing in COPD. *Chest* :Suppl. 291-293.

Demarco, F. J., Wynne, J. W., Boysen, P., and Taasan, V. C. (1981). Oxygen desaturation during sleep as a determinant of the blue and bloated syndrome. *Chest* **79**:621-625.

Dolly, F. R., and Block, A. M. (1983a). Increased ventricular ectopy and sleep apnea following ethanol ingestion in COPD. *Chest* **83**:469-472.

Dolly, F. R., and Block, A. J. (1983b). Medroxyprogesterone acetate and COPD. *Chest* **84**:394-398.

Douglass, N. J., Leggett, R. J., Calverley, P. M., Brash, H. M., Flenley, D. C., and Brezinova, V. (1979). Transient hypoxemia during sleep in chronic bronchitis and emphysema. *Lancet* Jan. 6, 1-4.

Findly, L., Barth, J., Wilhoit, S., Powers, D., Boyd, D., and Suratt, P. (1985). Nocturnal hypoxia and cognitive functions in sleep apnea patients. *Am. Rev. Respir. Dis.* **131**:Suppl. A105.

Fletcher, E. C., and Levin, D. C. (1984). Cardiopulmonary hemodynamics during sleep in patients with COPD: The effect of long and short term oxygen. *Chest* **85**:6-14.

Flick, M. R., and Block, A. J. (1977). Continuous in-vivo monitoring of arterial oxygenation in COPD. *Ann. Intern. Med.* **86**:725-730.

Gaultier, C., Praud, J. P., Clement, A., D'Allest, A., Khaita, M., Tournier, G., and Girard, F. (1985). Respiration during sleep in children with COPD. *Chest* **87**:168-173.

George, C. F., and Kryger, M. H. (1985). When is an apnea not an apnea? *Am. Rev. Respir. Dis.* **131**:485-486.

Goldstein, R. S., Ramcharan, V., Bowes, G., McNicholas, W. T., Bradley, D., and Phillipson, E. (1984). Effect of supplemental oxygen on gas exchange during sleep in patients with severe COPD. *N. Engl. J. Med.* **310**: 425-429.

Guilleminault, C., van den Hoed, J., and Mitler, M. (1978). Clinical overview of the sleep apnea syndromes. In *Sleep Apnea Syndromes.* Edited by C. Guilleminault and W. Dement. New York, Alan R. Liss, pp. 1-12.

Guilleminault, C., Cumminskey, J., and Motta, J. (1980). Chronic obstructive airflow disease and sleep studies. *Am. Rev. Respir. Dis.* **122**:397-406.

Harman, E. M., Wynne, J. W., and Block, A. J. (1982). The effect of weight loss on SDB and oxygen desaturation in morbidly obese men. *Chest* **82**:291-294.

Heaton, R. K., Grant, I., McSweeny, A. J., Adams, K. M., and Petty, T. L. (1983). Psychologic effects of continuous and nocturnal oxygen therapy in hypoxic COPD patients. *Arch. Intern. Med.* **134**:1941-1947.

Hudgel, D. W., Martin, R. J., Capehart, M., Johnson, B., and Hill, P. (1983). Contribution of hypoventilation to sleep oxygen desaturation in COPD. *J. Appl. Physiol.* **55**:669-677.

Kales, A., Bixler, E., Cadieux, R., Schneck, D., Shaw, L., Locke, T., Vela-Buena, M. A., and Soldatos, C. (1984). Sleep apnea in a hypertensive population. *Lancet* **2**:1005-1008.

Krieger, J., Turlot, J., Mangin, P., and Kurtz, D. (1983). Breathing during sleep in normal young and elderly subjects: hypopneas, apneas, and correlated factors. *Sleep* **6**:108-120.

Littner, M. R., McGinty, D. J., and Arnand, D. L. (1980). Determinants of nocturnal oxygen desaturations in the course of ventilation during sleep in COPD. *Am. Rev. Respir. Dis.* **122**:849-854.

Orr, W., Martin, R., Imes, N., Rogers, R., and Stahl, M. (1979). Hypersomnolent and nonhypersomnolent patients with upper airway obstruction during sleep. *Chest* **75**:418-422.

Phillipson, E. A., and Goldstein, R. S. (1984). Breathing during sleep in COPD. *Chest* **85**:Suppl. 24s-30s.

Reynolds, C., Coble, P., Kupfer, D., and Holzer, B. (1982). Applications of the MSLT in disorders of excessive somnolence. *Electroencephalogr. Clin. Neurophysiol.* **53**:445-452.

Roth, T., Hartse, K., Zorick, F., and Conway, W. (1980). Multiple naps in the evaluation of excessive somnolence. *Sleep* **3**:425-439.

Skatrud, J. B., and Dempsey, J. A. (1983). Relative efficiency of acetazolamide vs progesterone in correction of CO_2 retention in COPD. *Am. Rev. Respir. Dis.* **127**:405-412.

Smallwood, R., Vitiello, M., Giblin, E., and Prinz, P. (1983). Sleep apnea: Relationship to age, sex, and Alzheimers dementia. *Sleep* **6**:16-22.

Stradling, J. R., and Lane, D. J. (1983). Nocturnal hypoxia in COPD. *Clin. Sci.* **64**:213-222.

Sullivan, C. E., Issa, F. G., Berthon-Jones, M., and Saunders, N. A. (1984). Pathophysiology of sleep apnea. In *Sleep and Breathing.* C. E. Sullivan and N. A. Saunders. New York, Marcel Dekker, pp. 299-363.

Taylor, D. R., Klonoff, H., and Fleetham, J. A. (1985). Change in psychological status following corrective upper airway surgery in patients with obstructive sleep apnea. *Am. Rev. Respir. Dis.* **131**:Suppl. A105.

Tilkian, A., Motta, J., and Guilleminault, C. (1978). Cardiac arrhythmias in sleep apnea. In *Sleep Apnea Syndromes.* C. Guilleminault and W. C. Dement. New York, Alan R. Liss, pp. 197-210.

Tirlapur, V. G., and Mir, M. A. (1982). Nocturnal hypoxia and associated ECG changes in patients with COPD. *N. Engl. J. Med.* **306**:125-130.

Trask, C. H., and Cree, E. M. (1962). Oximeter studies on patients with chronic obstructive emphysema, awake and during sleep. *N. Engl. J. Med.* **266**:639-642.

Wynne, J. W., Block, A. J., Hemenway, J., Hunt, L., and Flick, M. R. (1979). Disordered breathing and oxygen desaturation during sleep in patients with COPD. *N. Engl. J. Med.* **66**:573-579.

Yesavage, J., Bliwise, D., Guilleminault, C., Carskadon, M., and Dement, W. C.
    (1985). Preliminary communication: intellectual deficit and sleep-
    related respiratory disturbance in the elderly. *Sleep* 8:30-33.
Zwillich, C., Devlin, T., White, D., Douglass, N., Weil, J., and Martin, R.
    (1982). Bradycardia during sleep apnea. *J. Clin. Invest.* 69:1286-1289.

3

Neuropsychological Correlates of COPD

GEORGE P. PRIGATANO

Barrow Neurological Institute
St. Joseph's Hospital and Medical Center
Phoenix, Arizona

IGOR GRANT

University of California, San Diego
San Diego Veterans Administration
    Medical Center
La Jolla, California

I. Introduction

In discussing the various causes underlying metabolic coma, Plum and Posner (1982) described the condition of anoxic anoxia. Their comments help introduce the notion that patients with chronic obstructive pulmonary disease (COPD) may indeed demonstrate subtle neuropsychological deficits that potentially reflect subacute or chronic diffuse hypoxia. They state:

> In *anoxic anoxia,* insufficient oxygen reaches the blood so that both arterial oxygen content and tension are low. This situation results from a low oxygen tension in the environment (e.g., high altitude or displacement of oxygen by an inert gas such as nitrogen) or from the inability of oxygen to reach and cross the alveolar capillary membrane (pulmonary disease and hyperventilation). With mild or moderate hypoxemia the cerebral blood flow increases to maintain the cerebral oxygen delivery, and no symptoms occur. However, clinical evidence suggests that in chronic conditions the cerebral blood flow can only increase to about

twice normal. When the increase is insufficient to compensate for the degree of hypoxia, the $CMRO_2$ begins to fall and symptoms of cerebral hypoxia occur (page 208).

This description highlights the point that biologic protective mechanisms that regulate oxygen metabolism in the brain are limited. This is true not only in the acute case but also in chronic conditions. In addition, while it has been traditional to be concerned about sudden drops in the level of PaO_2 at any single time, the clinical significance of small or moderate lowering of PaO_2 over long periods of time has generally not been appreciated. Most of the research and resultant information regarding anoxic anoxia comes from the study of young, healthy men exposed for time-limited periods to simulated altitude. The results of such work have been reviewed by Gibson et al. (1981), who summarize the alterations in cognitive functioning in relation to drop in arterial blood oxygen (Table 1). Recent neurobehavioral research on elderly COPD patients has, for the first time, allowed for an assessment of the effects of less dramatic but long-lasting lowering of PaO_2 on higher cerebral function. A complicating feature of such research has been the fact that COPD patients tend to be older and chronically ill, therefore it has been important to consider what alterations in cerebral function might be attributed to the aging process and/or to chronic illness. When these factors are controlled for, the effects of hypoxemia and, by inference, cerebral hypoxia on behavior can be determined.

In this chapter we will review research on the neuropsychological correlates of COPD. Because most COPD patients are older, we will pay specific attention to the effects of disease and aging. Before doing so, however, we will discuss briefly what is meant by the terms *neuropsychological function* and *dysfunction* and describe how these functions are measured.

II. Neuropsychological Function and Its Measurement

The term neuropsychological applies to those behaviors shown empirically to be adversely affected by pathoanatomic or pathophysiological brain changes (see extensive reviews of this topic in Filskov and Boll, 1981; Grant and Adams, 1986; Hecaen and Albert, 1978; Heilman and Valenstein, 1985). Systematic observation of these behaviors is generally accomplished by various neuropsychological tests, of which there is a great number, each differing in its sensitivity and specificity (Lezak, 1983). Because several neuropsychological functions often need to be assessed in concert (e.g., attention, language, perception, memory), batteries of tests are commonly administered

Table 1 Neuropsychological Changes at Altitude

Altitude (m)	PaO_2 (mmHg)	$PaCO_2$ (mmHg)	Possible neuropsychological changes/signs
Sea level	95	38	Normal
1500	85	38	Impaired dark adaptation
3000-4500	60-45	36-34	Impaired concentration; impaired short-term memory; hyperventilation
4500-6000	45-35	34-30	Lethargy, euphoria, irritability, hallucinations, impaired critical judgement, muscular incoordination
Above 6000	<35	<30	Loss of consciousness

Source: Grant and Heaton (1985), p. 357.

(Grant and Adams, 1986). Of these, the Halstead-Reitan Battery has been most extensively studied; this approach was used in the two largest investigations of the neuropsychological correlates of COPD: the Nocturnal Oxygen Therapy Trial (NOTT; Grant et al., 1982) and the Intermittent Positive Pressure Breathing Trial (IPPB; Prigatano et al., 1983).

A. The Halstead-Reitan Battery: Its Characteristics and Rationale for Its Use in Studies of COPD Patients

The Halstead-Reitan Battery (HRB) is an ensemble of tests and procedures that includes measures of intelligence (the Wechsler Adult Intelligence Scale [WAIS] is part of the extended battery), attention, language, abstracting ability, complex perceptual motor skills, sensation, motor ability, and memory (Reitan, 1986; Reitan and Davison, 1974). In various studies, the success of the HRB in discriminating patients with brain disorders from others has been reported to be in the order of 70-90% (Parsons and Prigatano, 1978; Heaton et al., 1981).

Despite its obviously broad parametric coverage, the HRB has been criticized for lacking depth in assessment of certain specific functions (e.g., memory or language), and because its development was not rooted in any specific theory of brain-behavior relationships.

Although there is some merit to the concern that the HRB might not be the method of choice for certain hypothesis-testing experiments in neuropsychology, the Battery seemed ideally suited to descriptive clinical research aimed at ascertaining the prevalence, severity, and qualitative features of neuropsychological disturbance in a disease state such as COPD. Having established the fact of neuropsychological deficit in hypoxemic patients, investigators will then be in a position to move to the next step, that is, the effort to understand how certain neurophysiological changes translate into specific behavioral disturbances.

B. The Problems of Aging and Neuropsychological Measurement

As the central nervous system ages, there are predictable neuroanatomic and neuropsychological changes. Besides shrinking of neural density and enlargement of sulci and ventricles, older subjects (usually in their mid 60s or older) show less efficient memory, are slower in information processing, and generally have greater difficulty in developing novel approaches to solving problems (Horn, 1975). Thus, one would expect that as people get older they will do more poorly on a number of neuropsychological tests. Neuropsychological studies have shown, for example, that age negatively correlates with various measures of the Halstead-Reitan Battery (Heaton et al., 1986; Prigatano and Parsons, 1976). This is such a powerful relationship that if age is not taken into consideration, one can make erroneous conclusions about whether or not the test behaviors are indicative of brain dysfunction secondary to the disease under study. Figure 1 highlights this point. In 25 perfectly healthy control subjects (selected in the IPPB project), a computer program was used to evaluate their performance. The age variable was not taken into account. As one can see, at age 55 or above, approximately one-half of these normal subjects were misclassified as brain dysfunctional, when a standard cutoff score was used. This finding makes it imperative that age be considered both in the initial experimental design and in the later statistical analysis of data. The gradual development of age-education-sex-corrected test norms (e.g., Heaton et al., 1986) will greatly facilitate this sort of research in the future.

C. The Problem of Chronic Illness

A second variable that potentially could influence neuropsychological test performance is chronic illness. Patients who do not feel well may not be motivated to perform on various tests. This variable, unfortunately, has not been

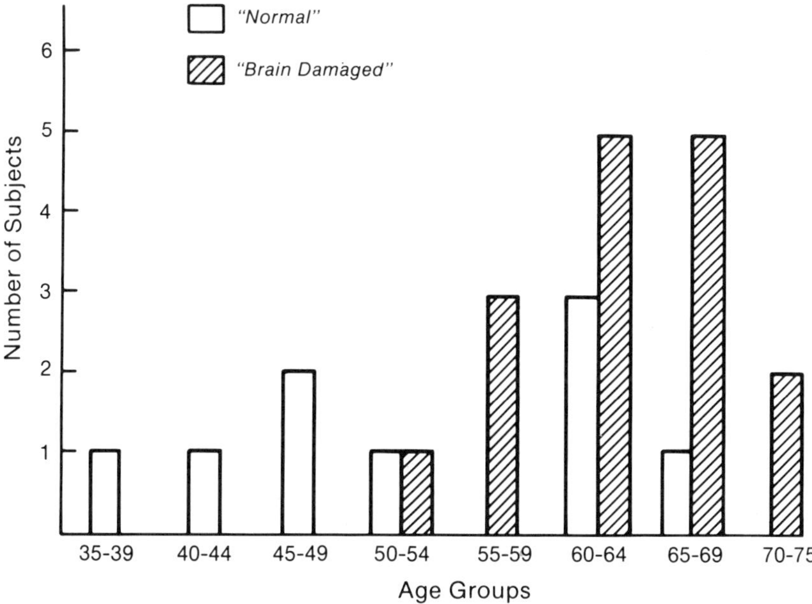

Figure 1 Computer-assisted classification of nonpatients using standard cutoff scores and disregarding age.

adequately dealt with in studies on COPD patients. However, specifically in the IPPB project, the patient's ability to carry on various exercise activities and severity of depressed mood were studied in relation to neuropsychological performance. Neither exercise tolerance nor depression significantly predicted neuropsychological test scores in the patient group (Prigatano et al., 1983). Nevertheless, future investigations should continue to examine the potential confounding effect of chronic illness on neuropsychological performance.

III. Review of Earlier Work

The first psychological studies of COPD patients were not neuropsychological in nature; they covered the emotional aspects of COPD. These are reviewed in the chapter by McSweeny. Perhaps the first modern neuropsychological study of COPD patients reported in the literature was that of Krop et al. (1973). Interested in the effects of continuous oxygen therapy on COPD patients, these authors studied a small group of patients with neuropsychological and personality measures before and after oxygen treatment. The patients' test scores suggested that hypoxemic COPD patients were impaired on measures of visual-spatial function and speed of simple motor movement. Overall measures of intelligence and memory were generally within the normal range for this relatively small group of patients. In addition, significant elevations on scales 1, 2, and 3 of the MMPI were reported prior to oxygen treatment. Improvement on the depression and social introversion scales of the MMPI was reported after oxygen treatment. The authors concluded that COPD patients with hypoxemia evidenced not only heightened depression but also impairment in certain neuropsychological functions that might be partially reversed with oxygen treatment.

Kass et al. (1975), in a study aimed at predicting vocational rehabilitation outcome in COPD patients, reported on the performance of COPD patients on several psychological tests, some of which had neuropsychological properties. They found that 85% of the patients had test scores that they suggested were indicative of brain dysfunction. However, these measures of brain dysfunction were not correlated with PaO_2 levels and adequate controls were not used. As a result it was unclear how nonpatients in their late 50s and early 60s would have performed on these tests.

The first major studies on the neuropsychological function of COPD patients that included adequate controls have just recently been completed. Sponsored by the National Heart, Lung, and Blood Institute, clinical trials on the effectiveness of nighttime oxygen (Nocturnal Oxygen Therapy Trial, NOTT) and Intermittent Positive Preassure Breathing (IPPB study) have been performed. In both of these studies neuropsychologists were allowed to examine patients using extensive neuropsychological measures. That data base has provided our first clear view of the neuropsychological correlates of COPD.

IV. Clinical Trial Data

The rationale, design, and overall results of these two clinical trials have been reported by the respective study groups (Intermittent Positive Pressure Breathing Trial Group, 1983; Nocturnal Oxygen Therapy Trial Group, 1980). In this chapter we will focus on their neurobehavioral findings.

A. The NOTT Study

In an attempt to assess the effectiveness of continuous versus only nighttime oxygen therapy in advanced COPD patients, 203 hypoxemic patients and 74

well-matched controls were studied with serial neuropsychological measures
(Grant et al., 1982). The Halstead-Reitan Battery and related tests were used
in this study as well as in the IPPB project.

These COPD patients had a mean PaO_2 of 51.2 with a mean age of
65.5 ± 8.4 years. Compared to controls, they performed worse on most of
the neuropsychological tests administered to them. While mean verbal IQ
scores of controls (108.6) and patients (104.6) were statistically different
(p = 0.05), this difference was small, and both mean scores were in the normal
range. There were, in contrast, many notable differences between COPD patients and controls on the Halstead-Reitan Battery. Highly reliable differences
were found on a number of psychomotor tests (e.g., Tactual Performance
Test), simple motor speed tests (e.g., Tapping Test), and strength measures
(Grip Strength). The overall average impairment rating was also significantly
different in the two groups. COPD patients had a mean score of 2.28 ± 0.78;
controls had a mean score of 1.72 ± 0.63. These findings make it clear that
these hypoxemic COPD patients showed a general pattern of impairment in
neuropsychological function. It is of some interest that this measure also
showed a modest but significant relationship with the level of PaO_2 (r = 0.20,
p = 0.008).

The authors concluded that although their findings showed "clearcut
quantitative differences" between the groups, the pattern of performance was
strikingly similar to that of controls. They suggested, therefore, "that COPD
may not be related to any specific brain pathological findings, but rather is
aggravating neuropsychological decline that occurs as part of aging" (pp. 1472-
1473).

In a subsequent study by the same authors (Heaton et al., 1983), these
severely hypoxemic COPD patients were compared to controls in terms of
their neuropsychological test scores at 6 months and 12 months after oxygen
treatment.

After 6 months 42% of patients and 6% of controls showed modest improvement in neuropsychological performance on the basis of case-by-case
ratings of initial and follow-up data (clinicians were blind to group member-
ship). At this point there were no differences between continuous and intermittent oxygen treatment. One year follow-up of a small group of patients
suggested that the continuous group was performing better than the nocturnal
group (see details in chapter by Heaton).

While the purpose of the study was to evaluate the relative effects of
continuous oxygen therapy versus nighttime oxygen therapy, this study provided one method of checking on the reliability of neuropsychological findings.

Despite modest improvement, the rate and nature of neuropsychological impairment observed in the patients at baseline were comparable to those observed on follow-up. These data are important insofar as they affirm the reliability of observed neuropsychological deficits in hypoxemic COPD patients.

B. The IPPB Study

In the second clinical trial on the effectiveness of IPPB (Prigatano et al., 1983), 100 mildly hypoxemic COPD patients and 25 well-matched controls were studied using the same neuropsychological measures as in the NOTT study. Moreover, controls were selected using the same identification procedures as in the prior investigation.

The IPPB patients had a mean PaO_2 of 66.3 (compared to 51.2 in the NOTT) and a mean age of 61.5 years (65.5 in the NOTT). As a group, therefore, the IPPB patients were slightly younger and substantially less hypoxemic than their NOTT counterparts.

The IPPB patients' average impairment rating (AIR) was 1.80 ± 0.59 compared to 1.42 ± 0.04 for controls. These mildly hypoxemic patients generally performed better on the Halstead-Reitan Neuropsychological Battery compared to the more severely hypoxemic patients studied in the Grant et al. (1982) study (AIR = 2.28 ± 0.78). It is interesting, however, that the IPPB and COPD patient groups were equally impaired on some measures. For example, number of errors on the Category Test was equivalent. This is a measure of abstract reasoning. Also, their errors on the Seashore Rhythm Test, which samples ability to concentrate and attend to nonverbal stimuli, were nearly identical. These findings suggest that certain tests on the Halstead-Reitan Battery are sensitive to the presence of hypoxemia, but do not predict its degree. On other tests, the more severely hypoxemic patients clearly showed worse performance than the mildly hypoxemic ones. For example, NOTT patients were much slower on simple speed of motor activity (Tapping Test) compared to IPPB patients. They also were slower in performing complex perceptual-motor tasks (Tactual Performance Test). Memory seemed to be worse in the NOTT group. Finally, the NOTT patients had greater difficulty in shifting their cognitive set (as measured by the Trail Making Test, Part B).

The authors of the IPPB study concluded that while the neuropsychological test findings were certainly compatible with enhanced aging, some of the results were more indicative of acquired brain dysfunction. For example, the hypoxemic patients in the IPPB study made more errors than would be expected of normal elderly on simple tests of language function; furthermore, other research has indicated that simple language skills generally do not worsen with aging (see Horn, 1975).

C. Combined NOTT-IPPB Data Bank

Given the above observations it became desirable to combine the data banks of both the NOTT and IPPB projects to investigate systematically the specific relationship of degree of hypoxemia with neuropsychological deficits. This type of investigation held the promise of identifying more precisely what types of neuropsychological deficits are most common in COPD, as well as defining the incidence of neuropsychological impairment in this heterogenous population. Since detailed findings of the combined data bank have been reported elsewhere (Grant et al., 1987), only an overview is provided here.

The combined data pool consisted of 302 patients and 99 controls. COPD patients were classified as being mildly hypoxemic (PaO_2 = 68), moderately hypoxemic (PaO_2 = 54), or severely hypoxemic (PaO_2 = 44).

Neuropsychological examination showed that, in general, the severely hypoxemic group performed more poorly than both the moderately and mildly hypoxemic groups. There were also significant differences between the mildly hypoxemic group and controls on some tests.

The AIR, a composite index that takes many WAIS and Halstead measures into account, illustrates the impact of hypoxemia on neuropsychological function. Table 2 shows that the controls performed significantly better than the mildly hypoxemic group, but that the moderately and severely hypoxemic groups were not significantly different from one another. The latter two patient groups were significantly impaired compared to both age-matched controls and mildly hypoxemic patients.

These findings suggest that even with mild hypoxemia there is overall impairment in higher cerebral functioning that may not be observed on more traditional intelligence testing. For example, the mildly hypoxemic group did not differ significantly from the control group in terms of the WAIS verbal IQ (see Table 2). This finding reaffirms that one cannot use general measures of intellectual functioning (which are heavily influenced by past educational experiences, cultural background, etc) in the hope of unraveling the neuropsychological sequelae associated with COPD. Tests more sensitive to underlying brain dysfunction are necessary.

It is also interesting to observe that a test of simple speed of associate learning reflected the most striking differences between patients and controls. The Digit Symbol subtest of the WAIS requires the patient to write a symbol

Table 2 Neuropsychological Test Performance of Patients in Three Hypoxemia Groupings and Nonpatient Controls

| Test | Nonpatient controls | | Patient hypoxemia category | | | | | |
| | | | Mild | | Moderate | | Severe | |
	Mean	s.d.	Mean	s.d.	Mean	s.d.	Mean	s.d.
Average impairment rating[a]	1.69	.62	1.81	.58	2.13	.72	2.38	.72
Verbal IQ	107.2	14.6	104.8	15.1	102.7	16.3	101.6	14.9
Digit symbol[b] (scale scores)	7.4	2.5	6.3	2.0	5.7	2.8	5.1	2.5
Trial making B[c]	122	62	124	60	156	78	183	81
Category test[d] (errors)	65.2	26.4	80.7	22.6	77.0	27.2	86.7	27.8

Significant (p < 0.05) differences on post hoc testing:

[a]Controls better than mild; controls and mild better than moderate and severe, which are indistinguishable.
[b]Controls better than mild; controls and mild better than severe; mild and moderate indistinguishable.
[c]Controls better than mild; controls and mild better than moderate and severe which are indistinguishable.
[d]Controls better than mild, moderate and severe; latter three indistinguishable.

Note: A complete listing of test results is provided in Grant et al. (1987).

or mark that goes with a number. Nine number-symbol pairs are used. The patient is asked to do this under time pressure and the number correctly transcribed during a 90-sec interval determines the score. On this very simple test, which has been shown in other research to be highly sensitive to the effects of brain injury (see Prigatano et al., 1984a) we see striking differences. As shown in Table 2, controls significantly outperformed mildly and moderately hypoxemic patients, whereas the latter two groups performed better than the severely hypoxemic patients.

Another very sensitive measure was the Trail Making Test, Part B (Reitan and Davison, 1974). This test requires patients rapidly to shift their cognitive set between numbers and letters and draw a line connecting them in alternating fashion. The score is based on how fast the individual can complete this task. Controls and mildly hypoxemic patients did not differ. However, the mildly hypoxemic group was reliably different from the moderate and severe groups (see Table 2).

While previous investigations have suggested that abstract reasoning capacity is significantly compromised in hypoxemic COPD patients, it is interesting to note that this measure did not reliably separate the groups when they were classified according to degree of hypoxemia. Errors on the Category Test did not differentiate the mild, moderate, and severe hypoxemia groups. However, as a group, *all* COPD patients performed worse than controls (Table 2). This finding suggests that the neuropsychological sequelae of COPD may have both general and specific effects. That is, if one has COPD, some generalized deficits may exist, one of which appears to be decreased performance on the abstract reasoning measure. However, when one looks particularly at speed of motor activity and psychomotor activity, there seems to be a more monotonic relationship between the level of hypoxemia and neuropsychological sequelae.

D. Risk of Neuropsychological Impairment Attributable to COPD

While the two clinical trials make it clear that COPD patients have impairment in higher cerebral functioning, a very practical question for clinicians is the risk of such impairment.

Neuropsychologists consider a diagnostic measure to possess adequate sensitivity and specificity if it can properly classify 80% of the population under investigation. Since 99 nonpatient subjects were given the extended Halstead-Reitan Battery as part of NOTT-IPPB studies, an opportunity was available to classify this elderly comparison group using an empirical criterion.

Table 3 Risk of Neuropsychological Impairment Attributable to Progressive Levels of Hypoxemia

Hypoxemia category	Total NP risk (%)	Risk attributable to age (%)	Risk attributable to hypoxemic category (%)
Mild n = 86	26.7	20.6	6.1
Moderate n = 155	44.5	20.6	23.9
Severe n = 61	61.5	20.6	40.9

It was observed that nearly 80% of these controls obtained an AIR of 2.1 or below. This suggests that if patients obtained scores higher (i.e., in the direction of worse performance) than this value substantially more frequently than 20%, the probability that neuropsychological dysfunction was attributable to some process beyond aging would be increased.

The results of classifying patients using the AIR greater than 2.1 criterion are presented in Table 3. Approximately 21% of the controls had an AIR greater than 2.1. Subtracting this "age-risk" figure from the actual rate of impairment in the three groups of patients reveals that the risk of neuropsychological impairment attributable to different stages of disease rises from 6% in the mildly hypoxemic group to 41% in the severely hypoxemic patients.

What Aspects of the Disease Account for Increased Neuropsychological Risk

Beyond age and education, what characteristics of COPD patients help to predict neuropsychological impairment? To examine this question, the NOTT-IPPB investigators identified nine variables that are known to change as COPD evolves, and which individually or jointly might contribute to cerebral dysfunction. These variables are listed in Table 4.

Stepwise logistic regression was selected as the statistical technique to model these data (see Grant et al., 1987). This approach allows one to estimate whether selected predictor variables (i.e., those listed in Table 4, plus age and education) improve success at classifying patients as impaired or unimpaired, and if so, to determine which specific variables make a significant contribution.

Table 4 Medical Variables Entered into Logistic Regression Study to Predict Impaired Neuropsychological Status

---

$FEV_{1.0}$

PaO_2

$PaCO_2$

Respiratory rate

Exercise tolerance (bicycle ergometer)

Hemoglobin

pH

Systolic blood pressure

Diastolic blood pressure

A correct overall classification rate of 75% was achieved using a model with four predictors: education (p = 0.001), PaO_2 (p = 0.005), age (p = 0.001), and diastolic blood pressure (p = 0.05). As a practical matter, only three of these four variables are probably of importance, since the contribution of diastolic blood pressure is very much less than that of education PaO_2, and age.

The chi square statistic for the logistic regression was highly significant (chi square = 81.95; d.f. = 4; p = 0.0001), but did not provide a practical sense of how well the model actually performed. To get a better idea of this we compared results from the model to those expected from an educated guesser who did not know the neuropsychological status of any particular patient, but was aware of the overall rate of impairment in COPD patients. Since 58% of the patients were unimpaired and 42% were impaired, the probability that an educated observer would classify patients correctly by chance would be $(0.58)^2$ + $(0.42)^2$ or 52%. Thus, the model represents a modest but not spectacular improvement of 23% over base-rate adjusted chance.

These findings confirm that the clinician's index of suspicion that a patient with COPD might have subtle cerebral dysfunction should be heightened in the case of the patient who is hypoxemic, older, and less well educated.

V. Implications for the Pulmonary Clinician

In addition to alerting pulmonary clinicians in a general way that severely hypoxemic COPD patients have a relatively high prevalence of neuropsychological deficit, the present data have specific implications. COPD patients may have mild difficulties in abstract reasoning and problem-solving, even when the IQ appears to be normal. As a group, they will experience a relatively high rate of psychomotor disturbance expressing itself in slowed speed of simple motor activity, and even more so when abstract reasoning or problem-solving is involved in the motor task. This means that patients are generally going to be slower in carrying out these tasks, and this slowness will not simply be a product of easy fatigability.

At the same time these data also suggest that some functions are relatively spared. Memory is one of these. In fact, in the combined IPPB-NOTT study, ability to recall short stories read to patients was not different for the three levels of hypoxemia. While all COPD patients differed from controls in this measure, the difference was relatively small. One clinical implication is that even patients with some neuropsychological deficit should generally have the capacity to remember simple instructions concerning their treatment regimen.

Patients and controls did not differ in their basic verbal skills. This means that their communication skills will tend to be intact, even if there are other neurobehavioral disturbances. At the same time, preservation of language skills should not obscure other types of impairment. For example, while verbal IQ does not differ between patients and controls, performance IQ does. This suggests that when patients are asked to carry out tasks under time pressure, they will have difficulty. To some degree, these defects in speed of information processing are related to degree of hypoxemia. For example, on the performance IQ, whereas controls were not different from the mildly hypoxemic patients, they performed significantly better than moderately and severely hypoxemic patients. The mildly hypoxemic patients could not be distinguished from the moderate, but were significantly better than the severely hypoxemic patients (Grant et al., 1987).

These examples suggest that members of the pulmonary care team must be prepared to follow their clinical intuition if, through personal observation, or reports by family members, it appears that neuropsychological deficit might be present. Preserved verbal skills should not reassure treatment personnel that all is well. If neuropsychological or neuropsychiatric consultation is not readily available, clinicians can perform a simple screening with procedure such as the Trail Making Test. This simple paper and pencil instrument is moderately sensitive to neuropsychological disorder, but should not be considered diagnostic. Rather, it can help confirm clinical judgment, and form a basis for requesting more detailed assessment.

VI. Summary and Areas for Future Research

The research to date has emphasized that *as a group,* COPD patients demonstrate signs of neuropsychological impairment. This impairment cannot be accounted for simply on the basis of age, physical infirmity, or depression. There is a relationship between degree of hypoxemia in COPD patients and severity of neuropsychological deficits. Abstract reasoning is affected even in mild hypoxemia. Speed of information processing and general psychomotor speed and accuracy decline with reduction in PaO_2. Memory is not severely impaired and language skills tend to be preserved.

Future research should investigate the parameters that influence psychomotor deterioration and problems in speed of information processing. The fact that tests that deal with motor function are most compromised in COPD patients raises the possibility that brain structures subserving motor expression are at high risk in hypoxemia. After acute hypoxic insult, pathologic changes are known to occur in the basal ganglia (Brierley, 1976). Because movement disorders and extrapyramidal signs were rarely observed in the COPD patients, the mechanism underlying psychomotor deficit must be different. Further neuropsychological and neuropathologic investigation of COPD patients should help shed light on this important question.

Also, further research is needed to describe more clearly what the underlying nature of the neuropsychological deficits is and what medical parameters they relate to. Next, it is important to understand the changes in neuropsychological function that occur over time in these patients. The cross-sectional studies that have been reported make it clear that level of PaO_2 is related to certain neuropsychological deficits. Within the same patients, is there evidence of progressive decrease in certain neuropsychological functions as PaO_2 decreases? What is the natural history of cognitive decline in COPD?

Another question of importance to clinicians is the extent to which neuropsychological disturbance compromises the patient's ability to comply with rehabilitation. For example, research on treatment of alcoholics suggests that cognitively impaired patients adhere less well to therapy and have higher rates of relapse (Walker et al., in press). Could some of the noncompliance in COPD have a similar basis? In addition, it would be important to explore the potential interactions of neuropsychological deficit, affective disturbance (severe anxiety or depression), and social support in determining treatment outcome.

Related to this question is the issue of how neuropsychological deficits influence quality of life in COPD patients. Some initial studies have suggested

that neuropsychological status, in fact, is related to the quality of life (Mc-
Sweeny et al., 1985). Prigatano et al. (1984b), for example, noted that limitations in physical measures of quality of life were related to the overall
neuropsychological status of the patient. McSweeny and colleagues (1985)
have described two sets of associations between neuropsychological and life
quality variables. The physical dimension of health status is correlated with
performance on tests involving psychomotor speed and coordination, whereas
ability to communicate with family and friends is related to presence of subtle
aphasic signs.

In the studies reviewed above the role of chronic illness could not be
properly evaluated as one of the potential confounding variables in this research. While in the IPPB project, it was shown that depression and exercise
levels did not predict AIR, this is still not a convincing piece of evidence.
COPD patients should ideally be compared with other chronically ill patients
who have a similar level of physical disability, but no evidence of brain dysfunction (e.g., patients with moderate arthritis).

In conclusion, this review of the neuropsychology of COPD finds support for the comment made by the NOTT investigators during the initial
phases of their work, to the effect that COPD is a disease that affects the
brain as well as the lungs and heart (Grant et al., 1980).

Acknowledgments

Writing of this chapter was supported in part by award SA325 to Dr. I. Grant
from the Medical Research Service of the Veterans Administration. The
NOTT/IPPB data were gathered through work supported by contracts NOI-
HR-6-2942, 2943, 2944, 2945, 2946, 2947 and NOI-RH-72901, 72903,
72904, 72905, and 72906 from the National Heart, Lung, and Blood Institute.

The authors thank Joanne McCoy, Debi Taylor, Megan Cunningham,
and Robert Reed for their help in preparing the manuscript.

References

Brierley, J. D. (1976). Cerebral hypoxia. In *Greenfield's Neuropathology*.
    Edited by W. Blackwood and J. A. Corsellis. Year Book Medical Pub-
    lishers, Inc., Chicago, pp. 43-85.
Filskov, S. B., and Boll, T. A. (1981). *Handbook of Clinical Neuropsychol-
    ogy*. New York, John Wiley and Sons.

Gibson, G. E., Pulsinelli, W., Blass, J. P., and Duffy, T. E. (1981). Brain dysfunction in mild to moderate hypoxia. *Am. J. Med.* **70**:1247-1254.

Grant, I., and Adams, K. M. (1986). *Neuropsychological Assessment of Neuropsychiatric Disorders.* New York, Oxford University Press.

Grant, I., and Heaton, R. K. (1985). Neuropsychiatric abnormalities in advanced COPD. In *Chronic Obstructive Pulmonary Disease,* 2nd ed. Edited by T. L. Petty. New York, Marcel Dekker, pp. 355-373.

Grant, I., Heaton, R. K., McSweeny, A. J., Adams, K. M., and Timms, R. M. (1980). Brain dysfunction in COPD. *Chest* **77**(suppl.):308-309.

Grant, I., Heaton, R. K., McSweeny, A. J., Adams, K. M., and Timms, R. M. (1982). Neuropsychologic findings in hypoxemic chronic obstructive pulmonary disease. *Arch. Intern. Med.* **142**:1470-1476.

Grant, I., Prigatano, G. P., Heaton, R. K., McSweeny, A. J., Wright, E. C., and Adams, K. M. (1987). Progressive neuropsychological impairment in relation to hypoxemia in chronic obstructive pulmonary disease. *Arch. Gen. Psychiatry* **44**:999-1006.

Heaton, R. K., Grant, I., Anthony, W. Z., and Lehman, R. A. W. (1981). A comparison of clinical and automated interpretation of the Halstead-Reitan Battery. *J. C.in. Neuropsychol.* **3**:121-141.

Heaton, R. K., Grant, I., McSweeny, A. J., Adams, K. M., and Petty, T. L. (1983). Psychologic effects of continuous and nocturnal oxygen therapy in hypoxemic chronic obstructive pulmonary disease. *Arch. Intern. Med.* **143**:1941-1947.

Heaton, R. K., Grant, I., and Matthews, C. G. (1986). Differences in neuropsychological test performances associated with age, education, and sex. In *Neuropsychological Assessment of Neuropsychiatric Disorders.* Edited by I. Grant and K. M. Adams. New York, Oxford University Press, pp. 100-120.

Hecaen, H., and Albert, M. L. (1978). *Human Neuropsychology.* New York, John Wiley and Sons.

Heilman, K. M., and Valenstein, E. (1985). *Clinical Neuropsychology.* New York, Oxford University Press.

Horn, J. L. (1975). Psychometric studies of aging and intelligence. In *Aging,* vol. 2. Edited by S. Gershon and A. Raskin. New York, Raven Press.

Intermittent Positive Pressure Breathing Trial Group (1983). Intermittent positive pressure breathing therapy of chronic obstructive pulmonary disease: a clinical trial. *Ann. Intern. Med.* **99**:612-620.

Kass, I., Dyksterhuis, J. E., Rubin, H., and Patil, K. D. (1975). Correlation of psychophysiologic variables with vocational rehabilitation outcome in patients with chronic obstructive pulmonary disease. *Chest* **67**:433-439.

Krop, H., Block, A. J., and Cohen, E. (1973). Neuropsychologic effects of continuous oxygen therapy in chronic obstructive pulmonary disease. *Chest* **64**:317-322.

Lezak, M. D. (1983). *Neuropsychological Assessment.* New York, Oxford University Press.

McSweeny, A. J., Grant, I., Heaton, R. K., Prigatano, G. P., and Adams, K. M. (1985). Relationship of neuropsychological status to everyday functioning in healthy and chronically ill persons. *J. Clin. Exp. Neuropsychol.* **7**(3):281-291.

Nocturnal Oxygen Therapy Trial Group (1980). Continuous or nocturnal oxygen therapy in hypoxic chronic obstructive lung disease: a clinical trial. *Ann. Intern. Med.* **93**:391-398.

Parsons, O. A., and Prigatano, G. P. (1978). Methodological considerations in clinical neuropsychological research. *J. Consult. Clin. Psychol.* **7**(3); 281-291.

Plum, F., and Posner, J. B. (1982). *The Diagnosis of Stupor and Coma.* Philadelphia, F. A. Davis.

Prigatano, G. P., and Parsons, O. A. (1976). Relationship of age and education to Halstead Test performance in different patient populations. *J. Consult. Clin. Psychol.* **44**:527-533.

Prigatano, G. P., Parsons, O. A., Wright, E. C., Levin, D. C., and Hawryluk, G. (1983). Neuropsychological test performance in mildly hypoxemic patients with chronic obstructive pulmonary disease. *J. Consult. Clin. Psychol.* **51**:108-116.

Prigatano, G. P., Fordyce, D. J., Zeiner, H. K., Roueche, J. R., Pepping, M., and Wood, B. C. (1984a). Neuropsychological rehabilitation after closed head injury. *J. Neurol. Neruosurg. Psychiatry* **47**:505-513.

Prigatano, G. P., Wright, E. C., and Levin, D. C. (1984b). Quality of life and its predictors in mildly hypoxemic COPD patients. *Arch. Intern. Med.* **144**:1613-1619.

Reitan, R. M. (1986). Theoretical and Methodological bases of the Halstead-Reitan Neuropsychological Test Battery. In *Neuropsychological Assessment of Neuropsychiatric Disorders.* Edited by I. Grant and K. M. Adams. New York, Oxford University Press, pp. 3-30.

Reitan, R. M., and Davison, L. A. (1974). *Clinical Neuropsychology: Current Status and Applications.* Washington, D.C., V. H. Winston and Sons.

Walker, R. D., Donovan, D. M., Kivlahan, D. R., Roszell, D. K. (1986). Prediction of alcoholism treatment outcome: multiple assessment domains. In *Neuropsychiatric Correlates of Alcoholism.* Edited by I. Grant. Washington, D.C., American Psychiatric Association. pp. 110-125.

4

Quality of Life in Relation to COPD

A. JOHN McSWEENY

Medical College of Ohio
Toledo, Ohio

I. Introduction

The term *quality of life* has enjoyed colloquial use in the fields of medicine
and health for a long time, although its use as a scientific concept is relatively
recent. A major conceptual impetus to the scientific application of psychosocial concepts in medicine was provided by the publication of George Engel's
(1980) paper on the biopsychosocial model of medicine. Using a systems
theory framework, Engel argued that the inclusion of psychosocial information in the formulation of medical concepts, research, and patient care serves
to make medicine a more "scientific" enterprise when compared with more
narrow biomedical models or with nonscientific "holistic" models. Engel's
viewpoint has been widely embraced by medical schools, and a new genera-
tion of physicians and medical investigators is being trained within the biopsychosocial model.

II. Issues in Life Quality Research

A. Definitions of Life Quality

One result of the intensified interest in psychosocial issues in medicine is the development of the concept of quality of life or "life quality." As might be expected with any relatively new concept, several definitions have been offered. A review of alternative definitions of life quality reveals some commonalities but some variation as well, particularly in terms of comprehensiveness, specificity, and theoretical relevance. Levine and Croog (1984), for example, note that many medical researchers have utilized a single variable of human functioning, such as employment, general happiness, or sexual functioning, as an indicator of life quality in an ad hoc fashion. In contrast, Wenger et al. (1984a) have provided a detailed definition of life quality that incorporates three basic dimensions (functional capacity, perceptions, and symptoms) and nine subdimensions (daily routine, social functioning, intellectual functioning, emotional functioning, economic status, health status, well-being or life satisfaction, and symptoms related to the disease under study as well as other diseases). Wenger et al. also provide a fairly detailed set of rationale for the inclusion of each life-quality criterion.

Most definitions fall somewhere between the extremes, as just described, and demonstrate some commonality of content. The definition provided by McSweeny et al. (1982) is fairly typical. McSweeny and his colleagues composed their definition after a review of the limited literature on the psychosocial aspects of chronic obstructive pulmonary disease (COPD) but without the detailed consideration of the definition issues as exemplified by Wenger et al. Four dimensions of life quality are included in McSweeny et al.'s definition: (1) emotional functioning, including mood changes and other psychiatric symptoms; (2) social role functioning, including employment, home management, and social/family relationships; (3) daily-living activities, such as self-care skills and mobility; and (4) the ability to engage in enjoyable activities, such as hobbies and recreational activities.

Another issue in the definition of life quality is the perspective from which it is defined. Pearlman and Jonsen (1985) note that definition of life quality changes when it is defined from the perspectives of the patient, of an "onlooker of another's life situation" (i.e., a relative or physician), or society in general. Many times the perspective issue is reduced to a debate concerning the relative value of "subjective" versus "objective" viewpoints on life quality, with the usual conclusion that both viewpoints should be considered, although the latter viewpoint is more amenable to scientific study.

McCullough (1984) concludes that the perspective issue is quite complex and reflects a more general value issue. He notes that the use of objective measures by clinicians and researchers stems from a "beneficence model" of health care that assumes that health professionals know "what promotes or protects the best interests of patients." This is a "remarkable claim" according to McCullough. The beneficence model is contrasted with the "autonomy model," which depends upon the patients to provide knowledge about what is in their best interests. McCullough concludes that the beneficence and autonomy models have the same final goal: "seeking the greater balance of good over harm for the patient." However, the two models differ in terms of who should decide how to define what *good* or what *harm* is, how the goal should be reached (i.e., what treatments should be used), and how the outcome should be measured.

McCullough's work on alternative models of health care and life quality should sensitize those of us who work with patients to the concept that the patient's viewpoint of what constitutes a good quality of life is at least as valid as what a researcher or clinician might suggest. Pearlman and Jonsen's discussion (1985) points out that the patient's "significant others," and even society in general, may hold additional viewpoints on an appropriate definition of life quality. From a practical aspect, researchers and clinicians should try to incorporate these different perspectives in their definitions of life quality. This is particularly important when the definition of life quality has potential impact on the treatment of patients.

The preceding discussion points to some of the complexities in the definition of life quality. The reader is advised to consult Wenger et al. (1984a,b) or Levine and Croog (1984) for more detailed discussions of these issues.

B. Measurement of Life Quality

McSweeny et al. (1982) reported that the validity and range of measurement devices represented serious methodological problems in the research conducted before 1980 on life quality and COPD. The authors noted a common failure to specify the assessment procedures other than in vague terms such as "psychiatric interview" or "nursing interview." One must suspect that here the interview procedures were as vague as the descriptions. Although an unstructured clinical interview might provide rich clinical information about a single patient it does not have the requisite psychometric characteristics, e.g., validity and reliability, to permit sound research.

Those studies that did use formal psychometric procedures often used only one or two instruments to assess emotional status, one of which usually was the Minnesota Multiphasic Personality Inventory (MMPI; Dahlstrom et al., 1972). The MMPI has a long history of use in medical research and is the instrument that many medical researchers turn to first when investigating the psychosocial aspects of a medical problem. Unfortunately, this "old favorite" of medical psychologists is inadequate as a single instrument of life quality. The MMPI is concerned primarily with symptoms of personality and emotional disturbance, which makes it useful for psychiatric diagnosis but less useful as a measure of general life quality. Other aspects of life quality, as described earlier, including social adjustment, daily activities, and recreational activities, are not addressed by the MMPI or by the studies that used it as a single psychosocial measure. In addition, the original clinical scales of the MMPI are heterogeneous in their content, and several, particularly that of depression (scale 2), include a variety of physical symptoms. Thus, the meaning of an elevated scale is not always clear without additional analysis (McSweeny, 1984). This is especially relevant when one considers the frequent finding of depression in COPD from the MMPI-based studies.

The history of life quality measurement follows the history of the development of the concept of life quality quite closely. Much of the important work in this area has been accomplished in the last 10 years. Most authors now recommend that several aspects of life quality should be assessed in any study of the concept given its multidimensional nature. In addition, assessment from multiple perspectives, i.e., those of the patient, the care givers, and the relatives, are suggested. Single perspective, unidimensional, single-instrument evaluations of life quality are now recognized as inadequate and are becoming rarer.

Psychometricians interested in medical research recently have developed several instruments designed specifically to measure life quality or similar concepts. This has made it easier for life quality researchers to conduct investigations in the area. These instruments vary in their content, comprehensiveness, and established psychometric characteristics, but several, such as the Sickness Impact Profile (SIP; Bergner et al., 1981) and the McMaster Health Index Questionnaire (Chambers et al., 1982), show considerable promise. Six of these instruments are reviewed in Wenger et al. (1984a), and the basic characteristics of those instruments are illustrated in Table 1.

The availability of "ready-made" measures of life quality does not relieve investigators from the necessity of a careful consideration of the aforementioned issues. Usually, it will still be necessary to supplement one of the ready-made life quality measures with other measures to assess the concept adequately.

Our study of life quality in COPD (McSweeny et al., 1982) illustrates a typical life quality assessment battery as used in current research. As noted before, we assessed four dimensions of life quality: (1) emotional functioning, (2) social role functioning, (3) daily-living activities, and (4) recreational activities. These four dimensions were assessed with data from self-reports and reports from the patient's spouse or a close relative of the patient. The three self-report measures included the MMPI, the Profile of Mood States (POMS; McNair et al., 1971), and the SIP. The MMPI served as a measure of psychiatric disturbance, whereas the POMS indicated general mood. The SIP, which contains 12 sections, served as a "broad-band" measure of life quality. The Katz Adjustment Scale-Relative's version (KAS-R; Katz and Lyerly, 1963) was used to assess functioning from the perspective of someone who interacted with the patient on a regular basis. These instruments and their use in COPD studies are described in more detail elsewhere (McSweeny, 1984; McSweeny et al., 1982).

Investigators and clinicians who wish to use life quality measures may wish to consult Ware (1984) for specific criteria to guide their choice of instruments.

C. Methodological Issues in Life Quality Research

We have noted (McSweeny et al., 1982) several methodological problems with previous life quality research in addition to problems with measurement. First, many of the studies were restricted by sample size and representativeness. All of the studies that we reviewed had sample sizes of less than 50; most other studies investigated even smaller samples. This fact limits the statistical conclusion validity and external validity (Cook and Campbell, 1979) of the studies. In less technical terms, conclusions drawn from these studies may not be considered to be reliable and cannot be generalized to other patients and settings.

A second methodological issue that was noted by McSweeny et al., in all but one of the reports they reviewed, was the lack of a comparison group matched in terms of age, sex, social position, and other factors that must be assessed separately from the effects of the disease to ensure internal validity (Cook and Campbell, 1978). Related to this is the fact that patients with various chronic diseases have very similar psychosocial profiles. Cassileth et al. (1984), for example, studied 758 patients from six different diagnostic groups (arthritis, diabetes, cancer, renal disease, dermatological disorders, and depression) using the Mental Health Index, a multiscale instrument concerned with different aspects of psychological distress and well-being (Veit and Ware, 1983). Cassileth et al. found no significant differences among the five groups

of patients with a diagnosis of a chronic physical disease which, in turn, did show some significant differences from the depressed group. Their findings raise the question of how much uniqueness there is to the psychosocial consequences of COPD, at least when compared with other chronic diseases. Although more recent studies of life quality and COPD (e.g., McSweeny et al., 1982; Prigatano et al., 1984) have employed control groups matched for the sociodemographic variables mentioned previously, they have not included a control group of patients with other chronic diseases. Thus, the uniqueness of the psychosocial aspects of COPD remains an open question.

A final problem noted by McSweeny et al. concerned data analysis. Most of the studies in their review contained no formal data analyses or only simple statistics, once again limiting the statistical conclusion validity of the studies. Fortunately, more recent studies have included appropriate methods of statistical data analysis.

III. Review of Current Findings

A. Emotional Disturbances Associated with Chronic Obstructive Pulmonary Disease

Depression

By far the most commonly reported emotional consequence associated with COPD is depression. Depressive symptoms, including pessimism, hopelessness, and feelings of hopelessness, have been reported in virtually every study of the psychological aspects of COPD as well as in reviews of the literature (Dudley et al., 1980; Greenberg et al., 1985; Sandhu, 1986). To some extent, this consistency across studies may reflect the fact that many used the MMPI as the measure of depression and, as noted earlier, the MMPI depression scale contains several items concerned with somatic symptoms. However, depression has been noted to be the predominant emotional difficulty in studies that have used instruments other than the MMPI, including those that have utilized the perspective of a relative (McSweeny et al., 1982; Prigatano et al., 1984). Depression appears to be a relatively common problem among COPD patients. Agle and Baum (1977) reported "significant" depression in 74% of their patients, whereas McSweeny et al. reported that 42% of their patients were primarily depressed and an additional 7% had symptoms of depression combined with other psychiatric symptoms. The differences between the two studies are probably due to differences in patient samples and measurement methods, but the basic finding of COPD patients being at high risk for depression is consistent.

Differing opinions exist about the causal factors in depression in COPD. Most writers have focused on the psychosocial consequences of COPD such as the loss of pleasurable activities, economic hardship, and difficulties in coping (Barstow, 1974; Dudley et al., 1980a; Post and Collins, 1981-1982). Others have suggested that physiological factors, including the hypoxygenation of the limbic system and related brain mechanisms, might also be relevant factors (McSweeny et al., 1982). Labuhn and McSweeny (1987) tested the relative importance of a variety of psychosocial and mediophysiological factors in the development of depression in a group of 303 COPD patients using path analytic, causal-modeling methods. Their results led them to conclude that although physiological factors did play an important role in the development of depression, the depression that COPD patients experience is largely a reaction to their situation. This study is described in more detail later.

Other Emotional Disturbances

A variety of other emotional disturbances have been reported in addition to depression. These include anxiety, irritability, hysterical disorders, somatic preoccupation, dependency, and aggressive behavior (Agle and Baum, 1977; Burns and Howell, 1969; Dudley et al., 1980a; Greenberg et al., 1985; Kinsman et al., 1983; McSweeny et al., 1982; Prigatano et al., 1984; Sandhu, 1986). The findings of anxiety and somatic preoccupation appear to be fairly reliable across studies. To some extent, this is because many studies have used the MMPI. However, it is not difficult to imagine that anxiety and concern about one's bodily condition would be a common occurrence in COPD. Agle and Baum (1977), for example, reported disabling anxiety in 96% of their patients, and McSweeny et al. (1982) reported somatic preoccupation in 8.7% of their patients in contrast to 0% in the demographically matched control group.

The findings of hysterical disorders, suspiciousness, and aggressive behavior have been less reliable. Although some of the earlier studies reported hysterical tendencies (e.g., Burns and Howell, 1969), later studies have not consistently confirmed these results. McSweeny et al. (1982) found that 2.7% of their COPD patients exhibited primarily hysterical symptoms compared with 1.5% of the older normal individuals. In addition, the MMPI hysteria scale, which is often used as the criterion of hysterical complaints, contains a high number of somatic symptoms. McSweeny et al. also failed to find unusual degrees of suspiciousness or anger, although relatives of the patients did report a moderate degree of oppositional behavior. The lack of overt hostility is consistent with the clinical picture of the "emotional straight-jacket" as described by Dudley et al. (1973). On the basis of Dudley's classic studies of the psychophysiology of breathing (Dudley, 1969), Dudley et al. (1973) suggested that the COPD patient learns to avoid the expression of strong emotions, including anger, to prevent the excessive oxygen uptake that occurs in conjunction with physiological arousal. This relationship between dyspnea and emotional status was also observed in a study by Burns and Howell (1969), who found that "disproportionately breathless" COPD patients had higher rates of emotional distress than the remaining COPD patients. In addition, the dyspnea improved with the resolution of emotional disturbance.

B. Social Role Functioning and Activities of Daily Living

General Discussion

The performance of basic social roles (SR) and activities of daily living (ADL) is often used as a standard for the impact of a disease entity. However, this area is less well represented in the COPD literature than that of emotional functioning, primarily because of the lack, until recently, of appropriate methods of assessment.

Barstow (1974) reported that "major changes" were evident in the "style of living" manifested by the COPD patients in her study. These included alterations in bathing, grooming, dressing, eating, sleeping, and mobility. She noticed, for example, that "the mode of dress was altered in favor of less restrictive clothing that was easily slipped on and off." Food intake was decreased by many of the patients because an overdistended stomach would interfere with diaphragmatic breathing. Sleep/rest difficulties received particular attention in Barstow's report. Disruptions of sleep because of cough, dyspnea, or restlessness were common. In addition, Barstow reported some sleep changes that were apparently related to endogenous depression.

McSweeny et al. (1982) also reported a broad range of SR and ADL dysfunction. The SIP was used to present the patient's self-evaluation. In all categories of the SIP except one, COPD patients reported a much higher percentage of impairment than did control subjects. The only category not affected differentially was employment, presumably because the COPD and control groups both contained many elderly retired persons. The areas of functioning found most severely affected were home management and sleep/rest. Eating and communication, on the other hand, seemed to be only mod-

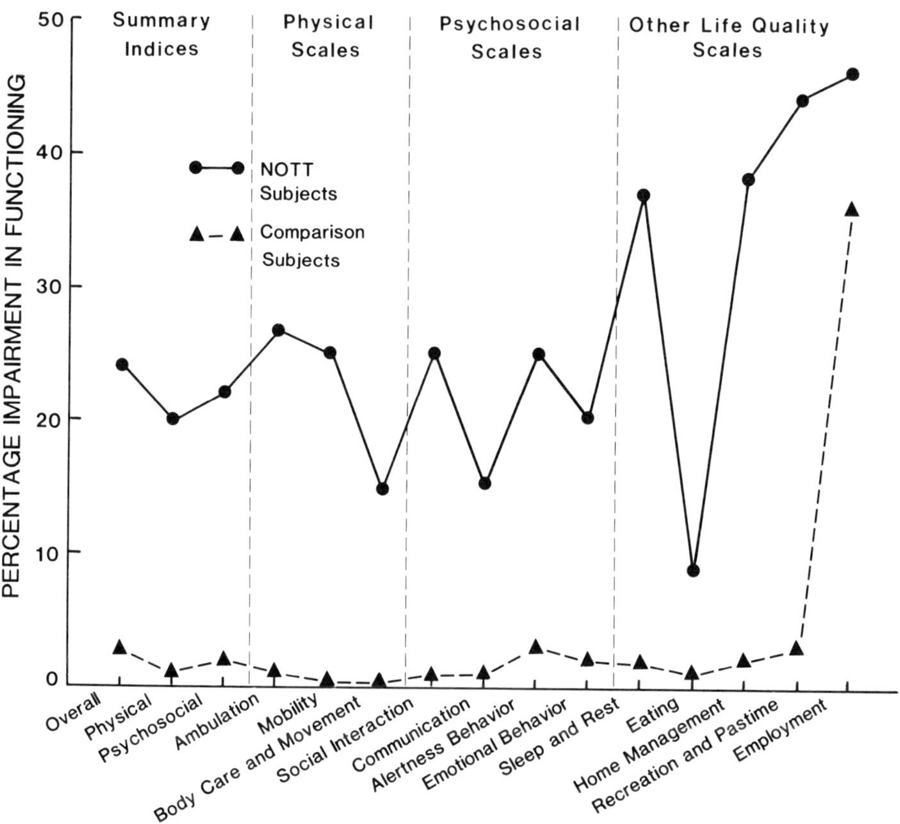

Figure 1 Mean sickness impact profiles for patients with chronic obstructive pulmonary disease (COPD) and control subjects. Patients with COPD are significantly ($p < 0.001$) more impaired on all scales except employment using paired t tests ($n = 66$). NOTT = nocturnal oxygen therapy trial. (From McSweeny et al., 1982. Copyright, American Medical Association. Reprinted with permission.)

erately affected by the disease (Fig. 1). The results from the KAS-R, which presented the relative's viewpoint, indicated that relatives regarded the patient's social role functioning as deficient; they expected less of the patients but still felt dissatisfied with the patients' performance of social roles.

Prigatano et al. (1984) also utilized the SIP and KAS-R with their mildly hypoxemic COPD patients. Their findings were quite similar to those from McSweeny et al.'s severely hypoxemic patients, although, as might be expected, the degree of impairment was proportionately less. One interesting exception was that Prigatano et al. did find significant differences in employment status between COPD patients and controls. This appears to be because the control subjects in Prigatano et al.'s study were much more likely to be employed than those in that of McSweeny et al. (1982). This, in turn, is the result of a greater proportion of persons younger than 65 among the patients and controls in the Prigatano et al. study. In summary, employment status is more likely to be a significant issue for younger patients than for older patients and may be affected even in those who have small reductions in PaO_2.

One final noteworthy study is a questionnaire survey of approximately 130 COPD patients conducted by Hanson (1982). Her survey included 40 questions about 11 areas, including several aspects of social role functioning and activities of daily living such as employment, self-care, home/personal business, marriage, care of grandchildren, and dependency on others. Hanson's results were consistent with those from McSweeny et al. (1982) and Prigatano et al. (1984) in that she found a general negative effect of COPD across the different categories in her survey. One interesting aspect of her study is that her questionnaire was bipolar, i.e., it allowed respondents to indicate a positive impact of COPD on different life areas as well as a negative impact. In fact, a few individuals did indicate a positive effect, ranging from 28% for care of grandchildren to 40% for marriage. One might be tempted to conclude that there is some benefit to adversity, but the meaning of her results are unclear given the lack of a comparison sample. The seemingly positive results could also be due to confusion or differing interpretations of the questions. Hanson also studied sexuality and those results are discussed in the following section.

Sexual Functioning

One topic not assessed in detail in the McSweeny et al. (1982) and Prigatano et al. (1984) studies is that of sexual functioning. Other investigators, however, have paid more attention to this important aspect of human function. In one of the earlier studies on the topic, Kass et al (1972) reported that 19% of their male COPD patients were impotent. More recent studies have suggested even higher rates of sexual dysfunction among men. Fletcher and Martin (1982), for example, reported that 30% of their COPD patients were impotent and that an additional 5% had ceased intercourse because of dyspnea. Frequency of intercourse for the remaining 65% of their patients was only 16% of predisease levels.

Sadly, no objective data appear to exist concerning sexual functioning in female COPD patients, although it is probably safe to assume that the factors that affect sexual function in men affect sexual functioning in women as well. One self-report study concerning sexual functioning in a mixed sex (62% men, 38% women) sample that does exist is the previously described one by Hanson (1982). She found that among the 11 life areas assessed in her study, sexual functioning was the area most consistently rated as being negatively affected by COPD. Thus, Hanson's results are consistent with the more objective findings from Fletcher and Martin (1982) and Kass et al. (1972) and also suggest that COPD presents problems for sexual functioning for women as well as for men. Unfortunately, Hanson did not report results separately for men and women, and we are still left in some doubt. Clearly, the sexuality of female COPD patients is a neglected area and in need of further research.

One controversy in the area of sexuality and COPD concerns whether the problems that are observed are largely secondary to a past history of marital and sexual difficulties or to the relatively immediate physical effects of the disease. Kass et al. (1972) reported on a sample of 90 men and 10 women and concluded that the sexual problems associated with COPD patients were *not* primarily due to the effects of the disease. Rather, such problems were the result of life-long patterns of behavior. The presence of a wife who was angered by the level of support required by her husband was also mentioned as a common problem in the maintenance of good sexual functioning. The authors provided five case histories (all were of men) to illustrate their conclusions.

In contrast to Kass et al.'s report are the more recent findings of Fletcher and Martin (1982). Fletcher and Martin carefully assessed erectile dysfunction in relation to cardiopulmonary, hormonal, and neurovascular dysfunction. They concluded that

> Data from this study suggest that sexual dysfunction and erectile impotence can accompany COPD in the absence of other known causes of sexual problems. Furthermore, sexual dysfunction tended to be worse in those subjects with more severe pulmonary function impairment as assessed by pulmonary function tests, blood gases, and exercise tests [p. 420].

Fletcher and Martin did note that several of their subjects who were impotent by nocturnal penile tumescence had high T-scores on some **MMPI** scales, but the effects of the disease of COPD appeared to underly both the emotional and sexual dysfunction in these patients. Only one of their 20 subjects had clearly psychogenic impotence.

In summary, COPD has a documented negative effect on sexual functioning in men and possibly in women as well. Although psychosocial factors play an important role in sexual functioning, the sexual dysfunctioning associated with COPD is closely linked with cardiopulmonary dysfunction and hypoxemia.

C. Hobbies and Recreational Activities

As was true for social role functioning and activities of daily living, only limited data exist concerning hobbies and recreational activities. McSweeny et al. (1982) noted that their patients with COPD reported severe restrictions in recreation and other leisure time activities. The SIP results suggested a reduction of 40 to 50% in pleasurable activities, which is certainly an important aspect of life quality. Indeed, the category of recreation and pastimes showed the greatest level of impairment relative to the other categroies on the SIP when compared with the control group. The results from the KAS-R indicated the relatives also recognized decrements in the free-time activities of the patients.

The study by Prigatano et al. (1984) produced results quite similar to those of McSweeny et al., with the exception that the effects were less severe. A reduction of 30 to 40% in pleasurable activities was seen in the mildly hypoxemic patients on the SIP. This was, again, the most impaired category on this test. In addition the KAS-R results indicated that the relatives were aware of the problem.

That there is a significant loss of pleasurable activities in COPD is relevant to theories of depression that suggest that the loss of reinforcers is a major contributory factor in the development of depression (Costello, 1972). Therefore, helping COPD patients to maintain old hobbies and develop new ones might help ameliorate the negative impact of COPD on emotional status.

IV. Life Quality and Its Relationship to Other Factors

A. Basic Research

McSweeny et al. (1982) noted that there was considerable variability in the life quality of patients with COPD. This raises the question of what factors might improve or worsen emotional functioning and other aspects of life quality in COPD patients.

Writers in the area have made several suggestions. Sandhu (1986) defined psychosocial assets as "those individual characteristics and social supports that allow coping with or modifying one's environment." In a review of the literature Sandhu noted that psychosocial assets "play a major, perhaps central, role in the patient's ability to cope adoptively." He concluded that high assets have correlated with positive outcome in medical treatment, whereas low assets have typically been associated with a variety of poor outcomes, including increased morbidity and mortality.

DeAruajo et al. (1973) assessed psychosocial assets in a sample of 36 patients with chronic asthma and found that patients with high assets required less medication and adapted to life changes more readily than did patients with lower psychosocial assets. Pattison et al. (1971) found that COPD patients with high assets also responded more positively to group therapy. Dudley et al. (1980a) have also found psychosocial assets to be associated with patient response to dyspnea, treatment program compliance, and survival time. More recently, Jensen (1983) found that lack of social assets, as well as life stress, predicted subsequent hospitalizations in a group of COPD patients better than did demographic characteristics, severity of illness, or history of previous hospitalizations.

Two other studies have focused on specific psychosocial assets. Barstow (1974) noted that patients identified the presence of a supportive spouse as the most important factor for successful coping, and Young (1982) found that material resources, such as monetary savings and health insurance, to predict positive adjustment.

McSweeny et al. (1982) and Prigatano et al. (1984) examined a variety of factors relation to life quality by using simple correlations and multiple regression techniques. McSweeny et al. found relatively strong correlations between life quality and age, neuropsychological status, socioeconomic status, and exercise capability. Less robust, but significant, relationships were noted between life quality and overall disease severity as well as did specific indicators of COPD such as oxygen transport. McSweeny et al. offered the heuristic model pictured in Figure 2 to aid in the explanation of the interrelation of COPD and other variables in life quality.

Prigatano et al.'s investigation confirmed the results of McSweeny et al. and produced several additional findings of interest. Life quality was also found to be significantly related (negatively) to smoking history but not to recent life changes. In addition, Prigatano et al. discovered that neuropsychological functioning, exercise capability, and pulmonary variables were more strongly related to physical aspects of life quality than to psychosocial aspects

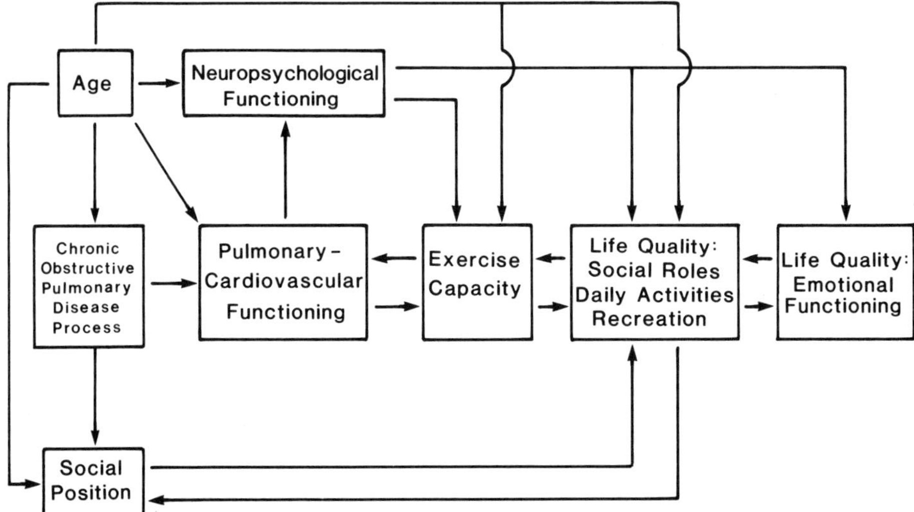

Figure 2 Heuristic model for interrelation of chronic obstructive pulmonary disease and other variables affecting life quality. (From McSweeny et al., 1982. Copyright, American Medical Association. Reprinted with permission.)

as measured by the physical and psychosocial scales of the SIP, respectively. In contrast, mood and emotional functioning, as measured by the MMPI and POMS were more strongly related to the psychosocial aspects than to the physical aspects of life quality. In summary, Prigatano and his colleagues have demonstrated some of the complex interrelationships that exist between various aspects of life quality as well as between life quality and other spheres of functioning in COPD patients.

Labuhn and McSweeny (1987) sought to investigate in more detail the interrelationships between life quality and other aspects of functioning in COPD. To accomplish their goal, they combined the data from McSweeny et al. and Prigatano et al. into one set of data and applied a multivariate statistical technique known as path analysis (Asher, 1976). Specifically, Labuhn and McSweeny attempted to develop and test a multivariate model for explaining depression in COPD. The model represented an attempt to integrate the various biological, psychological, and sociological explanations of depressed mood as applied to COPD patients. The path model (shown in Fig. 3) included five sociodemographic variables and five clinical or disease-related

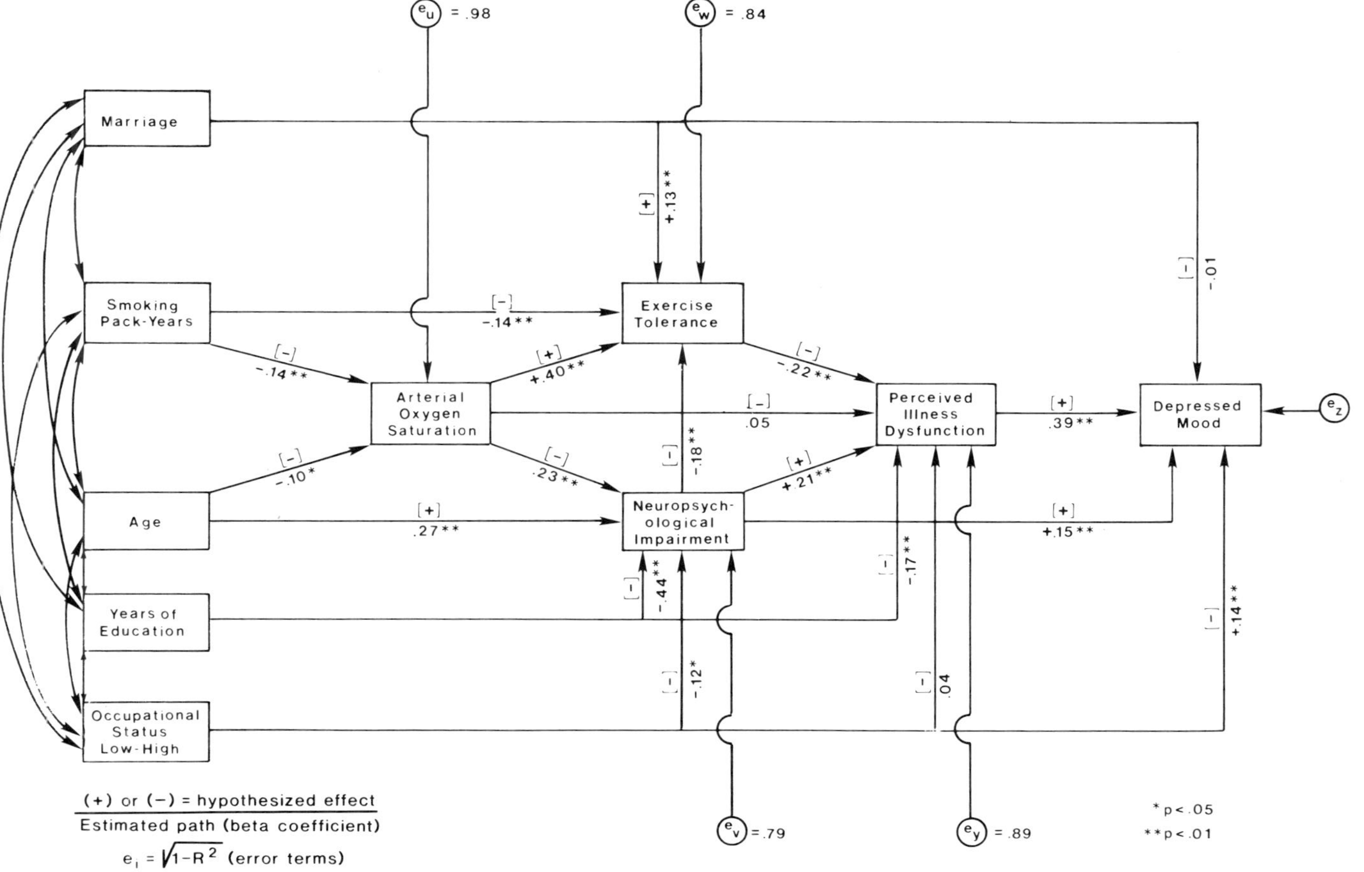

Figure 3 Path model for depressed mood in chronic obstructive pulmonary disease. (From Labuhn and McSweeny, 1987.)

Table 2 Direct, Indirect, and Total Effects of Predictors on the NOTT and IPPB Patients' Depressed Mood Scores

Predictor variable	Direct effect	Indirect effect	Total effect
Perceived illness dysfunction	+0.39	0.0000	+0.3900
Neuropsychological impairment	+0.15	+0.0973	+0.2473
Exercise tolerance	0.00	−0.0858	−0.0858
Arterial oxygen saturation	0.00	−0.1007	−0.1007
Occupational status (low-high)	+0.14	−0.0453	+0.0947
Education (low-high)	0.00	−0.0751	−0.0751
Age	0.00	+0.0834	+0.0834
Smoking pack-years	0.00	+0.0274	+0.0274
Marriage	−0.01	−0.0112	−0.0212

Source: Adapted from Labuhn and McSweeny, 1987.

variables. According to the model, one variable—perceived illness dysfunction (self-reported physical and psychosocial deficits as measured by the SIP)—directly impacts on mood, with more dysfunctional patients having higher levels of depressed moode (POMS—depression/dejection). Five variables, exercise tolerance, smoking, age, education, and arterial oxygen saturation, indirectly influence depressed mood through their effects on other variables in the model. Three variables, neuropsychological impairment (Average Impairment Rating; Russell et al., 1970), occupational status, and marital status were hypothesized to have both direct and indirect effects on depressed mood.

Ordinary least-squares, multiple-regression procedures were used to test the hypothesized linkages in the model. The resulting standardized β-coefficients are shown in Figure 3 and are listed in Table 2. Table 2 also offers a summary of the direct, indirect, and total effects of each predictor variable to depressed mood.

Perceived illness dysfunction, which reflects patient dysfunction, which in turn reflects the patient's ability to carry out physical and psychosocial activities, clearly makes the largest contribution to emotional disturbance in the form of depression. Neuropsychological impairment contributes heavily to depressed mood by impacting on exercise tolerance, physical functioning, and psychosocial functioning. Neuropsychological impairment also serves as an important intervening variable between depressed mood, oxygen saturation, education, and age. Exercise tolerance comes in third in order of importance to depressed mood, although much of its contribution is through perceived illness dysfunction. Arterial oxygen saturation is fourth in order of importance and is followed by the sociodemographic variables that contribute relatively small amounts of variance.

Additional analyses by Labuhn and McSweeny revealed that the relative order of the predictor variables changes as the disease of COPD becomes more advanced. Psychosocial factors were relatively more important in early stages of the disease, physiological and neuropsychological factors gained in importance during later stages. However, emotional status was never a simple function of disease severity. Indeed, a wide range of adjustment was seen at all stages of the disease.

B. Practical Applications

The fact that there is an interrelationship between psychosocial and physiological factors in COPD has been exploited infrequently in the clinical situation, if we are to judge from the number of published reports. Those reports that I was able to locate all came from the United Kingdom. This flies in the face of the popular stereotype of the erudite, but impractical, British as contrasted with the practical, down-to-earth Americans!

The earliest report is by Clark and Cochrane (1970), who employed the personality theory, and assessment procedures of Eysenck (1960; Eysenck and Eysenck, 1964) to help predict which COPD patients would show higher-than-expected CO_2 retention. Indeed, a significant correlation was found between extraversion and the departure of observed CO_2 tension (P_{CO_2}) from that predicted from forced expired volume in one second (FEV_1). The authors noted that according to Eysenck, extraversion is related to the degree of excitation in the central nervous system. Thus, they reasoned that extraversion should be related to the excitability of respiratory neurons. This hypothesis remains untested, however.

Rutter (1979) examined the usefulness of several psychological and physiological variables to predict outcome in an evaluation of a management program for COPD patients that included medical treatment, physical therapy, and breathing training. She found that the psychological variables had significant but limited value for predicting outcome as assessed by medical measures of disease severity. Psychological variables, in contrast, were highly useful in predicting the vocational adjustment and work record after management, whereas the physiological variables had very limited prognostic value.

Four relatively recent articles (Geddes, 1984; Morgan et al., 1983a,b;

Webber, 1981) have focused on exercise capability as an outcome of treatment and rehabilitation. These studies have produced remarkably consistent results. Psychological factors, including mood, attitudes, and beliefs, are important predictors of outcome as assessed by exercise-capability tests. Indeed, the reports indicate that psychological variables are at least as important, and perhaps even more so, than initial ventilatory status. Patients who feel better about themselves, their situation, and the future will participate more actively in therapies and will subsequently benefit more.

V. Implications of Life Quality Research

A. Implications for Research in Chronic Obstructive Pulmonary Disease

The investigations reviewed in the preceding sections underline the importance of psychological factors in the experience of COPD, the patient's ability to cope with life and to benefit from rehabilitation and treatment. Thus, it would seem axiomatic that psychological variables should be included as outcome variables in most patients and predictor or moderator variables in some patients, when medical and rehabilitative interventions for COPD are evaluated. In addition, as the research by Dudley (1969) and Clark and Cochrane (1970) demonstrates, psychological factors may also be useful in explaining some aspects of respiration in COPD that cannot be otherwise explained. Fortunately, this book demonstrates and documents the maturation of behavioral research in relation to COPD. Future research should include formal evaluations of psychological interventions for COPD patients that are aimed at ameliorating the psychological consequences of COPD as well as at improving the process and outcome of treatment and rehabilitation programs.

B. Clinical Implications

General Comments

Clinicians who care regularly for patients with COPD will not be surprised that researchers have found that many of their patients are unhappy, anxious, obstreperous, and unable to manage social transactions appropriate to their age and socioeconomic situation. Perhaps the more important finding, however, is that life quality is not simply a function of the patient's cardiopulmonary pathophysiology. Rather, the ability of the COPD patient to cope is influenced by age, social position, and neuropsychological status as well. Thus, the older and more disadvantaged patient is likely to have more social impairment and subjective distress. At the same time, changes in mental abilities may make the patient less able to understand treatment and less cooperative and flexible in seeking alternative sources of satisfaction in life.

Current research leads to the prediction that the patient with the poorest life quality would be the least likely to respond to traditional intervention because of the COPD-associated features of advanced age, low social position, and neuropsychological deficit. This prediction is borne out by one study by Pattison et al. (1971) that attempted to use insight-oriented group psychotherapy with COPD patients. Several of the persons in this program became openly hostile to the implication that they might have a "psychological problem," and others showed little or no benefit.

A more fruitful approach might be to integrate psychosocial supports into a multimodal pulmonary rehabilitation program, a suggestion also made by Dudley et al. (1980b). Psychological interventions that are part of standard patient education and rehabilitation programs are less obtrusive, more acceptable to patients, and have greater potential for success than does traditional psychotherapy. A program devised by the American Lung Association of West Virginia (Carlson et al., 1981), for example, includes both didactic lectures concerning the psychosocial effects of COPD and how to cope with them and structured group exercises for patients with COPD and their families. This program puts a particular emphasis on "depersonalizing" the emotional effects of COPD by attributing them to the disease process and teaching patients how to maximize access to activities that would yield psychological reinforcement. I have adopted this program for use with patient support groups (Better Breathers Clubs) in the Toledo area and have found it to be enthusiastically received.

Some Suggestions for Pulmonary Clinicians

A goal of this chapter has been to point out the importance of psychosocial factors in the lives of COPD patients. At the beginning of the chapter, I noted that this was consistent with Engel's (1980) biopsychosocial model for the science and profession of medicine. As Sandhu (1986) has noted, this model may also be used fruitfully as a guide to the management of the patient with COPD. To begin with, the physician will want to assume an empathetic and understanding, but encouraging (when appropriate) attitude toward patients and their families. Patients and family members should feel confident that their doctor will listen to their concerns, respond to questions about the psychosocial issues, and give them advice (or provide for other health care professionals to do so) on how to best cope with the "slings and arrows of [their] outrageous fortune" (Shakespeare, 1603/

1952) as well as to maximize the rewards and pleasures that are available to
them. This requires regular appointments, even when the patient appears
to be functioning well; recognizing and dealing with psychological defenses;
good interpersonal skills, as well as the time, willingness, and ability to listen.

Pulmonary clinicians may find it useful to include an assessment of
psychosocial functioning in their patients. This should always include an
interview of the patient and, if possible, relatives concerning emotional functioning, social role functioning, activities of daily living, sexuality, and recreational pastimes. Current smoking behavior should also be periodically
assessed and addressed. For some patients it may be useful to consult a clinical psychologist or psychiatrist for suggestions concerning a formal assessment that includes psychometric measures. The areas assessed and specific
instruments to be used could include several of those mentioned in earlier
sections of this chapter. The MMPI could be used to provide a good overview
of psychological adjustment and psychopathology, whereas the SIP may be
used to obtain a broad view of the patient's psychosocial and physical behavioral functioning. The POMS may be used to assess mood, and the Berle
Index may be employed to assess psychosocial status (see also Chap. 9 by
Dudley and Sitzman). The Millon Behavioral Health Inventory (MBHI; Millon et al., 1982) is a relatively new instrument that has not been used systematically in research with COPD patients but has demonstrated utility with
adult medical patients in general. It is a relatively brief (150 items vs. 566
for the MMPI) test of personality and emotional functioning developed specifically for use with physically ill patients. Twenty scales are grouped into
four basic categories: basic coping styles, psychogenic attitudes, psychosomatic correlates, and prognostic indices.

Computer scoring and interpretation programs exist for several psychological tests including the MMPI and MBHI, and many can be used on a personal computer. Most of these programs have the patina of validity but, in
fact, their quality varies greatly. As an experienced computer user and
psychometrician, I would strongly recommend against using a computerized
interpretation of a psychological test unless the reader is already well familiar with the test instrument and its interpretation. If this is not the case, a
psychologist or psychiatrist who is familiar with the test should be consulted.

Once the assessment is completed, an intervention plan should be developed. Many times, patients and relatives may be already functioning
relatively well and may only require simple advice and reassurance from their

physician concerning the conduct of their lives. Many patients and relatives will also find support groups, such as the Better Breathers Clubs, that are supported by the local chapters of the American Lung Association, to be very helpful. These groups usually include discussions of psychosocial issues as well as educational programs concerning medical aspects of COPD. Practical information, such as the location of restaurants with no-smoking policies, is often available through these groups. The location and time of the meetings may be obtained by contacting the local chapter of the American Lung Association.

As noted previously, psychosocial issues may also be handled efficaciously in a rehabilitation or patient education program. These are usually based in the respiratory therapy department of a local hospital. Many, but not all, of these programs do address psychosocial issues. Therefore, the physician or nurse may wish to visit the program and review it before referring patients to it.

A few patients (and relatives) will require referral to a mental health professional. Because the problems of the COPD patient are unique and somewhat different from the typical psychiatric patient, it will be important to choose a mental health professional who is familiar with medical illness and the problems it presents. If psychotropic medication is indicated, familiarity with the interaction between psychotropic drugs and the drugs used in the management of COPD is essential as is knowledge of the effects of the psychotropic drugs on respiration. The reader should consult Chapter 9 by Dudley and Sitzman for further details on the use of psychotropic medications.

VI. Conclusion

The goal of this chapter has been to underline the importance of psychosocial factors in COPD. It is my hope that pulmonary physicians will wish to incorporate a biopsychosocial model in their clinical and research efforts. Similarly, I hope that the chapter may encourage interested behavioral scientists and clinicians to bring their talents to bear on understanding and ameliorating the many problems faced by the COPD patient.

The psychosocial management of the COPD patient has received brief treatment in this chapter. For further suggestions the reader is advised to consult Dudley et al. (1980b,c), Grant and Timms (1985), and Sandhu (1986), as well as other chapters in this book.

References

Agle, D. P., and Baum, G. L. (1977). Psychosocial aspects of chronic obstructive pulmonary disease. *Med. Clin. N. A.* **61**:749-758.

Asher, H. B. (1976). *Causal Modeling.* Beverly Hills, Sage.

Barstow, R. E. (1974). Coping with emphysema. *Nurs. Clin. N. A.* **9**:137-145.

Bergner, M., Bobbitt, R. A., Carter, W., and Gilson, B. S. (1981). The Sickness Impact Profile: Development and final revision of a health status measure. *Med. Care* **12**:787-805.

Burns, B. H., and Howell, J. B. L. (1969). Disproportionately severe breathlessness in chronic bronchitis. *Q. J. Med.* **38**:277-294.

Carlson, J., Hoy, R., McSweeny, A. J., Rhodes, R., and Zaldivar, G. (1981). *Your Guide to Better Breathing: Instructor's Manual.* Charleston, WV, American Lung Association of West Virginia.

Casselith, B. R., Luck, E. J., Strouse, T. B., Miller, D. S., Brown, L. L., Cross, P. A., and Tenaglia, B. S. (1984). Psychosocial status in chronic illness: a comparative analysis of six diagnostic groups. *N. Engl. J. Med.* **311**: 506-511.

Chambers, L. W., MacDonald, L. A., and Tugwell, P. (1982). The McMaster Health Index Questionnaire as a measure of the quality of life for patients with rheumatoid disease. *J. Rheumatol.* **9**:780-784.

Clark, R. J. H., and Cochrane, G. M. (1970). Effect of personality on alveolar ventilation in patients with chronic airways obstruction. *Br. Med. J.* **1**:273-275.

Cook, T. D., and Campbell, D. T. (1979). *Quasi-Experimentation: and Analysis Issues for the Field Settings.* Chicago, Rand-McNally.

Costello, C. G. (1972). Depression: loss of reinforcers or loss of reinforcer effectiveness? *Behav. Ther.* **2**:240-247.

Dahlstrom, W. G., Welsh, G. S., and Dahlstrom, L. E. (1972). *An MMPI Handbook,* Rev. Ed. Minneapolis, University of Minnesota.

De Araujo, G., Van Arsdel, P. P., Holmes, T. H., and Dudley, D. L. (1973). Life change, coping ability and chronic intrinsic asthma. *J. Psychosom. Res.* **17**:359-363.

Dudley, D. L. (1969). *Psychophysiology of Respiration in Health and Disease.* New York, Appleton-Century-Crofts.

Dudley, D. L., Glaser, E. M., Jorgenson, B. N., and Logan, D. L. (1980a). Psychosocial concomitants to rehabilitation in chronic obstructive pulmonary disease, part I: Psychosocial and psychological considerations. *Chest* **77**:413-420.

Dudley, D. L., Glaser, E. M., Jorgenson, B. N., and Logan, D. L. (1980b). Psychosocial concomitants to rehabilitation in chronic obstructive pulmonary disease, part II: Psychosocial treatment. *Chest* 77:544-551.

Dudley, D. L., Glaser, E. M., Jorgenson, B. N., and Logan, D. L. (1980c). Psychosocial concomitants to rehabilitation in chronic obstructive pulmonary disease, part III: Dealing with psychiatric disease. *Chest* 77: 667-684.

Dudley, D. L., Wermuth, C., and Hague, W. (1973). Psychosocial aspects of care in the chronic obstructive pulmonary disease patient. *Heart Lung* 2:289-303.

Engel, G. E. (1980). The clinical application of the biopsychosocial model. *Am. J. Psychiatry* 137:535-543.

Eysenck, H. J. (1960). *The Structure of Human Personality*, 2nd ed. London, Methuen.

Eysenck, H. J., and Eysenck, S. B. G. (1964). *Manual of the Eysenck Personality Inventory*. London, University of London Press.

Fletcher, E. C., and Martin, R. J. (1982). Sexual dysfunction and erectile impotence in chronic obstructive pulmonary disease. *Chest* 81:413-421.

Geddes, D. M. (1984). Chronic airflow obstruction. *Postgrad. Med. J.* 60: 194-200.

Grant, I., And Timms, R. M. (1985). Psychiatric disturbances in chronic obstructive pulmonary disease. In *Manual of Clinical Problems in Chronic Obstructive Pulmonary Disease*. Edited by R. A. Bondow and K. M. Moses. Boston, Little, Brown.

Greenberg, G. D., Ryan, J. J., and Bourlier, P. E. (1985). Psychological and neuropsychological aspects of COPD. *Psychosomatics* 26:29-33.

Hanson, E. I. (1982). Effects of chronic lung disease on life in general and sexuality: perceptions of adult patients. *Heart Lung* 11:435-441.

Jensen, P. S. (1983). Risk, protective factors, and supportive interventions in chronic airway obstruction. *Arch. Gen. Psychiatry* 40:1203-1207.

Kass, I., Updegraff, K., and Muffly, R. B. (1972). Sex in chronic obstructive pulmonary disease. *Med. Aspects Hum. Sex.* 6:33-42.

Katz, M. M., and Lyerly, S. B. (1963). Methods of measuring adjustment and behavior in the community: I. Rationale, description, discriminative validity, and scale development. *Psychol. Rep.* 13:503-535.

Kinsman, R. A., Yaroush, R. A., Fernandez, E., Dirks, J. F., Schocket, M., and Fukuhara, J. (1983). Symptoms and experiences in chronic bronchitis and emphysema. *Chest* 83:755-761.

Labuhn, K. T., and McSweeny, A. J. (1987). A causal modeling study of determinants of depressed mood in chronic obstructive pulmonary disease. (submitted for publication).

Levine, S., and Croog, S. H. (1984). What constitutes quality of life?: a conceptualization of the dimensions of life quality in healthy populations and patients with cardiovascular disease. In *Assessment of Quality of Life in Clinical Trials of Cardiovascular Therapies.* Edited by N. K. Wenger, M. E. Mattson, C. D. Furberg, and J. Elinson. New York, LeJacq.

McCullough, L. B. (1984). The concept of quality of life: a philosophical analysis. In *Assessment of Quality of Life in Clinical Trials of Cardiovascular Therapies.* Edited by N. K. Wenger, M. E. Mattson, C. D. Furberg, and J. Elinson. New York, LeJacq.

McNair, D. M., Lorr, M., and Droppleman, L. F. (1971). *Manual for the Profile of Mood States.* San Diego, Educational and Industrial Testing Service.

McSweeny, A. J. (1984). Assessing the quality of life in patients with chronic obstructive pulmonary disease. In *Assessment of Quality of Life in Clinical Trials of Cardiovascular Therapies.* Edited by N. K. Wenger, M. E. Mattson, C. D. Furberg, and J. Elinson. New York, LeJacq.

McSweeny, A. J., Grant, I., Heaton, R. K., Adams, K. M., and Timms, R. M. (1982). Life quality of patients with chronic obstructive pulmonary disease. *Arch. Intern. Med.* **142**:473-478.

Millon, T., Green, C. J., and Meagher, R. B. (1982). *Millon Behavioral Health Inventory Manual.* 3rd ed. Minneapolis, National Computer Systems.

Morgan, A. D., Peck, D. F., Buchanan, D. R., and McHardy, G. J. R. (1983a). Effects of attitudes and beliefs on exercise tolerance in chronic bronchitis. *Br. Med. J.* **286**:171-173.

Morgan, A. D., Peck, D. F., Buchanan, D. R., and McHardy, G. J. R. (1983b). Psychological factors contributing to disproportionate disability in chronic bronchitis. *J. Psychosom. Res.* **27**:259-261.

Pattison, E. M., Rhodes, R. J., and Dudley, D. L. (1971). Response to group treatment in patients with severe chronic lung disease. *Int. J. Group Psychother.* **21**:214-255.

Pearlman, R. A., and Jonsen, A. (1985). The use of quality-of-life considerations in medical decision making. *J. Am. Geriatr. Soc.* **33**:344-352.

Post, L., and Collins, C. (1981-82). The poorly coping COPD patient: a psychotherapeutic perspective. *J. Psychiatry Med.* **11**:173-182.

Prigatano, G. P., Wright, E. C., and Levin, D. (1984). Quality of life and its predictors in patients with mild hypoxemia and chronic obstructive pulmonary disease. *Arch. Intern. Med.* **144**:1613-1619.

Russell, E. W., Neuringer, C., and Goldstein, G. (1970). *Assessment of Brain Damage: A Neuropsychological Key Approach.* New York, Wiley-Interscience.

Rutter, B. M. (1979). The prognostic significance of psychological factors in the management of chronic bronchitis. *Psychol. Med.* **9**:63-70.

Sandhu, H. S. (1986). Psychosocial issues in chronic obstructive pulmonary disease. *Clin. Chest Med.* **7**:629-642.

Shakespeare, W. (1603/1952). The tragedy of Hamlet, Prince of Denmark. In *Shakespeare: The Complete Works.* Edited by G. B. Harrison. New York, Harcourt, Brace and World.

Veit, C. T., and Ware, J. E. (1983). The structure of psychological distress and well-being in general populations. *J. Consult. Clin. Psychol.* **51**: 730-742.

Ware, J. E. (1984). Methodological considerations in the selection of health status assessment procedures. In *Assessment of Quality of Life in Clinical Trials of Cardiovascular Therapies.* Edited by N. K. Wenger, M. E. Mattson, C. D. Furberg, and J. Elinson. New York, LeJacq.

Webber, B. A. (1981). Living to the limit: exercise for the chronic breathless patient. *Physiotherapy* **67**:128-130.

Wenger, N. K., Mattson, M. E., Furberg, C. D., and Elinson, J. (1984a). Preface and overview: assessment of quality of life in clinical trials of cardiovascular therapies. In *Assessment of Quality of Life in Clinical Trials of Cardiovascular Therapies.* Edited by N. K. Wenger, M. E. Mattson, C. D. Furberg, and J. Elinson. New York, LeJacq.

Wenger, N. K., Mattson, M. E., Furberg, C. D., and Elinson, J. (1984b). Assessment of quality of life in clinical trials of cardiovascular therapies. *Am. J. Cardiol.* **54**:908-913.

Young, R. F. (1982). Marital adaptation and response in chronic illness: the case of COPD. Doctoral dissertation, Wayne State University, 1981. *Diss. Abstr. Int.* **42**:4947A.

5

Medical Management of COPD

THOMAS L. PETTY

Webb-Waring Lung Institute
University of Colorado
  Health Sciences Center
Denver, Colorado

I. Introduction

The problem of emphysema and chronic bronchitis, together called chronic
obstructive pulmonary disease (COPD), has reached immense proportions.
At least 15,000,000 symptomatic patients live in the United States and probably the overall prevalence of disease in our country is 30 million. More than
500,000 are receiving Social Security Disability payments for advanced disease (Roberts, 1980).

In a carefully performed prevalence study in a small Colorado resort
community with no significant industry or air pollution, 13% of the men over
the age of 20 had significant chronic airflow obstruction judged by spirometry
and 4% ofthe women had the same degree of abnormality (Mueller et al., 1971).
Subsequent evaluation of these patients indicated both premature morbidity
and mortality in those found originally abnormal by spirometric testing (see
below). In fact, this indicator of disease proved to be effective in identifying
patients at high risk, but it likely identified patients who were relatively ad-

vanced in their development of COPD. The natural history of chronic obstructive pulmonary disease is now known to cover approximately 30 years and begins with some cellular or biochemical events leading to damage and destruction of alveolar walls and airway inflamation and fibrosis. As the process advances clinical signs and symptoms occur, resulting in a disease state that can be readily identified and treated. The systematic approach to the identification and treatment is the subject of this chapter.

II. Assessment of the Symptomatic Patient

The cardinal symptoms of COPD are dyspnea on exertion, cough, and expectoration. Wheeze may or may not be present. Dyspnea on exertion is by far the most important symptom and correlates roughly with the degree of airflow obstruction as judged by spirometry. Cough, though common, is not at accurate indicator of disease severity since many patients with "simple bronchitis," that is, with cough and expectoration, but *without* airflow obstruction are present in North America, and these individuals do not suffer premature mortality. The most useful indicator of disease severity, across all stages of disease is spirometry, with the FEV_1 being the best indicator of abnormality. The rate of deterioration in FEV_1 is a potent prognostic indicator.

III. Management of COPD

A. Preventive Measures

We can view COPD as a disease caused by smoking in susceptible individuals, that is, those with a family history of COPD. Certain work environments and probably air pollution play an additional modifying role, but nothing is as important as smoking as an external controllable factor. Stopping smoking is of fundamental importance to the successful management of all stages of COPD. Stopping earlier in the natural course of disease will slow the rate of decline in ventilatory function to a rate equivalent to the age-related change (Fletcher and Peto, 1977).

Hazards in the work environment should also be eliminated. Dusts inhaled by grain and cotton workers, fumes from solvents such as isocyanates used in the urethane and paint industries and probably other work environmental hazards should be identified and eliminated if possible. It is doubtful whether common ground dust sometimes inhaled in arid areas or even coal dust causes harm in terms of damage to alveoli or airways in nonsmokers.

B. Vaccines

The patient with chronic obstructive pulmonary disease is more susceptible
to influenza and also more vulnerable to its damaging effects to the conducting airways. Thus, influenza virus vaccine should be given each fall, particularly if epidemics are likely. Progressively pure and potent multivalent (i.e.,
addressing several viral strains simultaneously) vaccines are now widely used.
Each fall generally requires a change in antigenic properties of the vaccine because the influenza virus mutates rapidly, rendering previous vaccines ineffective. The use of antiviral drugs such as amantadine by mouth during the
influenza season is an effective alternative. In fact, amantadine might be more
effective in preventing or modifying early states of diseases than the vaccine
itself. The two can be used concurrently.

Even though somewhat controversial, polyvalent (addressing several
strains of the bacterium) pneumococcal vaccine is also useful in affording at
least some degree of protection against these common pneumonia organisms.
Pneumococcal vaccine is now recommended to be given only once in a lifetime. The pneumococcal and influenza vaccines can be given at the same
time for convenience and efficiency.

C. Pharmacologic Therapy

The classes of drugs that are most useful in the management of COPD are the
antimicrobials (antibiotics), bronchodilators, and corticosteroids. These drugs
are widely used and the role of each class of drug as well as certain brief speci-
fics are considered below.

Antimicrobials (Antibiotics)

Numerous studies have attempted to define the role of bacterial infection on
the course and prognosis of COPD. Although it is well-known that bacterial
invasion of the normally sterile lower airways occurs commonly, the importance of this infestation or infection apart from causing exacerbations of symptoms (i.e., increased cough and expectoration) remains unknown. The most
common organisms that invade the lower airway are *Hemophilus* species, the
pneumococcus, occasionally mycoplasma, and, less frequently, the *Legionella*
bacillus and anaerobic bacteria.

With this knowledge and with the certainty that culture of expectorated
sputum is not likely to be practical or accurate in identifying which of the
several organisms is actually producing an infection, the clinician generally re-
lies on the empiric use of antibiotics based upon epidemiologic considerations.

Table 1 Common Antimicrobial (Antibiotic) Drugs Used for Flare-ups of Chronic Bronchitis

Name	Usual dose	Side effects
Ampicillin	250 or 500 mg 4 times a day	Rash, diarrhea
Erythromycin	250 or 500 mg 4 times a day	Stomach upset
Tetracycline	250 mg 4 times a day; some other preparations once a day	Stomach upset, diarrhea, vaginal yeast infections
Trimethoprim-sulfamethoxazole (Bactrim, Septra)	1 capsule twice a day	Rare gastrointestinal upset

Thus, most physicians would prescribe an antimicrobial at the first sign of sputum purulence (i.e., yellow or green sputum) with accompanying increased cough and fever.

Table 1 lists the antibiotics most commonly used and comments about each. It is probably best to have the patient initiate therapy at the first sign of infection and to report to the physician about the response. It is known that the use of antimicrobials will shorten the symptomatic period, reduce days lost from work, and probably prevent or shorten hospitalizations. For these reasons antimicrobials should be used in patients with exacerbations of purulent bronchitis. In many instances no infectious agent can be found to explain an exacerbation of purulent bronchitis. In these cases a virus infection is the most likely causative agent.

Bronchodilators

Bronchodilators are used because many patients with COPD have a degree of bronchial hyperreactivity. Bronchodilators promote airflow by combating increased muscular tension (bronchospasm), thereby dilating obstructed airways, and may also help in preventing reflex bronchoconstriction that occurs as a response to a variety of nonspecific stimuli. The two major classes of bronchodilators are the beta agonists and the theophylline preparations.

Beta agonists are commonly administered by the inhalational route. The

most convenient method of delivering a beta agonist aerosol is by a metered
dose device. Although this system of drug delivery has been under criticism
in some circles, no scientific evidence indicates that any better system exists.
The metered dose device can be kept in the pocket or purse and used for
emergencies to overcome shortness of breath.

A more useful role of these drugs is in maintenance management, which
involves regular dosing three or four times a day. In either instance patients
need detailed instructions in the proper use of the metered dose aerosol.
This can be provided by a nurse, therapist or physician. Figure 1 shows a
nurse teaching a patient the proper method of bronchodilator administration. Note that the mouth is open in preparation of inhalation of the bronchodilating aerosol. In fact, the mouthpiece could be placed further in front
of the mouth than the example in Figure 1 suggests. Three or 4 inches is a
proper distance. Some physicians prefer the use of a 4-6 inch tube spacer.
This distance allows for the precipitation of large particles that only land in
the mouth and are absorbed via the mucosa causing systemic effects. The
desired strategy of giving a bronchodilating aerosol is to deliver a minuscule
amount of active agent into the airways for effective bronchodilatation. Patients should be taught to inhale from midlung volume so that the airways
are open to allow deep penetration and deposition. Inhalation should be at
a slow flow rate with a pause at the end of inspiration followed by exhalation
against pursed lips, again to promote deposition of small particles. Separating
the two inhalations by 10-20 min also offers better bronchodilatation than
rapidly sequencing the two inhalations, which tends to be the common
practice.

Many patients use their metered dose aerosols incorrectly (Shim and
Williams, 1980). This fact underscores the importance of instructing patients
concerning proper use of their metered dose devices, and the dangers of excessive use. In this way it should be possible to capitalize upon the benefits of
these potent agents and minimize side effects or abuse.

Table 2 lists some of the beta agonist aerosols available both over the
counter and by prescription. An increasing number of products have been
released recently. The longest acting and most specific agents are albuterol,
bitolterol, and terbutaline. Although all bronchodilators are efficacious, there
are some individual differences in response and the possibility of relative tolerance or subsensitivity to one or another agent. For this reason it may be wise
to rotate the brand of bronchodilator aerosol, particularly if previous beneficial responses are no longer achieved.

Table 3 lists the solution of some of the same beta agonists available by

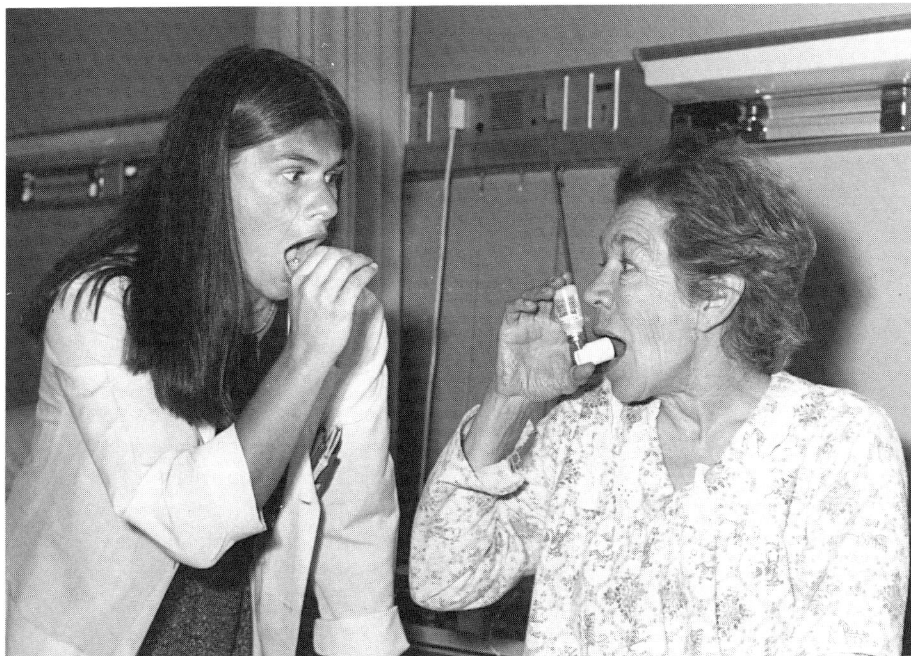

Figure 1 Nurse teaching patient how to use a metered-dose device. Inhalation should be from midlung volume with the mouth open. The mouthpiece should not be grasped with the lips. It would be even better, as the nurse is suggesting, to place the device 2 or 3 inches in front of the mouth to allow rain-out of large particles.

prescription for use in hand bulb or pump-driven nebulizers. These can also be used in intermittent positive-pressure breathing (IPPB) devices. Thus far no evidence exists that bronchodilator delivery via IPPB offers any advantage over other methods and, in fact, the high flow rate produced by the IPPB machine might actually interfere with deposition of particles. Pump-driven nebulizers are more convenient than hand bulb devices and offer a smaller particle size which, might suggest a theoretic advantage. However, small particles tend to coalesce when they encounter the warm moist air of the trachea forming larger particles. Thus the hand bulb or powered nebulizer probably offers no advantage over the metered dose device.

Table 2 Selected Bronchodilator Aerosols
(Metered-Dose Device)

Nonprescription
  Epinephrine (Bronkaid, Primatene)
Prescription
  Albuterol (Proventil, Ventolin)
  Bitolterol (Tornalate)
  Fenoterol (Berotec)*
  Isoetharine (Bronkometer)
  Isoproterenol (Isuprel)
  Metaproterenol (Alupent, Metaprel)
  Terbutaline (Brethaire)

*Not available in the United States.

Table 3 Beta Agonist Solutions for Hand
Bulb or Powered Nebulizers

Albuterol (Proventil, Ventolin)
Epinephrine (Vaponefrin or generic)
Isoetharine (Bronkosol or generic)
Isoproterenol (Isuprel or generic)
Metaproterenol (Alupent, Metaprel)

The beta agonist preparations are also available in oral form. Examples of commonly used oral beta agonists, and their usual dosages are metaproterenol (Alupent), 10-20 mg four times daily (qid); terbutaline (Brethine or Bricanyl) 2.5-5 mg three times a day (tid); albuterol (Proventil or Ventolin) 2 or 4 mg tid or qid. Considerable debate exists as to the role of oral beta agonists when patients are already receiving the same product by the inhaled route. It is unlikely that an additional degree of bronchodilitation can be produced with an oral agent, however.

The other popular class of oral agents used for bronchodilatation are theophylline salts or theophylline itself. Both short-acting and long-acting

Table 4 Common Oral Theophylline Products

Short-acting products (usually taken 3 or 4 times a day)	Long-acting products[a] (usually taken only twice a day)
Aminophylline (generic)	
	Choledyl SA
Choledyl	Constant T
	Resbid
Theophylline USP	Theo-Dur
	Ultra long-acting products (usually taken once a day)
	Theo-24
	Uniphyl

[a]Only a partial list.

preparations are widely used. Some of the commonly used products are listed in Table 4.

Theophylline is not only a bronchodilator but also has a beneficial effect on respiratory muscle fatigue. The clinical significance of this effect is not known. A small, but statistically significant improvement in cardiac function is also achieved in some patients (Matthay et al., 1982). Finally, theophylline is a mild respiratory stimulant that might be useful in patients with decreased respiratory center responsiveness.

A Suggested Bronchodilator Regimen

A typical strategy I use is to begin with an inhaled beta agonist morning, night, and at noontime if symptoms require more frequent dosing. The next step is an oral sustained release theophylline given once daily. The continuation of these products is guided by symptomatic improvement, objective functional improvement and lack of side effects. Many drug interactions affect the blood level of theophylline and thus the use of serum determinations is common, though I believe that there might be too much preoccupation with these determinations. Serious complications from oral theophylline are almost nonexistent in the absence of drug abuse or serious gastrointestinal symptoms.

Oral beta agonists are used in patients who will not or cannot use an inhaled beta agonist. Oral beta agonists have few drug interactions and blood level measurements are not required.

The beta agonists may also be preferred in some patients with gastrointestinal disease. Theophylline can aggravate peptic ulcer disease and gastrointestinal reflux. Furthermore, clearance of theophylline can be impaired by cimetidine and other H_2 blockers, which are used commonly to treat peptic ulcers.

Corticosteroids

Recent evidence clearly indicates that corticosteroids offer both subjective and objective benefit to a substantial number of patients. For example, a significant number of patients with advanced emphysema or chronic bronchitis participating in the Nocturnal Oxygen Therapy Trial (NOTT Group, 1980) achieved benefit with the equivalent of 40 mg prednisone given each morning for 2 weeks (Mandella et al., 1982). I have long believed that a therapeutic trial of corticosteroids in this dosage for this duration guided by symptoms and objective measurements focusing on *both* FEV_1 and FVC is wise. If objective benefit is gained, corticosteroids should be continued until maximum benefit occurs. After maximum benefit is reached, corticosteroids should be tapered to the lowest dosage that will maintain this predetermined benefit. This might be alternate day steroids or a small daily morning dose. It is unlikely that inhaled corticosteroids will be as effective as oral preparations in advanced COPD. Even moderate doses of daily corticosteroids are well tolerated by men and some women. Long-term complications include osteopenia (bone demineralization), premature cataract formation, and increased intraocular pressures associated with glaucoma. Men have far less osteopenia than women and large-boned, darker-skinned women have much less osteopenia than smaller-framed, light-skinned women. Most men and large women can tolerate 10-15 mg prednisone in a single morning dosage without symptomatic osteopenia.

Osteopenia is better prevented than treated. Patients should receive 1 g calcium daily in the form of a quart of skim milk or appropriate calcium supplements if the use of long-term corticosteroids is required. Exercise also mitigates osteopenia. Since the bronchodilator effect of corticosteroids will tend to increase exercise tolerance, this therapeutic action can offset the adverse osteopenic effect. Estrogen replacement is recommended for postmenopausal women.

Anticholinergics

Anticholinergics will soon be widely used in COPD. The recent release of ipratropium bromide (Atrovent) now provides a convenient product which

is available in a metered dose inhaler. Ipratropium bromide is frequently
more potent as a bronchodilator than an inhaled beta agonist in patients
with advanced COPD. Many patients respond more in volume, i.e., FVC than
in flow, i.e., FEV_1. Atropine derivatives probably work by interfering with
irritant vagally mediated reflexes. Ipratropium bromide is also compatible
with all inhaled beta agonists.

Other Pharmacologic Agents

Very few other drugs are useful in the management of COPD. Those patients
that are intensely anxious might benefit from small doses of benzodiazopenes,
but one must recognize the possibility of respiratory center depression. Two
mg diazepam (Valium) given occasionally almost never causes harm. Also
dihydrocodeine has been used to relieve dyspnea in the "pink puffer" type of
COPD; those patients with the highest respiratory drives and most intense
dyspnea (Johnson et al., 1983). An effective dose is 5 to 15 mg three or four
times daily.

Diuretics are useful for edema formation that may occur with or without heart failure. Thiazides are preferable to loop diuretics because they do
not promote calcium wasting. Digitalis is not useful in isolated right heart
failure, but can be used to combat supraventricular tachyarrhythmias. Calcium channel blockers are probably more effective than cardiac glycosides
and do not cause bronchospasm. Beta blockers (e.g., propranolol) of course
are contraindicated in patients with any bronchospastic disorder.

Mucoevacuants such as organic iodides are currently being reevaluated.

D. Pulmonary Rehabilitation

We have long been interested in the technique of pulmonary rehabilitation
(Petty, 1977, 1980). The definition of pulmonary rehabilitation adopted by
the Committee of the American College of Chest Physicians is as follows:

> Pulmonary rehabilitation may be defined as an art of medical practice
> wherein an individually tailored, multidisciplinary program is formu-
> lated which through accurate diagnosis, therapy, emotional support,
> and education, stabilizes or reverses both the physio- and psycho-
> pathology of pulmonary diseases and attempts to return the patient
> to the highest possible functional capacity allowed by his pulmonary
> handicap and overall life situation" (Petty, 1977).

Table 5 Essential Components of a Pulmonary
Rehabilitation Program

Patient and family education

Bronchial hygiene techniques

Breathing retraining and breathing exercises

Systematic exercise

Oxygen (selected patients)

In brief, the elements of a pulmonary rehabilitation program include
the factors listed on Table 5. Comments about each step in rehabilitation
follow.

Patient and family *education* is extremely important in any chronic
illness. The patient must understand the nature of the disease and the goals
of therapy. The realities of therapy in the long term must ultimately be understood. This requires that nurse, therapist, or physician sit with the patient to
explain about the disease, preferably with the aid of patient-oriented books
or pamphlets. Figure 2 shows the nurse using our first patient care manual
(*For Those Who Live and Breathe*, Charles C Thomas, Springfield, IL). A more
recent book, *Enjoying Life with Emphysema*, 2nd ed. (Lea & Febiger, 600
Washington Square, Philadelphia, PA 19106), is of additional value. Numerous other pamphlets can be used. Patients must understand the basics of
lung structure and function and the role of pharmacologic agents and understand basic health-oriented messages that are relevant to their own problem.
Above all, they must have a knowledge of their medications and become
realistic about the objectives of therapy.

Breathing training is also quite valuable to most patients. Relaxing the
abdomen during inspiration and exhaling against pursed lips as depicted in
Figure 3 has an established scientific basis. Slow breathing with exhalation
against pursed lips reduces the respiratory rate, increases the tidal volume,
and reduces the ventilation requires for oxygen transfer (Mueller et al.,
1970). Most importantly it relieves dyspnea. The leaning forward posture
also relieves dyspnea. It accomplishes this by relieving certain adverse reflexes of the respiratory muscles (mainly diaphragm). Recently new interest has focused on breathing exercises. Breathing against greater resistances
controlled by an orifice can improve muscular strength and relieve dyspnea
(Sonne and David, 1982). Performing a maximum voluntary ventilation

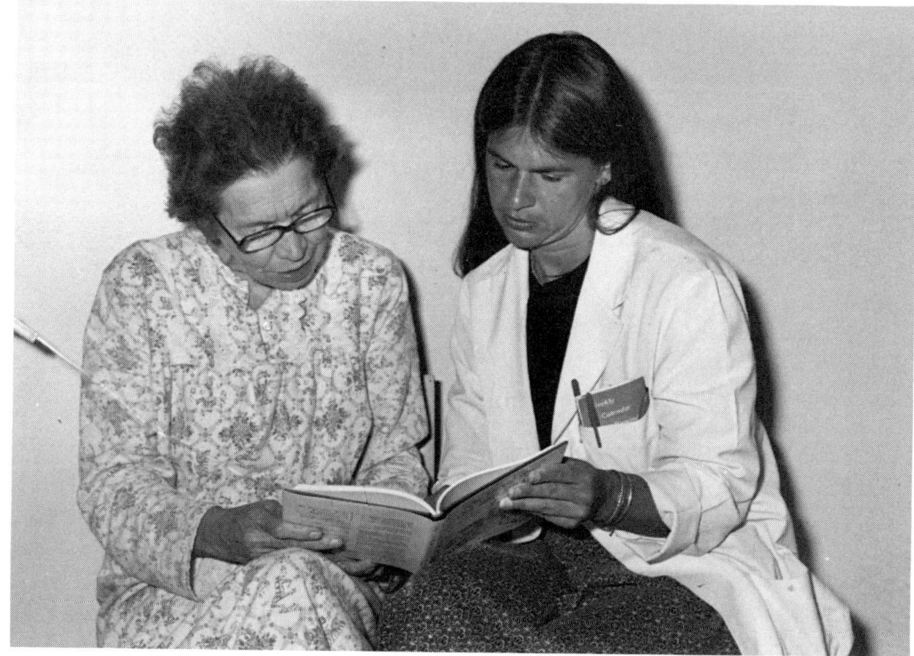

Figure 2 Nurse instructing patient in the details of care for advanced emphysema. She is using a book coauthored by the author, *For Those Who Live and Breathe* (Charles C Thomas, Springfield, IL).

maneuver accomplishes the same thing. Probably exercising itself has similar benefit. In any case, some activity should be designed to improve muscle strength, coordination, and thus overall functioning of the individual.

Systematic exercises are also valuable for patients with advanced disease. Almost any patient can be taught to walk increased distances. Patients must coordinate their breathing pattern with the walking pattern. Exercise in corridors and on stairs is most useful. Treadmills are often used to make measurements and are necessary for research purposes. However, treadmill walking cannot be mastered by many patients and demands a skill not necessary for daily living. Stationary bicycle exercises help train the lower extremities. It must be remembered, however, that training is task-specific. Since this is so, bicycle riding may not be translated into normal walking or activities of daily living. Nevertheless, some form of regular graded exercise is valuable to most patients.

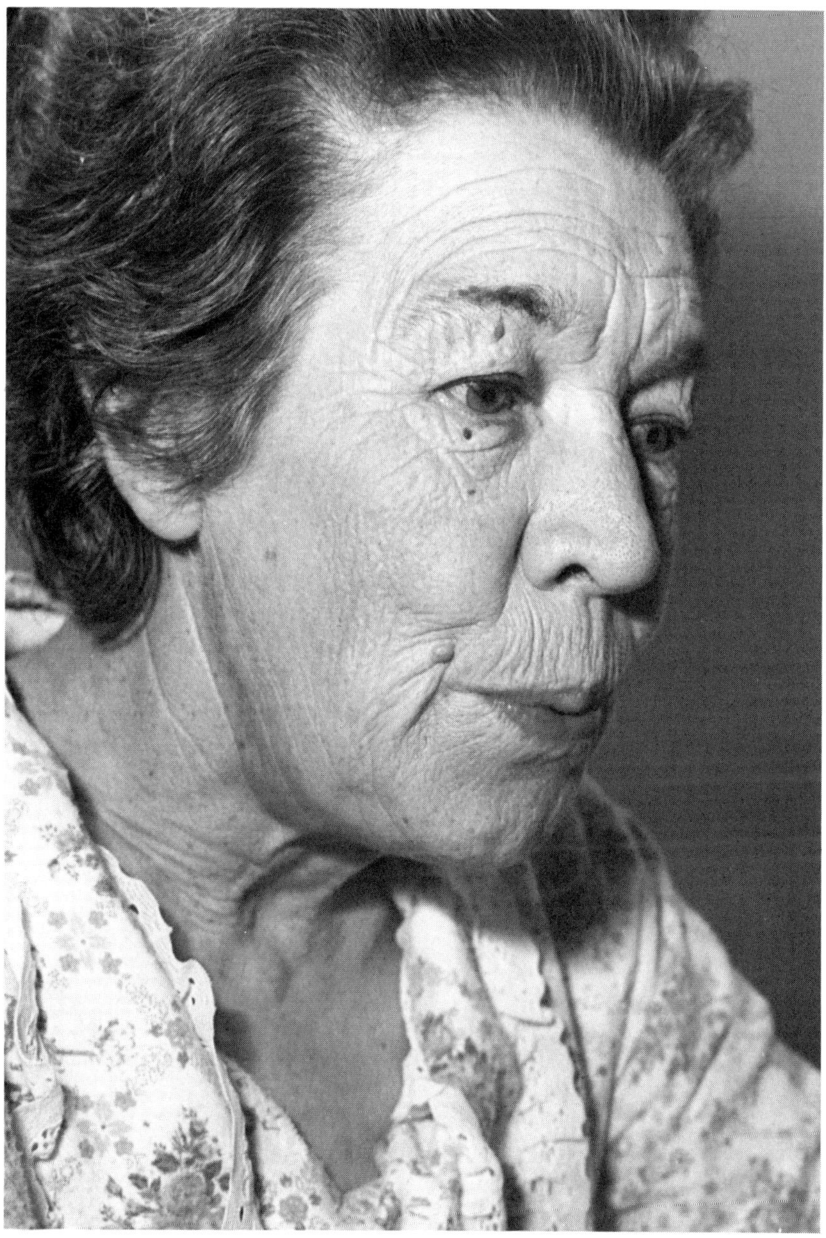

Figure 3 Technique of exhaling against pursed lips to provide more complete emptying of the lung and to slow the respiratory rate. This pursed-lip breathing technique has been shown to improve oxygen transfer across the lung (Mueller et al., 1970).

The mechanism underlying improvement in exercise tolerance has been widely debated. It is likely that improved use of muscles, better tolerance of dyspnea, and increased motivation are together helpful in improving exercise capability. One cannot exercise the patient with COPD to a predetermined heart rate such as in cardiac rehabilitation. Exercise is limited largely by ventilatory mechanics and the strength of the extremities.

E. Oxygen

Long-term home oxygen has emerged as an important method of treatment for selected patients with advanced COPD and hypoxemia. Oxygen improves exercise tolerance, reduces pulmonary artery pressures and pulmonary arteriolar resistance (in some, but not all patients), helps correct secondary polycythemia, and improves brain function. Overall, it improves the quality of life for many patients.

Two major controlled clinical trials have added to our understanding of the value of home oxygen. The Nocturnal Oxygen Therapy Trial focused upon the necessary duration of oxygen in advanced patients with COPD and hypoxemia. This study was conducted in Chicago, Denver, Detroit, Los Angeles, San Diego, and Winnipeg (NOTT Group, 1980). In all, 203 patients were randomized to receive either 12 or 24 hr per day oxygen. Outcomes included survival, neuropsychological function, quality of life indicators, detailed pulmonary function evaluations, and hemodynamic and exercise measurements. The results of this study showed a much better survival rate at 1 and 2 years' follow-up from continuous oxygen therapy (COT) compared to nocturnal oxygen therapy (NOT). COT patients had fewer hospitalizations. Brain function was equally improved in COT and NOT patients at 6 months but further mental improvement occurred in COT patients at 12 months, but this did not occur with NOT (Heaton et al., 1983). This aspect is discussed in more detail in Chapter 6.

In the British MRC study, 15 hr oxygen (including the hours of sleep) was compared to no oxygen in matched patients. Survival was much better in the oxygen patients than in the no oxygen control group. The British MRC 15 hr survival curve equalled the American NOT survival curve. Thus, taking these two major controlled clinical trials together, one can conclude that without oxygen survival in advanced COPD with significant hypoxemia is poor. Some oxygen is better than none; more continuous oxygen is better than lesser amounts in terms of survival.

Home oxygen systems include liquid portable, high-pressure cylinders, and concentrators.

IV. Effect of Systematic Treatment on Disease Outcome

Our studies and others have clearly shown that the application of therapeutic principles described above has a major impact on disease outcome. Almost all patients have an improved quality of life and carefully performed psychological studies have revealed a reduction in anxiety, depression, and somatic preoccupation. Exercise tolerance is improved in most. Although there is no clear evidence that survival is improved in large series, data from our rehabilitation program compared to similar patients in the Denver area suggested a modest survival benefit from a rehabilitation program (Petty, 1980). Those patients selected for oxygen in the Nocturnal Oxygen Therapy Trial clearly had improved survival. It was estimated that approximately 3.75 years of life was "bought" with the use of continuous oxygen as part of a total care program. Data from our rehabilitation program showed that hospital needs could be markedly reduced for at least 4 years in surviving patients, strongly indicating a major economic impact of comprehensive care (Hudson et al., 1976). The most important facet, however, is improved quality of life, including return to gainful employment in some patients and a reduced symptom impact.

The overall outcome, however, is not satisfactory and a marked excess mortality in advanced COPD is present in spite of a tailor-made, personalized, pulmonary rehabilitation program. This fact, previously reported, is underscored by scrutiny of the long-term survival of patients, mostly men with an average age of 61, mean FEV_1 = 0.94 (Petty et al., 1969). Figure 4 shows the survival curve of patients participating in a pulmonary rehabilitation program as previously described during the early years of our experience (Petty et al., 1969). The actual survival curve (solid dots) compared to the predicted survival of normal individuals (open circles) gives graphic evidence of the excess mortality of advanced COPD in spite of systematic therapy (Sahn et al., 1980). Thus, although we remain highly enthusiastic about what can be accomplished via modern therapy, we recognize that this benefit is largely improved quality of life and reduced hospitalization (Hudson et al., 1976). Is there a more potent argument for early identification and intervention?

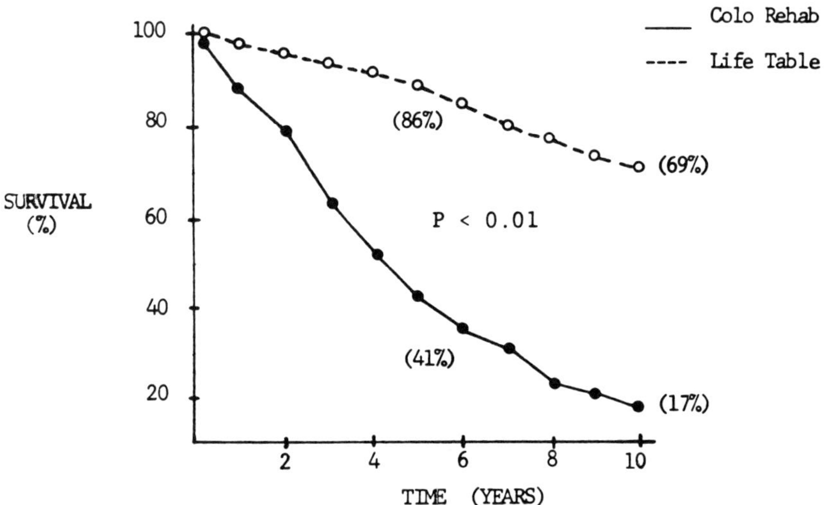

Figure 4 Survival curve from our rehabilitation program compared to predicted survival for normal males (open circles). The difference between the two survival curves is a crude estimate of excess mortality from COPD in spite of comprehensive therapy (reproduced with permission from Sahn et al., 1980).

References

Bates, D. V. (1973). The fate of the chronic bronchitis: a report of the ten year follow-up of the Canadian Department of Veterans Affairs coordinated study of chronic bronchitis. *Am. Rev. Respir. Dis.* **108**:1043-1065.

Fletcher, C., and Peto, R. (1977). The natural history of of chronic airflow obstruction. *Br. Med. J.* **1**:1645-1648.

Heaton, R. K., Grant, I., McSweeny, A. J., Adams, K. M., and Petty, T. L. (1983). Psychologic effects of continuous and nocturnal oxygen therapy in hypoxemic chronic obstructive pulmonary disease. *Arch. Intern. Med.* **143**:1941-1947.

Hudson, L. D., Tyler, M. L., and Petty, T. L. (1976). Hospitalization needs during an outpatient rehabilitation program for severe chronic airway obstruction. *Chest* **70**:606-615.

Johnson, J. A., Woolcock, A. A., and Geddes, D. M. (1983). Dihydrocodeine
   for breathless "pink puffer." *Br. Med. J.* **186**:675-677.
Mandella, L. A., Manfreda, J., and Warren, C. P. W. (1982). Steroid therapy
   in stable chronic obstructive pulmonary disease. *Ann. Intern. Med.* **96**:
   17-21.
Matthay, R. A., Berger, H. J., and Davies, R. (1982). Improvement in cardiac
   performance by oral long-acting theophylline in chronic obstructive pulmonary disease. *Am. Heart J.* **104**:1022-1026.
Mueller, R. E., Petty, T. L., and Filley, G. F. (1970). Ventilation and arterial
   blood gas changes induced by pursed lips breathing. *J. Appl. Physiol.*
   78:784-789.
Mueller, R. E., Kelble, D. L., and Plummer, J. (1971). The prevalence of
   chronic bronchitis, chronic airway obstruction and respiratory symptoms in a Colorado City. *Am. Rev. Respir. Dis.* **103**:209-229.
Nocturnal Oxygen Therapy Trial Group (1980). Continuous or nocturnal oxygen therapy in hypoxemic chronic obstructive lung disease. *Ann. Intern.
   Med.* **93**:391-398.
Petty, T. L. (1977). Pulmonary rehabilitation. *Respir. Care* **22**:68-77.
Petty, T. L. (1980). Pulmonary rehabilitation. *Am. Rev. Respir. Dis.* **12**:
   159-161 (Suppl: Conference on the Scientific Basis of in Hospital
   Respiratory Therapy).
Petty, T. L., Nett, L. M., and Finigan, M. M. (1969). A comprehensive care
   program for chronic airway obstruction. Methods and preliminary evaluation of symptomatic and functional improvement. *Ann. Intern. Med.*
   70:1109-1120.
Roberts, S. D. (1980). Cost effective oxygen therapy. *Ann. Intern. Med.*
   93:499-500.
Sahn, S. A., Nett, L. M., and Petty, T. L. (1980). Ten year followup of a
   comprehensive rehabilitation program for severe COPD. *Chest* **77**:
   suppl. 311-314.
Shim, C., and Williams, M. H. (1980). The adequacy of inhalation of aerosol
   from canister nebulizers. *Am. J. Med.* **69**:891-894.
Sonne, L. J., and Davis, J. A. (1982). Increased exercise performance in patients with severe COPD following inspiratory resistive training. *Chest*
   81:436-439.

6

Psychological Effects of Oxygen Therapy for COPD

ROBERT K. HEATON

University of California
San Diego, California

I. Introduction

In addition to their pulmonary and cardiovascular abnormalities, many patients who have hypoxemic COPD show neuropsychological impairment as well as emotional distress and reduced general life quality. These psychological disturbances are correlated with physiological measures of disease severity, and can become major concerns of patients, their families, and treating physicians. Therefore it is important to determine whether medical interventions in COPD result in psychological as well as physical benefits. This chapter considers the neuropsychological and life quality outcomes of patients who are treated with supplemental oxygen.

The psychological disturbances associated with COPD are described in detail in other chapters of this volume, so only a brief review will be given here. In the largest psychological investigation to date of patients with hypoxemic COPD (N = 203), 77% were found to have clinically significant neuropsychological impairment (Grant et al., 1982). In 42% of the cases this impairment was moderate or severe in degree, indicating profound limitations in basic adaptive abilities dependent upon brain function. The most serious deficits were noted on tests of conceptual skills, flexibility of thinking, and perceptual-motor integration, with milder impairment being demonstrated in simple sensory and motor skills, attention, learning and memory, and verbal abilities. Increasing hypoxemia was associated with more severe neuropsychological deficits. In terms of their emotional and social functioning, the patients tended to be tense, anxious, depressed, withdrawn, and somatically preoccupied. They also showed significant impairment in the areas of recreation and home management, ambulation, and sleep. These aspects of "life quality" were significantly related both to degree of neuropsychological impairment and to a composite physiological index of disease severity (McSweeny et al., 1982).

II. Effects of Supplemental Oxygen

Studies of supplemental O_2 administration in hypoxemic COPD have suggested several physical benefits. The most important of these is a reduced mortality rate, but decreased polycythemia, decreased pulmonary hypertension, and increased exercise tolerance have been reported as well (Chamberlain and Millard, 1963; Flenley et al., 1980; Neff and Petty, 1970; Petty and Finigan, 1968; Stewart et al., 1975). Two early studies by a group in Florida also suggested that supplemental O_2 may improve the neuropsychological and emotional disturbances associated with the disease (Block et al., 1974; Krop et al., 1973).

In the first of these psychological studies, 10 patients who had hypoxemic COPD were administered several behavioral tests before and after a 1-month period of ambulatory treatment with continuous supplemental O_2 (Krop et al., 1973). Baseline psychological testing was done while the patients breathed room air, whereas the follow-up testing was performed on supplemental O_2. In their follow-up evaluation, this group showed improved performance on the Wechsler Intelligence Scales (WAIS or Wechsler-Bellevue), the Wechsler Memory Scale, the Finger Tapping Test, and the Bender Gestalt Test (with and without the Background Interference Procedure). Furthermore, on the Minnesota Multiphasic Personality Inventory this group gave evidence of improved depression and reduced somatic preoccupation. An untreated control group of COPD patients (N = 12) did not show any improvement in neuropsychological functioning or in emotional status.

The second study of O_2 effects on neuropsychological functioning also included electroencephalographic (EEG) evaluations (Block et al., 1974). However, this investigation did not use an untreated group of patients or normals to help control for practice effects on the neuropsychological tests. The baseline EEG and neuropsychological testing were performed on room air, and the follow-up assessments were done on supplemental O_2. At baseline, 9 of the 12 patients with hypoxemic COPD showed mild, diffuse EEG abnormalities. After 1 month of continuous O_2 treatment, improvement was noted in the EEGs of four of the nine patients who had had abnormal tracings at baseline. Also, over the 1 month test-retest interval, the total patient group showed significant improvement on each of the neuropsychological tests mentioned above in relation to the Krop et al. (1973) study. Average Wechsler IQs and Memory Quotients increased by 7 and 9 points, respectively; even though an untreated control group was not included in this project, it is unlikely that the patients' improved performance was due to practice effects because alternative forms of the tests were given in counterbalanced order (i.e., Forms I vs. II of the Wechsler Memory Scale, and the Wechsler Bellevue vs. WAIS). Substantial improvement also was noted on the Finger Tapping Test of motor speed and on the Bender Gestalt Test of visuographic skills; little or no practice effect is expected on the former test, and the improvement on the Bender Gestalt appears too large to be explained on the basis of practice. Moreover, perhaps the most interesting finding in this study was a correlation between the changes on the neuropsychological testing and the EEG: the only patients who failed to show improved neuropsychological functioning after 1 month of supplemental O_2 also continued to have abnormal EEG tracings. It was concluded that these parallel neuropsychological and EEG findings suggest reversible cerebral hypoxia in many patients who have hypoxemic COPD.

A. Nocturnal Oxygen Therapy Trial

In 1978, the National Heart, Lung and Blood Institute funded a large, multicenter study to elucidate the effects of supplemental O_2 treatment in hypoxemic COPD. This study, called the Nocturnal Oxygen Therapy Trial (NOTT), provides the most definitive information currently available about the psychological as well as physical effects of O_2 treatment in COPD. Therefore its methods and results will be reviewed here in some detail.

In practice, supplemental O_2 often has been prescribed on a nocturnal basis rather than continuously. This is because hypoxemia tends to be worse during sleep, and because it seemed that nocturnal O_2 might provide similar benefits while avoiding the inconvenience and expense of using portable O_2 delivery systems during the day. Thus, the NOTT was designed to compare the effectiveness of continuous O_2 (COT; 20 hr/day) with that of nocturnal treatment (NOT; 12 hr/day).

Several other design features of the NOTT differed from those of the earlier studies by the Florida group. A much larger patient group was involved, and the effects of COT and NOT were compared over a minimum of 6 months (average was 19 months). Much more comprehensive neuropsychological and life-quality outcome measures were used. Potential subjects were excluded from the NOTT if they had any significant current illnesses other than COPD, and if they had any history of neurologic illness or alcohol or other substance abuse. Prior to the NOTT baseline evaluations, patients with COPD had to be free of exacerbations of their illness and had to show stable hypoxemia ($PaO_2 < 60$ mmHg) during a formal 3-week observation period. Baseline *and* follow-up psychological evaluations were performed while patients breathed room air. Finally, a carefully selected group of healthy elderly subjects was included in the study to control for practice effects on the neuropsychological testing.

Details of the medical evaluations in the NOTT are available elsewhere (NOTT Group, 1980). The neuropsychological evaluations included the Wechsler Adult Intelligence Scale (WAIS) and an expanded Halstead-Reitan Battery (HRB). This battery measures a wide range of abilities that can be affected by cerebral disorders, including conceptual abilities and flexiblity of thinking, concentration and attention, learning and memory, verbal language functions and academic skills, complex perceptual-motor integration, and simple sensory and simple motor skills (Grant et al., 1982). In addition to its sensitivity to changes in cerebral functioning, the battery measures strengths and deficits that are important in everyday living (Heaton and Pendleton, 1981). Outcome measures in the NOTT included neuropsychological summary scores and selected individual test scores, as well as clinical ratings of changes in global neuropsychological functioning and in the seven key ability areas listed above. These ratings of change were made independently by two experienced neuropsychologists, who were kept blind with respect to the patient or control status of the subjects being rated. A high degree of interrater reliability was demonstrated: using a five-point scale ranging from "much improved" to "much worse," the clinicians agreed totally on 85% of their ratings and differed by only 1 point on the remaining 15%. Clinical ratings such as these have been shown to be a valid means of data reduction and diagnostic interpretation in neuropsychology (Heaton et al., 1981, in press; Grant et al., 1982). In the NOTT these ratings had the advantage of detecting clinically significant changes that were apparent on varying combinations of tests within each ability domain. For example, two patients would be considered to have improved motor functioning, even though one showed the change on tests of speed and strength whereas the other showed improvement only in fine motor coordination. This avoids the unwarranted assumption that, to be significant, treatment-related improvements always have to occur on the same tests.

The NOTT "life quality" evaluation included the Minnesota Multiphasic Personality Inventory (MMPI; Dahlstrom et al., 1972), the Profile of Mood States (POMS; McNair et al., 1971), and the Sickness Impact Profile (SIP; Bergner et al., 1976). The MMPI and POMS assess emotional status and other dimensions of psychopathology. The SIP is a questionnaire that measures 12 dimensions of sickness-related behavioral dysfunction; the 12 subscales are then combined into summary scores reflecting physical, psychosocial, and overall behavioral dysfunction.

After completing 1 week of baseline physical and psychological evaluations, the patients were randomly assigned to receive COT or NOT. Oxygen was administered by nasal prongs, with a flow rate sufficient to relieve hypoxemia. Compliance with prescribed O_2 use was measured by logs kept by the patient and relatives and by times attached to some of the O_2 delivery systems. Average O_2 use was 11.9 (SD = 2.1) hr/day for the NOT group and 20.7 (SD = 3.7) hr/day for patients in the COT group.

The major psychological assessments took place at baseline and after 6 months of O_2 treatment. One hundred and fifty patients completed these two evaluations. In addition, 20 COT patients and 17 patients in the NOT condition completed 12 months of treatment while the neuropsychological laboratories were still in operation. These patients were therefore given a second follow-up evaluation to explore whether longer periods of NOT and COT result in different psychological outcomes.

The control group consisted of healthy elderly subjects who were individually matched to COPD patients with respect to sex, age, education, socioeconomic status, and neighborhood of residence. Fifty-three normals and 55 of the matched patients with COPD completed psychological evaluations at the baseline and 6-month points. Of course, the control group received no treatment between these two assessments.

Table 1 summarizes the baseline and 6-month neuropsychological test results of the controls and the matched COPD group. On most test measures average changes were comparable for the two groups, revealing no significant treatment effect. However, the patient group did show significantly greater improvement on tests of sequencing efficiency and flexibility of thinking (Trail Making Test, Part B), grip strength (Hand Dynamometer), and motor speed (Finger Tapping Test).

The clinicians' ratings of change provide more convincing evidence of

Table 1 Changes in Neuropsychological Functioning With 6 Months of O_2 Treatment (Patients) vs. No Treatment (Controls)

	Normal controls (N = 53)				Matched COPD group (N = 55)			
	Baseline		6 months		Baseline		6 months	
	Mean	SD	Mean	SD	Mean	SD	Mean	SD
Summary scores								
WAIS Verbal IQ	107.6	(15.1)	109.2	(15.1)	102.1	(15.3)	103.6	(13.6)
WAIS Performance IQ	108.1	(10.1)	111.7	(11.9)	98.2	(16.1)	102.5	(15.3)
Average impairment rating	1.72	(0.63)	1.59	(0.60)	2.20	(0.82)	2.04	(0.81)
Halstead impairment index	0.61	(0.25)	0.56	(0.29)	0.74	(0.24)	0.69	(0.28)
Brain-age quotient	91.1	(16.7)	96.8	(18.1)	76.6	(22.5)	83.4	(23.5)
Halstead-Reitan Tests								
Category errors	63.8	(25.3)	54.1	(25.0)	79.6	(26.5)	70.7	(29.1)
Trails, B, seconds	118.0	(61.9)	119.5	(68.4)	160.5	(90.3)	138.0	(84.8)[a]
Tactual performance test (min/blk)	0.88	(0.62)	0.71	(0.39)	1.78	(1.85)	1.58	(1.54)
Memory (correct)	6.5	(2.0)	6.7	(1.9)	5.4	(2.0)	5.5	(2.0)
Location (correct)	2.3	(2.2)	2.8	(2.1)	1.6	(1.5)	1.5	(1.5)

Speech perception errors	9.1	(8.3)	8.4	(6.3)	13.4	(10.8)	14.1	(15.1)
Seashore rhythm correct	23.2	(3.8)	24.6	(3.5)	22.6	(4.7)	22.3	(5.9)
Tapping (avg 2 hands)	44.2	(7.8)	44.1	(7.3)	40.3	(7.8)	43.1	(7.5)[a]
Sensory errors	9.1	(9.8)	6.4	(8.1)	14.7	(11.2)	14.4	(11.8)
Aphasia errors	6.8	(5.2)	6.4	(6.3)	8.9	(8.0)	8.1	(8.2)
Spatial relations errors	2.9	(1.6)	2.9	(1.5)	3.6	(2.3)	3.7	(2.1)
Added Neuropsychological Tests							
Grip strength (avg kg, 2 hands)	40.9	(12.5)	37.7	(11.7)	30.8	(11.0)	31.9	(11.9)[a]
Pegboard (avg sec, 2 hands)	86.1	(23.4)	85.8	(21.9)	121.0	(59.7)	113.9	(55.5)
Verbal learning (immed recall)	19.4	(6.2)	20.4	(5.9)	18.5	(7.1)	19.5	(7.7)
Verbal % forgetting ($>$ hr delay)	19.8	(19.7)	16.3	(18.1)	22.6	(23.0)	16.8	(22.3)
Nonverbal learning (immed recall)	7.9	(3.4)	8.5	(3.4)	5.4	(3.1)	6.2	(3.4)
Nonverbal % forgetting ($>$ hr delay)	19.8	(25.5)	15.6	(25.3)	34.6	(35.5)	25.1	(26.6)

[a]COPD group shows significantly more improvement than untreated controls ($p < 0.01$).

Table 2 Percentages of Subjects Rated as Improved from Baseline to 6-Month Neuropsychological Evaluations

	Untreated normal subjects (N = 53)	Matched subjects with COPD (N = 55)	χ^2
Simple motor	5.6	41.8	19.7***
Simple sensory	1.9	21.8	10.3**
Complex perceptual-motor	22.2	32.0	1.3
Attention	11.1	19.6	1.5
Memory	30.8	29.4	0.0
Abstraction/Flexibility	11.3	34.0	7.8***
Verbal	7.6	25.5	6.2*
Global judgment	5.6	41.8	19.7***

*p $<$ 0.05; **p $<$ 0.01; ***p $<$ 0.001.

neuropsychological improvement that can be attributed to supplemental O_2 therapy (see Table 2). After 6 months of treatment, 42% of the patients with COPD showed small but definite gains in neuropsychological functioning, whereas only 6% of the controls showed similar improvement. Ratings of individual abilities revealed that significantly more patients than controls showed improvement in verbal skills, abstraction and flexibility of thinking, simple sensory abilities, and simple motor skills. It is emphasized, however, that these changes were not very large; virtually all of the clinician ratings of improvement were in the category labelled "a little better."

The data in Table 3 indicate that, over 6 months of O_2 treatment, the patients with COPD did not improve more than the controls on any measure of emotional status, physical disability, or social functioning. Thus, no treatment-related change in life-quality could be demonstrated.

In considering the above findings in the psychological domain, it should be realized that 6 months of supplemental O_2 did not cause major changes on *physiological* measures of disease severity. From their baseline to their 6 month evaluations, the total patient group showed no improvement in lung function, arterial blood gases (tested on room air), cardiac output, or exercise capacity. There was an expected modest improvement in hematocrit, but the investigators considered this to be of dubious clinical significance (NOTT Study Group, 1980).

Table 3 Changes in "Life Quality" After 6 Months of O_2 Treatment (Patients) or No Treatment (Controls)

	Normal controls				Matched COPD group			
	Baseline		6 months		Baseline		6 months	
	Mean	(SD)	Mean	(SD)	Mean	(SD)	Mean	(SD)
MMPI (T-scores)								
Hypochondriasis	54.0	(8.2)	51.9	(7.4)	68.1	(14.1)	68.9	(14.3)
Depression	57.5	(10.8)	56.3	(9.8)	73.3	(11.9)	71.3	(13.1)
Hysteria	54.5	(8.2)	53.1	(7.5)	64.2	(10.2)	64.0	(11.1)
Psychopathic deviate	55.6	(9.8)	54.4	(9.3)	56.9	(10.1)	59.3	(10.2)[a]
Paranoia	54.3	(9.7)	52.5	(8.5)	50.8	(8.7)	50.7	(8.6)
Psychesthenia	52.0	(7.9)	52.7	(8.7)	60.3	(11.6)	59.7	(12.6)
Schizophrenia	54.3	(11.3)	52.8	(11.1)	58.1	(10.2)	59.9	(13.5)
Mania	52.4	(9.4)	51.2	(10.3)	54.3	(9.6)	56.9	(10.6)
Social introversion	53.7	(9.5)	53.8	(9.4)	58.1	(8.3)	58.1	(8.8)
Ego strength	44.0	(6.0)	43.0	(5.3)	37.2	(6.5)	37.6	(6.9)
POMS total mood disturbance	12.6	(20.1)	13.6	(18.9)	36.4	(28.4)	38.6	(31.7)
SIP (% impairment)								
Physical	0.4	(1.2)	0.9	(2.2)	18.6	(16.0)	17.3	(17.0)
Psychosocial	1.1	(1.9)	1.7	(3.3)	22.1	(18.8)	19.5	(17.9)
Total	2.9	(2.6)	2.7	(2.9)	23.4	(13.6)	21.7	(15.9)

[a]Matched COPD group shows significantly greater T-score increase than do untreated controls ($p < 0.05$).

MMPI, Minnesota Multiphasic Personality Inventory; POMS, Profile of Mood States; SIP, Sickness Impact Profile.
N for Controls is 47 on MMPI, 32 on SIP, 31 on POMS; N for COPD group is 45 on MMPI, 55 on SIP, 49 on POMS.

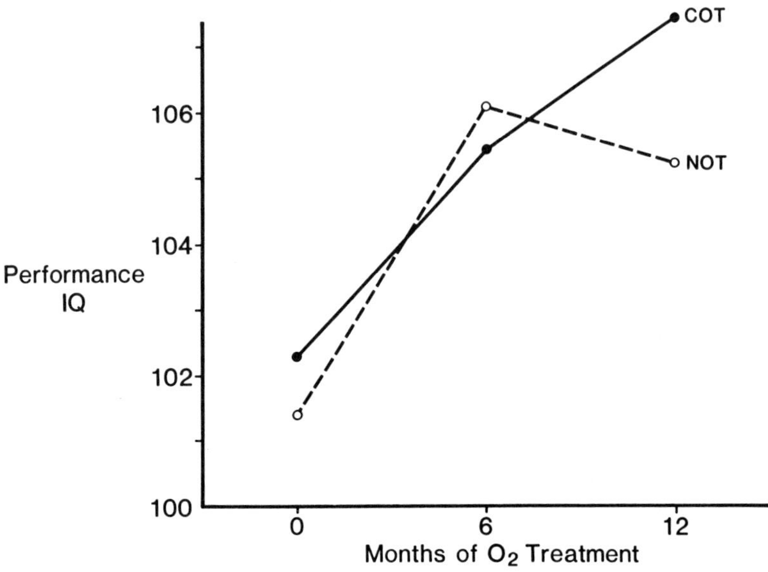

Figure 1 Mean WAIS Performance IQs for COT and NOT groups that completed neuropsychological evaluations at baseline and after 6 and 12 months of O_2 treatment (Heaton et al., 1983, by permission from Graftek Press, © 1983, American Medical Association).

Over the first 6 months of treatment, patients in the NOT and COT groups did not differ significantly in their changes on neuropsychological and life-quality testing. Clinician ratings of change in neuropsychological functioning also were comparable for the two groups. Moreover, at the 6-month point the NOT and COT groups had similar mortality rates and similar values on 13 of 14 physiological measures of disease severity. The only statistically significant difference was that the COT group improved in pulmonary vascular resistance, whereas the NOT group did not.

Twelve months after O_2 treatment was initiated, survivors in the NOT and COT groups again showed few differences on physiological measures of disease severity. However, at that point the mortality rate of the NOT group was almost twice that of the COT group (20.6% vs. 11.9%). The advantage in mortality rate achieved by COT generally was greater for patients who, at baseline, had worse mood disturbance, neuropsychological impairment, and physiological measures of disease severity.

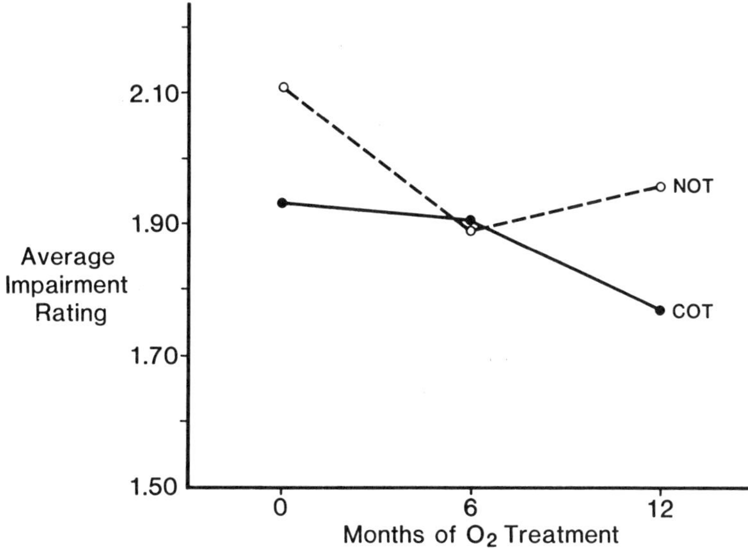

Figure 2 Mean average impairment ratings for COT and NOT groups that completed neuropsychological evaluations at baseline and after 6 and 12 months of O$_2$ treatment (Heaton et al., 1983, by permission from Graftek Press, © 1982, American Medical Association).

As noted above, 37 patients with COPD were given a third psychological evaluation after 12 months of supplemental O$_2$ treatment. Other than the fact that they were among the first patients recruited for the study, there was no bias involved in their selection; thus, this was considered a representative sample of the total patient group. At the 12 month point, clear differences had emerged between the COT and NOT groups on the neuropsychological battery: on four of the five summary measures from this battery, the patients who had been receiving COT did significantly better. The only summary score that did not reveal an advantage of COT over NOT was the WAIS Verbal IQ, and this measure is the least sensitive to cerebral dysfunction.

Figures 1 through 3 show the baseline, 6-month, and 12-month means for the two treatment groups on the WAIS Performance IQ, the Average Impairment Rating, and the Brain-Age Quotient. Both groups showed some improvement from the baseline to the 6-month point, but the results of the normal control group indicate that this change is mostly attributable to prac-

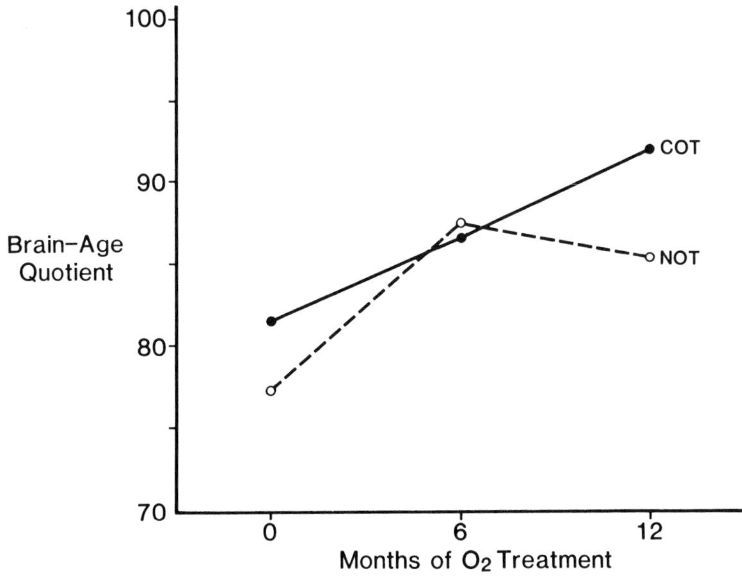

Figure 3 Mean brain-age quotients for COT and NOT groups that completed neuropsychological evaluations at baseline and after 6 and 12 months of O_2 treatment (Heaton et al., 1983, by permission from Graftek Press, © 1983, American Medical Association).

tice effect. However, between the 6-month and 12-month evaluations the COT group continued to improve, whereas the group that had received NOT did worse. This pattern of results can be interpreted in two ways that are not mutually exclusive. First, the improvement shown by the COT group between the 6 and 12-month points probably is not due to practice effect, becasue the NOT comparison group did not show such an effect. The 12-month results of the COT group are about the same as those of the healthy control group at baseline, and only part (perhaps half) of this improvement can be attributed to practice effect. The second point suggested by Figures 1 through 3 related to the NOT group's mild deterioration in functioning during the second 6 months of treatment. This finding reminds us that hypoxemic COPD is a progressive disease, and suggests that even no change in an aspect of disease severity may represent a treatment benefit. The absence of an untreated comparison group of COPD patients precludes direct testing of this hypotheses, but the results of the NOT group would predict that over a 6-12-month period untreated patients would show significantly worse neuropsychological functioning. From this perspective it seems likely that the use of a *normal* control group in the NOTT resulted in an underestimation of the benefits of supplemental O_2 on brain function and basic adaptive abilities.

Despite the fact that the COT group showed improved neuropsychological functioning after 12 months of treatment, they did not do any better than the NOT group on measures of emotional status or general life quality (i.e., the MMPI, POMS, and SIP). On the latter measures, little change has occurred since the patients' baseline evaluations 12 months earlier.

III. Conclusions

So far only three studies have evaluated psychological effects of supplemental O_2 treatment in patients who have hypoxemic COPD. All three found some benefit with respect to improving neuropsychological functioning, but the treatment-related gains were much greater in the two Florida studies (Block et al., 1974; Krop et al., 1973) than in the larger NOTT project. Although there are several methodologic differences between the NOTT and the other studies, factors most likely to have caused differences in study outcome are: (1) through its formal 3-week observation period the NOTT provided greater assurance that patients had stable hypoxemia and were not having exacerbations of their illnesses at the times of their baseline evaluations; and (2) follow-up neuropsychological evaluations were performed on room air in the NOTT and on supplemental O_2 in the Florida studies, so larger improvements in the latter studies may represent acute effects of O_2 on brain function.

Considering this second possibility, Heaton et al. (1983) speculated that supplemental O_2 may have multiple effects on the synthesis of neurotransmitters and on other aspects of CNS metabolic activity, some such effects being acute and short-lived, and others having a longer duration. The differing results of the NOTT and Florida studies raise the possibility that the *acute* effects of O_2 may have the most profound influence on brain function. On the other hand, Brezinova and co-workers (1979) found that acute O_2 administration had no effect on the EEGs of their patients, whereas chronic treatment with supplemental O_2 resulted in EEG improvements even when the patients' tracings were taken while they breathed room air.

Regardless of the mechanism responsible for such changes, it would be of considerable practical importance to determine whether acute O_2 effects on neuropsychological functioning are as substantial as the Florida studies suggest.

What is needed is a study that first ensures patients' disease stability at baseline, and then randomly assigns patients to be retested either on room air or on supplemental O_2. Between their baseline and follow-up evaluations, both patient groups would receive O_2 supplementation. Perhaps the study could use a double-blind placebo condition, in which patients assigned to breathe room air at follow-up do so through an identical O_2 delivery appartus. Ideally the study would use comprehensive neuropsychological evaluations, such as those in the NOTT, to elucidate O_2 effects on all major types of abilities. This type of study design would permit a direct comparison of the more stable effects of chronic O_2 administration (as in the NOTT) with the combined acute and longer-term effects (as in the Florida studies).

The NOTT project found that 6 months of nocturnal or continuous supplemental O_2 (NOT or COT) produced similar modest improvements in patients' neuropsychological functioning. Also after 6 months, little difference was noted in the NOT and COT groups' survival rates and physiological indices of disease severity. However, over the second 6 months of treatment important differences emerged in the outcomes achieved by the two O_2 regimens: the COT group showed a better survival rate, and survivors receiving COT showed improved neuropsychological functioning whereas those receiving NOT did not. Once again it should be recalled that the follow-up testing in this study was done on room air; thus, the COT groups' better neuropsychological results at the 12 month point would be due to the more stable (not the acute) O_2 effects postulated above. If future research does demonstrate more pronounced acute O_2 effects on neuropsychological functioning, an even greater advantage of the COT regimen is implied. This is because patients receiving COT would experience the benefits of both chronic and acute O_2 administration during the daytime hours when they are most active.

Because supplemental O_2 treatment is not known to enhance longevity in hypoxemic COPD, it is doubtful that any direct comparison can be made between effects of no O_2 treatment and either NOT or COT. However, the NOTT findings suggest that, if such a study were done, the untreated group would show deteriorating neuropsychological functioning within 12 months or less. Preventing such deterioration (i.e., no change) actually would represent a treatment benefit for such patients, but this cannot be detected in studies that use a control group of normals or of untreated patients who have less severe COPD. Thus, considerable benefit is implied when 12 months of COT not only prevents further deterioration but also even slightly improves neuropsychological functioning in hypoxemic patients.

Using the MMPI, Krop et al. (1973) found evidence of improved depression and reduced somatic preoccupation in patients who had received 1 month of COT. However, patients in the NOTT showed no changes in emotional status or general life quality after much lengthier periods of treatment with supplemental O_2 (either COT or NOT). This discrepancy in results cannot be attributed to the fact that the Krop et al. (1973) follow-up evaluations were performed while patients breathed supplemental O_2 ; this is because, unlike neuropsychological tests, the MMPI probably would not be sensitive to such short-term O_2 effects. Two other possible explanations seem more likely. First, if some of the Florida patients had baseline testing at times when their clinical condition were not stable, it is conceivable that their baseline MMPIs reflected some transient distress that would have improved without O_2 treatment. Another possible explanation for the discrepant results in the NOTT and Krop et al. (1973) studies relates to the large differences in duration of the follow-up periods. After only 1 month of their new treatment, the Florida patients may have maintained hopes for greater physical improvements than would actually occur; such optimism could be responsible for the changes noted on the MMPI. On the other hand, after 6 and 12 months of treatment NOTT patients may have given up hopes for major physical improvement; some of them even experienced additional deterioration in their conditions during this lengthier follow-up period. In any event, the NOTT findings indicate that patients who are receiving either NOT or COT over lengthy periods will continue to show significant depression, worry, somatic preoccupation, social withdrawal, and reduced participation in home and recreational activities. Although this is a disappointing conclusion, it is worth considering again that the expected course of these patients' illness is one of progressive deterioration. "No change" in life quality could represent a modest treatment benefit in patients who, without treatment, might well have gotten worse.

References

Bergner, M., Bobbit, R. A., Pollard, W. E., Martin, D. P., and Gilson, B. S. (1976). The Sickness Impact Profile: Validation of health status measure. *Med. Care* **14**:57-67.

Block, A. J., Castle, J. R., and Keitt, A. S. (1974). Chronic oxygen therapy treatment of chronic obstructive pulmonary disease at sea level. *Chest* **65**:279-288.

Brezinova, B., Calverley, P. M. A., Flenley, D. C., and Townsend, H. R. A.

(1979). The effect of long-term oxygen therapy on the EEG in patients with chronic stable ventilatory failure. *Bull. Europ. Physiopathol. Respir.* **15**:603-609.

Chamberlain, D. A., and Millard, F. J. C. (1963). The treatment of polycythemia secondary to hypoxic lung disease by continuous oxygen administration. *Q. J. Med.* **128**:341-350.

Dahlstrom, W. G., Welsh, G. S., and Dahlstrom, L. E. (1975). *An MMPI Handbook: Research Application,* Vol. 2. Minneapolis, University of Minnesota Press.

Flenley, D. C., Douglas, N. J., and Lamb, D. (1980). Nocturnal hypoxemia and long-term domiciliary oxygen in blue and bloated bronchitis. *Chest* **77**:305-307.

Grant, I., Heaton, R. K., McSweeny, A. J., Adams, K. M., and Timms, R. M. (1982). Neuropsychological findings in hypoxemic chronic obstructive pulmonary disease. *Arch. Intern. Med.* **142**:1470-1476.

Heaton, R. K., and Pendleton, M. G. (1981). Use of neuropsychological tests to predict adult patients' everyday functioning. *J. Counsult. Clin. Psychol.* (invited paper) **49**:807-821.

Heaton, R. K., Grant, I., Anthony, W. Z., and Lehman, R. A. W. (1981). A comparison of clinical and automated interpretation of the Halstead-Reitan Battery. *J. Clin. Neuropsychol.* **3**:121-141.

Heaton, R. K., Grant, I., McSweeny, A. J., Adams, K. M., and Petty, T. L. (1983). Psychologic effects of continuous and nocturnal oxygen theapy in hypoxemic chronic obstructive pulmonary disease. *Arch. Intern. Med.* **143**:1941-1947.

Heaton, R. K., Nelson, L. M., Thompson, D. S., Burks, J. S., and Franklin, G. M. (1985). Neuropsychological findings in relapsing-remitting and chronic progressive multiple sclerosis. *J. Consult. Clin. Psychol.* **53**:103-110.

Krop, H. D., Block, A. J., and Cohen, E. (1973). Neuropsychologic effects of continuous oxygen therapy in chronic obstructive pulmonary disease. *Chest* **64**:317-322.

McNair, D. M., Lorr, M., and Droppleman, L. F. (1971). *Manual for the Profile of Mood States.* San Diego, Educational and Industrial Testing Service.

McSweeny, A. J., Grant, I., Heaton, R. K., Adams, K. M., and Timms, R. M. (1982). Life quality of patients with chronic obstructive pulmonary disease. *Arch. Intern. Med.* **142**:473-478.

Neff, T. A., and Petty, T. L. (1970). Long-term continuous oxygen therapy in chronic airway obstruction. *Ann. Intern. Med.* **72**:621-626.

Nocturnal Oxygen therapy Trial Group (1980). Continuous or nocturnal oxygen therapy in hypoxemic chronic obstructive lung disease. A clinical trial. *Ann. Intern. Med.* **93**:391-398.

Petty, T. L., and Finigan, M. M. (1968). The clinical evaluation of prolonged ambulatory oxygen therapy in patients with chronic airway obstruction. *Am. J. Med.* **45**:242-252.

Stewart, B. N., Hood, C. I., and Block, A. J. (1975). Long-term results of continuous oxygen therapy at sea level. *Chest* **68**:486-496.

7

Behavioral Interventions for Patients with COPD

ROBERT M. KAPLAN

San Diego State University
University of California
San Diego, California

CATHERINE J. ATKINS

University of California
San Diego, California

I. Introduction

Behavior and chronic obstructive pulmonary disease (COPD) are inseparably intertwined. Extensive evidence suggests that smoking behavior is the major risk factor for the development of emphysema and chronic bronchitis (Higgins, 1958; Van der Lende, 1969; HIH, 1979; Lebowitz, 1982; Ravenholt, 1985; U.S. Department of Health and Human Services, 1984; Sawicki, 1972). In addition, several epidemiologic studies have shown that the rate of decline in pulmonary function for afflicted patients declines with cessation of smoking behavior (Astin, 1976; NIH, 1981). Thus, individual behavior is a major risk factor for development and maintenance of COPD.

Once a patient becomes afflicted with COPD, the disease comes to have a major effect upon behavior. Many of these effects are reviewed in this volume. For example, COPD may affect psychosocial function (McSweeny, Chap. 4) cognitive and psychomotor functions (Prigatano and Grant, Chap. 3), depression (McSweeny et al., 1982; Katz, 1982; Fix et al., 1981), and sexual behavior (Timms, 1982).

COPD has become an important public health problem for at least four reasons. First, COPD is among the top five leading causes of death. Second, it has a major impact upon activities of daily living. Third, it affects a large number of persons. And fourth, there is an increasing incidence of COPD. Currently, COPD represents this nation's most rapidly growing health problem (U.S. Government Task Force, 1977, 1979). Deaths due to COPD are rising at a rate of 1.4% per year, making it the most rapidly increasing of the top 10 leading causes of death in the United States (U.S. Government Task Force, 1979). From 1970 to 1975, the mortality rate from chronic obstructive pulmonary diseases increased from 16:100,000 of the population to 19:100,000 of the population (Brashear, 1980). COPD now ranks fifth as a cause of death in the United States and accounts for about 56,000 deaths per year (Lenfant, 1982).

Respiratory diseases are generally considered to be of greater importance as causes of disability and ill health than as causes of death. Studies that deal with the long-term course and prognosis of COPD indicate that the process covers a time span of at least 20-30 years and possibly longer (Petty, 1978). Morbidity from COPD results in approximately 34 days of restricted activity per 100 persons per year (Brashear, 1980). In the United States, from January, 1975, through December, 1976, an estimated 163.4 million office-based physician visits were attributed to respiratory diseases. These visits made up approximately 14% of all office visits for any condition during that period. COPD accounts for approximately one-fifth of these visits (Brashear, 1980; U.S. Government Task Force, 1977).

Some of the major impacts of COPD upon the daily lives of patients are summarized in Table 1. COPD is responsible for a substantial number of disability days, hospitalizations, and restrictions in performance of daily activities. These disease consequences translate into a serious economic burden.

Total costs for COPD were estimated to be $4.55 billion in 1972 (U.S. Government Task Force, 1977). By 1979, this estimate had jumped to $19 billion and current estimates go as high as $27 billion per year (Lenfant, 1972). COPD places an enormous demand upon the health care system. In the April 1984 issue of *Morbidity and Mortality Weekly Report,* it was estimated that COPD patients require well over 2 million visits to U.S. physicians each year.

In summary, COPD may in part result from a behavior pattern and may, in turn, come to affect other behavior patterns. Because of these interrelationships, behavioral programs may be important in the prevention and management of COPD. Numerous reports have called for programs to prevent COPD through smoking prevention and smoking cessation efforts (NIH, 1983; Cali-

Table 1 Prevalence, Disability, and Hospitalizations for COPD in 1979

	Chronic bronchitis	Emphysema	Total
Prevalence			
No. of cases	7,474,000	2,137,000	9,611,000
No. with limited activity	382,000	1,118,000	1,500,000
Percent limited activity	5.1	5.3	15
Disability			
Bed days	28,519,000	57,132,000	85,651,000
Restricted activity days	88,165,000	144,927,000	233,092,000
Work loss days	7,246,000	314,000	7,560,000
Hospitalizations			
Discharges	227,000	57,000	284,000
Hospital days	1,608,000	556,000	2,164,000

Health interview survey, NCHS unpublished data.
Source: Lenfant (1982), p. 755.

fornia Department of Health Services, 1982). As a result, research on anti-smoking programs has blossomed in recent years. This research is well summarized in several excellent reviews (Flaxman, this volume; Lichtenstein, 1982; Pederson, 1982). Therefore, the prevention of COPD through antismoking efforts will not be covered in this chapter. Instead, we will focus on behavioral programs for the management of patients with active COPD. Two separate aspects of this problem deserve consideration: the value of exercise and rehabilitation programs, and the problem of compliance with life style recommendations (Kaplan et al., 1985).

A. An Alternative Conceptualization of the Objective of Care

According to the American College of Chest Physicians, the goal of pulmonary rehabilitation is to ". . . return the patient to the highest possible functional capacity allowed by his pulmonary handicap and overall life situation" (Petty, 1977).

Some investigators have argued that the important variables to measure in COPD include dyspnea, decreased ventilatory capacity, respiratory muscle fatigue, and pulmonary hypertension leading to right ventricular dysfunction. Certainly these are the major characteristics of obstructive lung disease. However, these factors are important because they limit function or influence the probability of reduced function (including death) in the future. The objective of health care should be to extend life and provide the highest obtainable quality of life for the longest duration. Pulmonary hypertension should be treated because it may cause limitations in functioning and shortened life expectancy. Thus, pulmonary hypertension can be thought of as a mediator of health status. If pulmonary function did not affect health status, physicians and patients would be unconcerned about it. Our point is that producing the highest quality of life for the longest duration should be the object of health care and that various methods should be used to achieve this objective. These methods may or may not influence important mediating variables such as ventilatory capacity and respiratory muscle fatigue.

We have argued that programs for COPD patients should be evaluated using general health status measures (Kaplan et al., 1984a). These measures consider the impact of the disease upon function and life expectancy.

Over the course of the last decade, Bush and his colleagues have developed a comprehensive health decision model (Kaplan and Bush, 1982). The best known component in the model is a general health status index. One of the most important aspects of general health outcome measures is that they allow comparison between heterogeneous patient groups. For example, using these models, it is possible to evaluate the cost-effectiveness of a screening program for thyroid abnormalities (Epstein et al., 1981) with the cost-effectiveness of a treatment such as estrogen replacement for postmenopausal women (Weinstein, 1980). This method is in contrast to approaches that utilize a specific outcome measure for each disease entity.

Obtaining the highest level of function and extending the duration of life should define the objective of any intervention in health care. Medical management of COPD is essential for obtaining these objectives. However, other health status benefits may also result from behavioral interventions. Sometimes the behavioral interventions are directed at improving functioning without regard to the mediating physiological mechanism. For example, Fordyce (1983) has demonstrated that modifying the social environment may result in improved functioning for patients with back pain. There is also some evidence that COPD patients experience improved function following rehabilitation efforts, even though there is no change in traditional indicators of pulmonary function. We have been particularly interested in evaluating the health status benefits of adding behavioral programs as an adjunct to medical care for COPD patients.

B. Rehabilitation Programs in COPD

There is no medical cure for COPD and medical management includes the use of antibiotics, bronchodilators, corticosteroids, and a variety of other medications to prevent influenza and related medical complications (see Petty, Chap. 5). However, long-term use of these medications may cause side effects (Petty and Cherniak, 1981). Oxygen therapy increases survival and improves cognitive performance for COPD patients but is not advised for all patients (Anthonisen, 1983; NOTT, 1980). For most patients, behavioral programs for rehabilitation are highly advocated (Petty, 1985). Petty and Cherniak (1981) have argued that rehabilitation programs produce strong improvements in both survival and quality of life. They suggest that rehabilitation programs result in reduced symptoms, improved exercise tolerance, reduction in hospital days, more gainful employment, slowing of progress of disease, and increased survival. Pulmonary rehabilitation programs for patients with COPD have expanded substantially in the last 10 years (Unger et al., 1980). Most of the programs attempt to restore the patient to the highest possible level of health functioning and to reduce the frequency of hospital visits (Moser et al., 1980; Pulmonary Rehabilitation Study Group, 1974; Unger et al., 1980).

An important component of most pulmonary rehabilitation programs has been the establishment of a regular exercise regimen. Specific physical conditioning exercises, such as walking, can be undertaken by the patient to maintain lung functioning and improve the remainder of the oxygen delivery system (Bell and Jensen, 1977). In several published cases, the improvements in the condition of COPD patients following exercise training have been striking (Bass et al., 1970; Christie, 1968; Fishman and Petty, 1971; Mertens et al., 1978; Moser et al., 1980; Pierce et al., 1965; Unger et al.,1980). Specifically, appropriate physical conditioning exercises can improve oxygen consumption and utilization, reduce heart rate, improve ventilation, and increase tolerance for exercise.

There have been few systematic evaluations of COPD rehabilitation programs. Reports from nonexperimental studies typically suggest that these objectives can be achieved (Bass et al., 1970; Moser et al., 1980; Petty et al., 1969; Pierce et al., 1964; Unger et al., 1980).

Recently, two controlled trials documented the benefits of exercise pro-

grams for COPD patients. Cockcroft and co-workers (1981) randomly
assigned 39 patients to a 6-week exercise-training program or to a no-treatment control group. In comparison to the control group, patients in the exercise group experienced subjective benefits and increased the amount of distance they could walk in 12 min. Allison and colleagues (1981) documented
the benefits of a bicycle training program for COPD patients by obtaining
extensive physiological measures before and after a 12-week training program. However, it is difficult to draw conclusions from their study because
no control group was included. Furthermore, we are unable to link the results
of this work to important outcomes such as those suggested by Petty and
Cherniak (1981). Although the data on exercise for COPD patients appear
promising, the number of empirical studies is fewer than the number of review
articles claiming the benefits of exercise and rehabilitation programs. In 1981,
the American Thoracic Society (1981) officially set standards for physical rehabilitation and exercise training in COPD patients.

Although COPD patients can benefit greatly from exercise, motivating
them to comply to a physical regimen is difficult. In less disabled patients
there is no "critical incident" to convince them of the importance of exercise.
In contrast, the more severely disabled patients tend to think of their situation
as hopeless and one over which they have little control (Mertens et al., 1978).
In addition, long-term maintenance of physical exercise is rare even among patients who are initially motivated (Carmody et al., 1980). Most studies suggest
that the majority of these dropouts occur during the first 3 months of training
(Carmody et al., 1980; Oldridge et al., 1978; Wilhelmson et al., 1978). If the
patients are not conscientious in adhering to the regimen, it is difficult to measure the precise outcome of an exercise program.

II. Compliance

A burgeoning body of literature indicates that patient adherence to therapeutic regimens is typically poor (Christensen, 1978; Marston, 1970; Sackett and
Haynes, 1976; Windsor et al., 1980). Failure of patients to comply with medical regimens has now come to be recognized as a major problem hampering
the quality of medical care (Becker and Maimen, 1975). Published figures suggest rates of noncompliance that very from 15 to 93%, depending on the pa
tient population and the criteria used. In general, reviewers agree that at least
33% of the patient groups in most studies failed to adhere to the recommended
therapeutic regimen (Blackwell, 1973; Becker and Maimen, 1975; Davis, 1968;
Stimson, 1974). However, noncompliance rates appear to be much higher

among patients with chronic conditions who must undergo long-term therapy (Blackwell, 1973; Brody, 1980; Davis, 1968; Gillum and Barsky, 1974; Sackett, 1976; Stone, 1979).

Noncompliance rates are also very high for patients who must comply with regimens involving life style changes such as increasing physical exercise (Carmody et al., 1980; Hoepful-Harris, 1980; Kentala, 1972; Oldridge et al., 1978; Wilhelmson et al., 1975). Although compliance has not been studied directly with respect to COPD patients and their particular regimen, (Windsor et al., 1980), results with other patient populations can offer guidance in designing a compliance program for COPD sufferers.

III. An Experiment Comparing Behavioral Interventions

A. Introduction

Within the last few years, several authors have reported that behavioral and cognitive-behavioral methods may be very useful for helping patients adhere to life style changes. We have been particularly impressed with the work of Meichenbaum (1977) and Mahoney (1974) in the development of strategies for creating and maintaining behavior change. In the remainder of this chapter we will present evidence from our current research project on the efficacy of these types of interventions for increasing adherence to a behavioral regimen for COPD patients. The rationale for our interventions and research is as follows.

Patients with chronic obstructive pulmonary disease have been known to benefit greatly from exercise regimens. A major problem with this group is that they have high rates of noncompliance. Several cognitive and behavioral interventions based on current psychological theories appear promising for increasing compliance and these strategies were compared in the present study. The effectiveness of these interventions was evaluated using an outcome measure that reflects the quality of life for program participants. Other outcome measures were used to assess the behavioral and biological processes that mediated desirable outcomes. The effectiveness of the interventions was evaluated against their cost. The ultimate goal of the project was to identify strategies that would optimize the health status of COPD patients.

B. Method

Subjects

The subjects were 75 patients diagnosed as having COPD. The specific criteria for inclusion in the study include (1) a diagnosis of emphysema, chronic bronchitis, and/or asthma; (2) absence of other significant pulmonary disease (i.e., tuberculosis, fibrosis, or neoplasm); (3) freedom from chronic disabling nonpulmonary disease that would hinder participation (i.e., arthritis, retardation, etc); (4) absence of an acute cardiac disorder (i.e., myocardial infarction within the past 3 months); and (5) an ability to stand and walk unaided for at least 100 yards without complaints of severe dyspnea (shortness of breath).

Design

The patients were randomly assigned to one of five groups: behavior modification, cognitive-behavior modification, cognitive modification, attention control, and no-treatment control. In the experimental groups, patients participated in six sessions over the course of the first 3 months of the program. Patients were seen individually in their own home for these sessions. Behavioral treatment consisted of standard behavioral procedures including individualized daily scheduling of walks, self-recording of walking, charting of progress, goal setting, contracting, and self-reinforcement. Since anxiety can often exacerbate symptoms of dyspnea, patients in the behavioral treatment group were also given relaxation training. Cognitive treatment consisted of self-recording of cognitions and retraining in attitudes and self-statements related to exercise. Cognitive-behavior modification consisted of a combination of the behavioral and the cognitive interventions. The attention-control group received attention equal to that in other experimental groups, but did not receive any training designed to alter adherence. The no-treatment control group participated in the initial assessment and follow-up assessments but did not receive individual in-home instruction or attention. An expanded description of the treatment groups is included as an Appendix to this chapter.

Crude Evaluation Through Spirometry

Spirometry is a relatively simple method for evaluating pulmonary function. The test requires the patient to take a maximum inspiration, filling up the lungs with as much air as possible, and then blow out all of the air into a spirometer as forcefully and as rapidly as possible. A spirometer is a simple mechanical device for determining the volume of expired air and plotting it over time. Measurements are typically presented as volume versus time or flow versus volume.

In our research, a spirometer was used to measure each patient's forced vital capacity (FVC: the number of liters of air that can be expelled from fully inflated lungs) and forced expiratory volume (expressed in liters) at 1,

2, and 3 seconds (FEV_1, FEV_2, and FEV_3). Predicted spirometric values are expressed in terms of a normal range for age, sex, and height (Petty, 1978).

Chronic obstructive pulmonary disease is characterized by reduction in the forced expiratory volume, vital capacity, and forced expiratory volume as a percentage of vital capacity ($FEV_1/FVC\%$) (Petty, 1978; West, 1977). The ratio of forced expiratory volume at 1 sec (FEV_1) to forced vital capacity (FVC) appears to be the most useful measure for monitoring changes in moderate to severe obstructive disease (Petty, 1978; Sobel and Emirgil, 1977). In addition, $FEV_1/FVC\%$ has an advantage of having lower patient variability than other methods for measuring flow rate (Sobel and Emirgil, 1977).

Patients with normal lung function can usually expel 70% or more of their vital capacity in 1 sec. Figures 1 through 3 illustrate the comparison of the FVC tracing or flow-volume curves for three different women of approximately the same age and height. Figure 1 is an example of normal flow-volume curve. The flow-volume curve for Figure 2 indicates moderate obstruction. Figure 3 is illustrative of severe obstructive abnormality.

Development of an Exercise Prescription

A maximal graded exercise treadmill was used to determine exercise tolerance. The variables that were assessed during the test included (1) resting and exercise (after 3 min) blood pressure, (2) resting and exercise heart rate as measured by continuous electrocardiogram monitoring, (3) resting and exercise oxygen saturation as measured by a Hewlett-Packard Ear Oximeter, Model 47201A, and (4) walking tolerance on a treadmill (speed and duration).

The patient was placed on a treadmill with bipolar electrocardiogram (ECG) leads to monitor cardiac rhythm during exercise and a Hewlett-Packard Ear Oximeter to monitor oxygen saturation during exercise. All tests were conducted by either a licensed respiratory therapist or a trained nurse (R.N.). Exercise tests began at 0.6 miles/hr, at 0% grade. Speed was increased 0.2 miles/hr at 1 min intervals. For patients who demonstrated less than 85% resting arterial saturation (SaO_2), the treadmill was increased at 0.1 miles/ hr intervals each minute. Heart rate and SaO_2 arterial saturation were recorded during the last 15 sec of each speed increment. In addition, blood pressure was taken prior to the graded exercise test, and at 3 min of exercise. The endpoint of the exercise test was reached when any of the following occurred (1) the patient reached 85% of a predicted maximum heart rate, (2) the patient reported chest pain or dizziness, (3) the ECG displayed heart arrhythmias, (4) the patient reported being exhausted or severely short of breath. Shortness of breath was the most common cause for stopping the

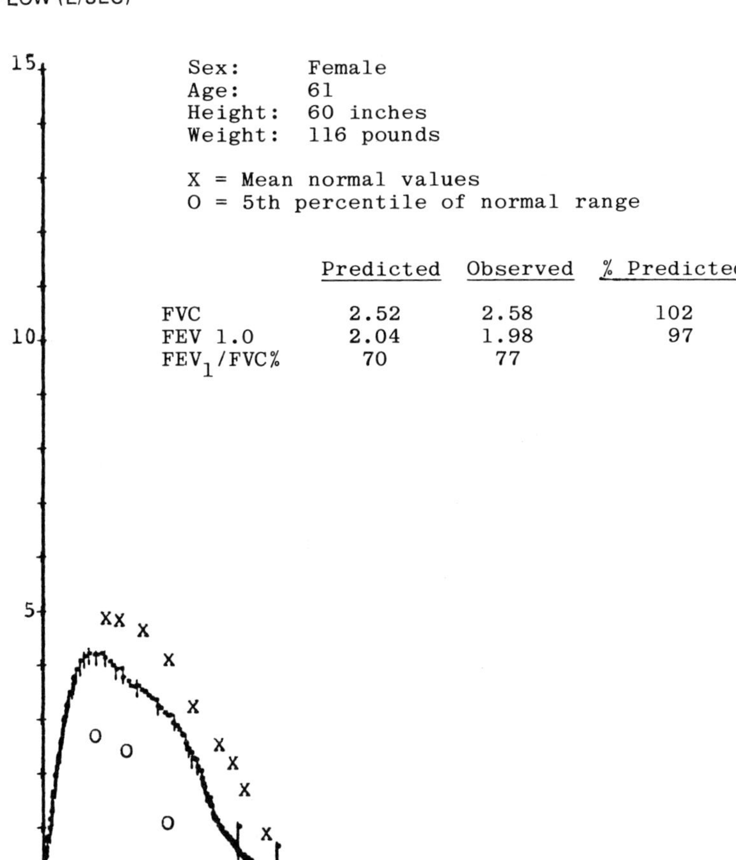

Figure 1 Spirogram depicting no obstructive abnormality.

FLOW (L/SEC)

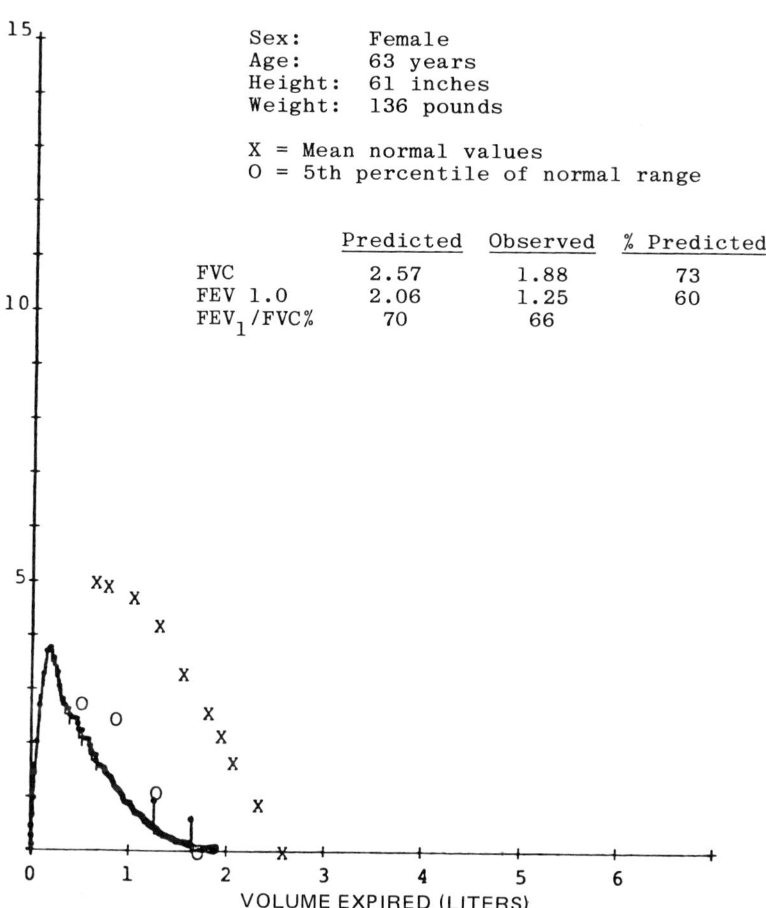

Figure 2 Spirogram depicting moderate obstructive abnormality.

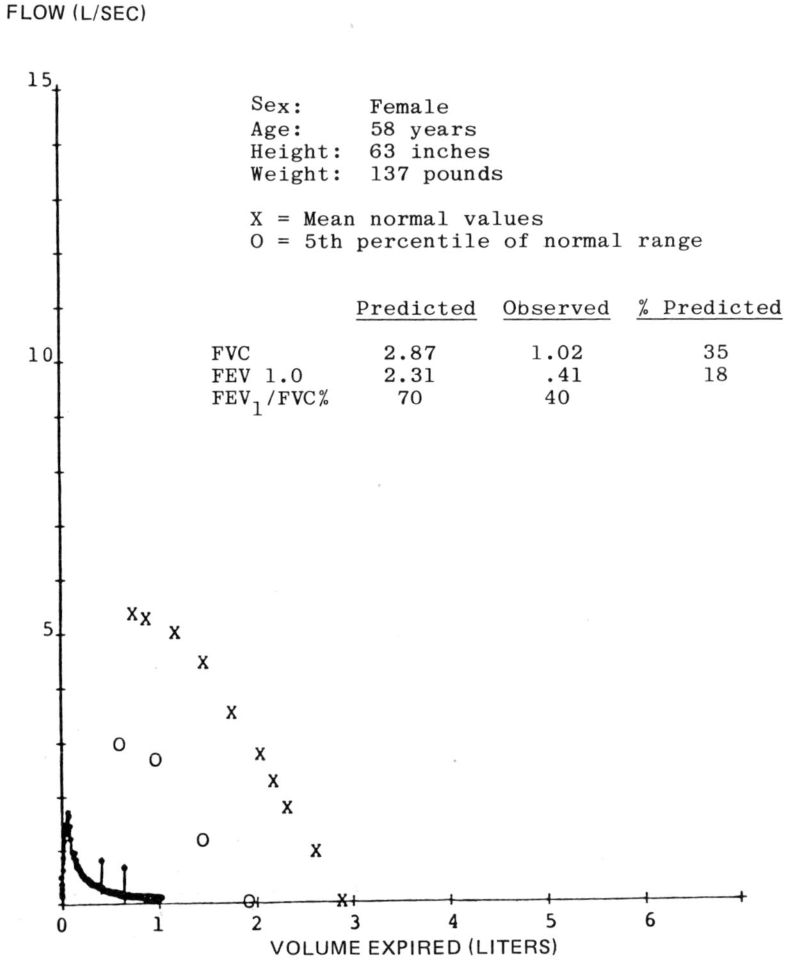

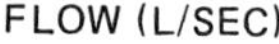

Figure 3 Spirogram depicting severe obstructive abnormality.

treadmill. A sample of a typical exercise data sheet is shown as Figure 4. The mean duration of treadmill exercise during the initial visit was 431.53 sec (S.D. = 242.66 sec).

Each patient was assigned an exercise prescription based upon the maxi-

Name: H. Schmidlapp
Age: 70
Date: 1-5-81
Session #: 1
Observer: C.J.A.

TIME	HEART RATE	BLOOD PRESSURE	SATURATION (%)	SPEED (MPH)
rest	80	128/60	94%	0
1	113		95%	.6
2	111		94%	.8
3	120	160/90	94%	1.0
4	110		93%	1.2
5	117		93%	1.4
6	113		93%	1.
7	108		92%	1.8
8	115		92%	2.0
9	127		92%	2.2
10		stopped at 9:24		
11				
12				
13				
14				
15				
16				
17				
18				

Exercise End Point: 85% max H.R.   Arrythmia   Chest Pain   (Exhaustion)   Muscular

(circle one)   Other ________________   (Dyspnea)

FVC   1. 2.65   2. 2.39   3. 2.92

FEV$_1$ 1. 1.07   2. 1.11   3. 1.27

85% predicted maximum heart rate 140

Exercise Assignment: Work Load (MPH): 1.3   % of Max. 60   Step/min 65

Frequency: once/day   (twice/day)

Duration: (5 min.)   10 min.   15 min   20 min

Other Observations: Patient reported his legs ached at around 5 minutes.

Figure 4 Sample of a typical exercise data sheet.

mum miles per hour (mph) he or she obtained on the treadmill. All assignments were made in terms of walking at defined speeds. Five progressive stages of exercise levels were assigned: stage 1—60% of maximum mph for 5 min twice daily; stage 2—60% of maximum mph for 10 min twice daily; stage 3—60% of maximum mph for 15 min twice daily; stage 4—60% of

Name: *Harvey Schmidlapp*   Date: *1-5-81*

The results of your exercise stress test show that you can walk
2.2 miles per hour. However in order not to overexercise an
exercise prescription has been developed for you which is based
on *60* percent of your maximum exercise tolerance. During the
Stage *I* of your exercise program you must walk *5* minutes,
2 times per day at a pace of *1.3* * miles per hour. Based
on the amount of distance you cover in one step, this means that
you should be taking an average of *65* steps per minute. Over
the course of the next few weeks, your exercise program will gradually be modified.

+ can cover ≈ 572 ft. in 5 min.

Figure 5 Sample of a typical exercise prescription.

maximum mph for 20 min twice daily; stage 5—70% of maximum mph for
20 min twice daily. Most of the patients were started at stage 1 of the exercise prescription. However, if exercise was well tolerated, stage 2 was determined to be the more appropriate exercise prescription. After a 10 min rest,
each patient was tested at his or her prescribed exercise level for 5 min. The
purpose of the testing was to determine the number of steps per minute the
patient would take at the assigned walking speed. The steps were counted
and recorded so that the appropriate pace could be replicated during the home
program. In addition, each patient was given information defining the appropriate distance he or she could expect to cover in 5 min walking at the prescribed pace. Patients were told to progress on to the next step of exercise as

they felt able to, and they were encouraged not to move too quickly through the stages. A walking exercise program was chosen because of familiarity, cost consideration, and convenience. Figure 5 shows a typical walking prescription.

Outcome Measures

In addition to data obtained as part of the exercise test (i.e., exercise tolerance, SaO_2, blood pressure, heart rate, etc.), several measures were taken at each clinic visit.

Health Status Index

All patients were classified on the Quality of Well-being scale of a general health index (Kaplan and Bush, 1982). This index is the point in time component of the general health decision model developed by Kaplan and Bush (1982). The index places each individual into 1 of 43 mutually exclusive and collectively exhaustive levels of functioning. The levels are obtained from three separate scales of functioning, mobility (with five levels), physical activity (with four levels), and social activity (with five levels, see Table 2). In addition, symptomatic disturbances are noted. The 43 levels of functioning are unique combinations of the steps of scales shown in Table 3. Although there are theoretically 100 possible combinations of these items, only 43 have been observed to date.

In addition to these levels of function, each patient is classified according to the symptom or problem that bothered him or her the most. There are 36 such complexes of symptoms and problems. In summary, each patient is classified according to objective functional limitation and subjective symptomatic complaint to provide a description of functioning. In previous research, each combination of function level and symptom/problem complex has been rated by random samples from the community to determine the weight or preference associated with the classification. Arrival at the correct function level classification requires the use of a survey instrument that is specific for age and employment status. The questionnaire has been validated in previous studies (Anderson and Bush, 1983).

As an example item characteristic of moderate to severe COPD patients, consider the following. At time 1, patient M.R. was described by the following scale steps:

Description	Level
In house	Mobility 3
In bed or chair	Physical activity 1
Had help with self-care activities	Social activity 1
Coughing, wheezing, or shortness of breath	Symptom/problem 11

The weight the community associates with this level of functioning is 0.5129 with the adjustment of –0.0075 for symptom/problem 11. Thus, the preference weight for this case description is 0.5054. In other words, an actual patient has classified into this level of function at time 1. A random sample of community members rated this as 0.5054. This means that community members value this objective level of function of about half-way between

Table 2 Dimensions and Steps for Function Levels in the Quality of Well-Being Scale

Mobility	Physical activity	Social activity
Drove car and used bus or train without help (5)	Walked without physical problems (4)	Did work, school, or housework and other activities (5)
Did not drive, or had help to use bus or train (4)	Walked with physical limitations (3)	Did work, school, or housework but other activities limited (4)
In house (3)	Moved own wheelchair without help (2)	Limited in amount or kind of work, school, or housework (3)
In hospital (2)	In bed or chair (1)	Performed self-care but not work, school, or housework (2)
In special care unit (1)		Had help with self-care (1)

Table 3 Ten Sample Symptom or Problem Complexes and Adjustments (W_i) for Level of Well-Being Scores

Complex number	Symptom or problem complex	Adjustment
C 1	Any trouble seeing: includes wearing glasses or contact lenses	0.0190
C 9	Pain in chest, stomach, side, back, or hips	−0.0382
C 11	Cough, wheezing, or shortness of breath	−0.0075
C 13	Fever or chills with aching all over and vomiting or diarrhea	−0.0722
C 15	Painful, burning or frequent urination	−0.0327
C 19	Pain, stiffness, numbness, or discomfort of neck, hands, feet, arms, legs, ankles, or several joints together	−0.0344
C 23	Two legs deformed (crooked), paralyzed (unable to move), or broken: includes wearing artificial limbs or braces	−0.0881
C 32	Loss of consciousness such as seizures (fits), fainting, or coma (out cold or knocked out)	−0.1507
C 33	Taking medication or staying on a pre-scribed diet for health reasons	0.1124
C 35	No symptom or problem	0.2567

Adapted from Kaplan et al. (1976).

optimal function (1.0) and death (0.0). Now consider the same patient at time 2. This time, M.R. is classified as:

Description	Level
In house	Mobility 3
In bed or chair	Physical activity 1
Performed self-care but not work, school, or housework	Social activity 2
Coughing, wheezing, or shortness of breath	Symptom/problem 11

The preference associated with this state of functioning is 0.5715. The adjustment for the symptom/problem is -0.0075, and the preference weight is 0.5640.

The difference between the two states described above is 0.0586 units of well-being. If this difference is maintained for 1 year, 0.0586 well years have been gained. If this benefit accrued for 100 people, the benefit would be 5.86 well years. Or, if it affected 1 person for 10 years, the benefit would be 0.586 well years. Another way to think of this benefit is that it is a perceived 5.86% improvement in the quality of life.

Since the index is used in a variety of medical studies, it is possible to compare changes produced by our interventions with changes on the same measure that might result from very different medical or health care interventions. Another advantage of the index is that it is linked directly to a general health policy model that is often used for cost-effectiveness studies (Kaplan, 1982; Kaplan and Bush, 1982). The validity and reliability of the index is described in several published papers (Kaplan et al., 1976, 1978, 1979; Kaplan and Ernst, 1983).

Efficacy Expectations

Efficacy expectations were assessed for each patient using an instrument adapted from studies by Bandura (1982). The patients were presented with a list of walking distances from 1 block to 3 miles. They were instructed to designate how far they thought they could walk right now. For each distance the patient designated, he or she was asked to rate the strength of the expectation to walk that distance on a 100-point probability scale ranging in 10-point intervals from high uncertainty through moderate certainty to complete certainty. Studies have shown that efficacy expectations are predictive of performance of patients in cardiac rehabilitation studies (summarized in Bandura, 1982). Further, our own validity data demonstrate that efficacy expectations correlate significantly with health status ($r = 0.49$), pulmonary function ($r = 0.44$), and exercise tolerance ($r = 0.61$).

Walking Logs

Each patient was asked to keep a daily log of walking and exercise activities. The patients were requested to record the time of day of each walk, the distance covered, total minutes spent walking, their heart rate, and any reason for not walking (i.e., illness, travel, guests, etc.). Patients were given a runner's wrist stop watch to time their walks. In behavioral conditions they could earn the watch for completing the walking log. Although walking data were based on self-report, we have some evidence for the validity. For instance, some of

WEEK NO. 1

DATE	DAY	TIME BEGAN	TIME END	TOTAL TIME	DISTANCE	PULSE RATE	COMMENTS:
1/12	MON	7:50ₐ	7:56ₐ	5:30	≈550′	82/110	drank coffee & read newspaper after walk.
		2:15	2:22	6:03	≈570′	80/105	read my novel after walk. Felt short of breath.
1/13	TUE	7:52ₐ	8:01ₐ	8:02	≈600′	85/115	drank coffee after walk Felt pretty good today
		—	—	—			Had unexpected visitors
1/14	WED	7:51ₐ	7:56ₐ	5:05	≈550′	81/99	read newspaper after walk Felt winded after walk.
		2:50	2:57	7:03	≈600′	86/104	Watched 3:00 movie after walk
	THU						
	FRI						
	SAT						
	SUN						
TOTAL TIME FOR WEEK:							
TOTAL NUMBER OF WALKS FOR WEEK:							

Figure 6 Sample of a typical walking log sheet.

the walks were completed under the supervision of project staff and reporting accuracy was validated. Records demonstrated that patients consistently reported decreased or no walking activity on sick days. In addition, self-reported walking was significantly correlated with improved exercise tolerance determined in an objective graded exercise test administered by a technician blind to the patients' experimental condition and walking history ($r = 0.34$ $p < 0.02$). An example of a page from the walking log is shown as Figure 6.

Dropouts

Five patients dropped out of the study before they could be evaluated at the 3-month testing session. Two patients dropped out of the behavior modification group complaining that they did not like to be regimented. One patient dropped out of the attention control group because she thought the questions were too personal and because she had too many other problems in her life. Two patients dropped out of the no-treatment control group. One of these patients moved away and could not be located. The other patient was not able to comply with the walking prescription and refused to be reevaluated. All of these patients were replaced. In addition, two patients, one from the attention-control group and one from the behavior modification group, refused to appear for the treadmill test and the pulmonary function testing. These patients were not dropped from the study because they agreed to participate in all of the other 3-month evaluation procedures if the experimenter came to their home.

C. Results

Analysis of Walking Data

Self-reported walking compliance was a major outcome variable in the study. Data collection began on week 3 and walking logs were evaluated for weeks 3-12 of the program. The experimental groups differed significantly in number of minutes walked per week during all except the first week. Week 12 was the last time at which there was monitoring of the walking log. The planned comparison contrasting the three experimental groups against the two control groups was statistically significant for all 9 weeks. The attention and no-treatment controls did not significantly differ for any week of the experiment.

Significant differences between the cognitive-behavior modification and the other two experimental groups began to emerge during the eighth week of the program. Thereafter, differences between these groups were statistically significant each week except week 11 (for the week, $p < 0.07$). The behavior modification and cognitive modification groups did not differ during any week of the experiment. The mean cumulative number of minutes each group spent in weekly walking is presented pictorially in Figure 7. Significance tests for these data revealed that (1) the combination of the three treatment groups produces greater adherence to walking than the control groups, (2) cognitive-behavior modification produces greater adherence to walking than either behavior modification or cognitive modification, and (3) although each treatment is superior to the no treatment control, only the cognitive-behavioral combination is significantly more effective than the attention control.

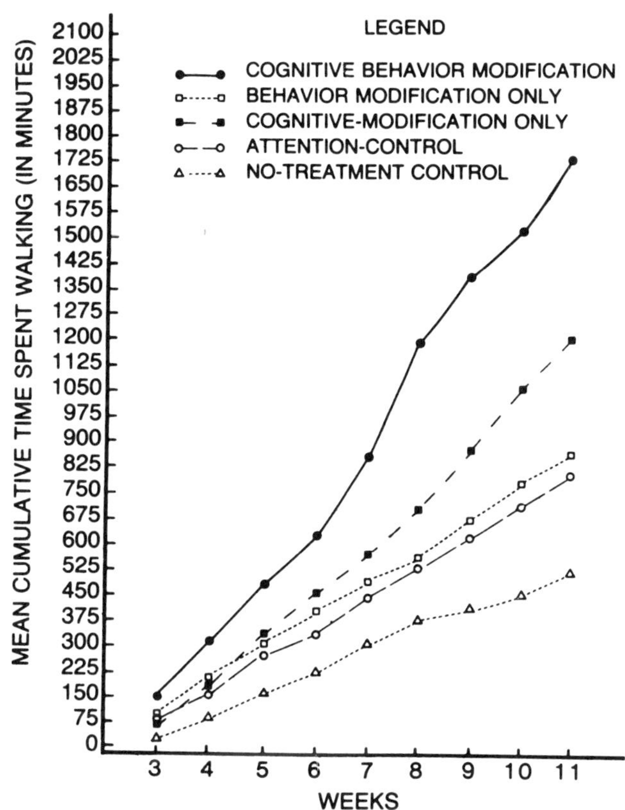

Figure 7 Cumulative weekly walking for each group.

Exercise Tolerance

An exercise tolerance score was created by dividing seconds of treadmill exercise tolerance at 3 months by the seconds of exercise tolerance at the initial visit. This ratio gives the percentage increase in exercise tolerance. Figure 8 displays percentage increases in exercise tolerance for the five groups participating in the study. The greatest average increase in exercise tolerance was obtained for the cognitive-behavior modification group (45%). There was a 36% average increase in exercise tolerance for the cognitive

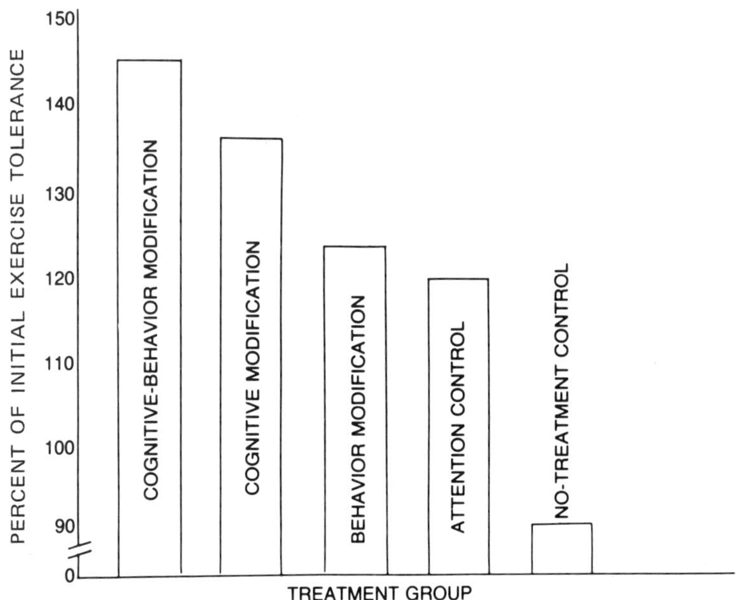

Figure 8 Exercise tolerance for the five groups at 3 months (percent of baseline).

group, a 123% average increase for the behavioral group, 117% average increase in exercise tolerance for the attention control groups, and a 9% decrease in exercise tolerance for the no-treatment group.

The three experimental groups differed significantly from the two control groups. However, the three treatment groups did not differ significantly from one another and differences between the two control groups were not significant.

Health Status Index

Data on the health index were obtained at the initial interview and at all follow-up sessions. Kaplan and colleagues (1978) have shown that the mean Quality of Well-being value over 4 days is more reliable than the value obtained on any one day. Therefore, Quality of Well-being data were obtained for the 4 days preceding each visit, and the mean value across the 4 days was used in all calculations. A one-way analysis of variance for Quality of Well-being scores

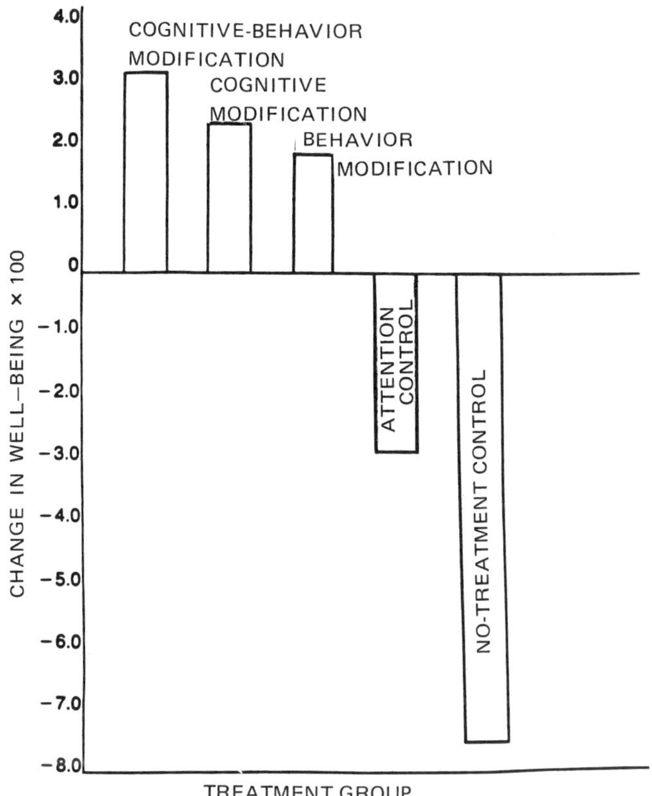

Figure 9 Mean change in index of well-being scores (multiplied by 100).

demonstrated groups did not differ prior to the interventions. For all other analyses, changes in Well-being scores from the initial 3-month assessment were used.

Differences in well-being scores are displayed in Figure 9. The cognitive-behavior modification group shows a 0.032 increase in well-being over the 3-month period while the cognitive and behavior modification groups each showed 0.024 and 0.019 increases, respectively. The attention-control group showed a decline in well-being of -0.029 units while the no-treatment group showed a decline of -0.075. Significance tests showed that the combination of the three treatment groups differed from the combination of the two control groups. Further, the three experimental groups did not differ from one another, but each differed from the no-treatment control. The cognitive and cognitive-behavioral groups showed significant improvements over the attention control while differences between the behavior modification and the attention control groups were nonsignificant. The correlation between changes in exercise tolerance and changes in Quality of Well-being was 0.40 (p < 0.01). Changes on the quality of well-being were also substantially correlated with walking compliance (r = 0.42, p < 0.01).

Changes in Physiological Parameters

Extensive evidence suggests that COPD cannot be cured through exercise. Thus, differences were not expected for spirometric variables. Indeed, there were no changes over time and no significant differences across groups for changes in vital capacity for forced expiratory volume in 1 sec (FEV_1). In addition, the groups did not change for resting diastolic blood pressure or change in systolic blood pressure. Although there were no differences between groups in mean arterial saturation of oxygen in blood after exercise, there was a nonsignificant trend suggesting that the two control groups became more desaturated upon retesting than did the experimental groups. These data confirm the work of many investigators who have demonstrated that exercise cannot reverse the physiological characteristics of COPD. Exercise may improve oxygen delivery as evidenced by the weak change in exercise SaO_2.

Self-Efficacy

In order to explain differences between groups in exercise tolerance and in walking compliance, self-efficacy ratings were studied. In particular, changes in efficacy ratings were evaluated for walking. Change scores were created by subtracting the efficacy rating obtained at the original visit from the efficacy rating obtained at the 3-month assessment. Efficacy ratings were not obtained from members of the no-treatment control group. There was a significant difference between groups for changes in self-efficacy (p < 0.01), with the experimental groups gaining more in walking efficacy judgment than the attention control group. Although the correlation between *changes* in efficacy and *changes* in exercise tolerance was nonsignificant (r = 0.10), the correlation between efficacy changes and changes on the Quality of Well-being was statistically significant (r = 0.28, p < 0.02). At each testing session there was a strong correlation between efficacy and exercise tolerance (session 1, r = 0.47; 3-month assessment, r = 0.61). Similarly, efficacy was strongly

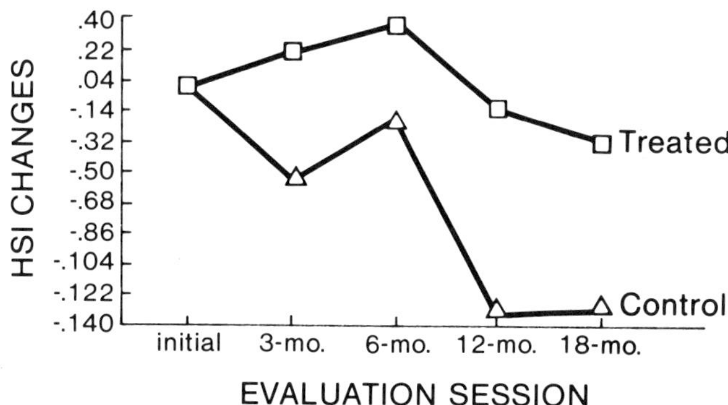

Figure 10 Differences in well-being scores between treated and control groups.

correlated with health status at both the initial (r = 0.50) and the 3-month assessment (r = 0.49).

Longer-Term Effects on Well-Being

Following the 3-month assessment, the experimental and control groups continued to differ at each assessment period (see Fig. 10). However, by the last follow-up, the differences were only marginally statistically significant. The reduction in statistical significance results from increased variability in both groups across follow-up sessions.

Table 4 summarizes the observed well-year benefits for the experiment. The first column shows the follow-up periods. The second column shows the change in Well-being score for the treated group while the third column shows the mean change in Well-being for the control subjects. The fourth column shows the difference between the treated and control group defined as mean treated minus mean control. The next column displays the number of patients available at that follow-up period. The second column from the right of the table shows the duration for which the assessment was based. For example, 0.25 means that the data represent assumed average well-being difference over a 3-month period. The final column shows the well-year yield for that period. It is calculated by obtaining the product of the difference in well-being between treated and control groups times the number of patients available for observation. That product is then multiplied by the proportion of the year the assessment represents. For example, at the 3-month follow-up, the

4 Observed and Projected Well-Year Benefits

w-up	(M) Treated	(M) Control	Difference	N	Duration	Well-years
onth	0.021	-0.055	0.076	70	0.25	1.33
onth	0.036	-0.021	0.056	55	0.25	0.77
onth	-0.012	-0.134	0.114	50	0.50	2.85
onth	-0.032	-0.131	0.099	48	0.50	2.38
			Total well-year production over project period			7.33
			Discounted (at 5%)			6.92
cted Benefits for Sensitivity Analysis						
-month (1 year after 18-month follow-up)			0.050	50	1.00	2.50
			Total well-year production			9.83
			Discounted (at 5%)			9.13
-month (2 years after 18-month follow-up)			0.025	25	1.00	1.25
			Total well-year production			11.08
			Discounted (at 5%)			10.18

ce: Toevs et al. (1984).

treated and control groups differed by 0.076 units of well-being. Multiplying this value by the 70 patients included in the analysis yields 5.32. The entire 70 patients were used for this calculation because the program costs accrued equally to the experimental *and* the control groups. However, this value is obtained only after one quarter of 1 year. To estimate the well-year production, we multiply 5.32 by 0.25 to obtain 1.33. Similar assessments were made for the 6-month, 12-month, and 18-month follow-ups. The total well year production is the sum of the well year produced at each assessment interval. According to this analysis, 7.33 well years were produced. Discounting this figure at 5% gives a well-year production of 6.92 years.

This analysis makes several assumptions including (1) that differences between treated and control means at the assessment date are representative of differences during the preceding interval, and (2) that the number of patients available for follow-up is a representative sample of the original participants. All known deaths are included in the analysis. The reduction in N at successive follow-ups represents drop-outs and those who have moved from the area. There were significant losses after the first follow-up, probably because project staff no longer had regular contact with the patients. The number of patients shown in the table are used because they are the ones upon whom project resources were devoted.

One potential problem is that dropouts could be unequal from the experimental and control groups. In order to evaluate this question, we systematically studied dropouts at each phase of the experiment. Although the number of dropouts accumulated over the 18-month study, there was no evidence for differential dropout rates between treated and control population. Chi square tests for 2 X 2 contingency tables (experimental-control versus dropout-continuer) were statistically nonsignificant at each follow-up period. Thus, differential dropouts would not cause systematic underestimation or overestimation of cost-effectiveness.

It is important to note that the benefits of a behavioral program should continue beyond a final assessment period. An important implication of the health index model is that it tracks patients over the remainder of their life expectancy. In other words, we would expect benefits to continue to accrue far beyond the treatment period. However, we are hesitant to estimate benefits we have not observed. For this reason, we projected future benefits to use in a sensitivity analysis. Even though future benefits continue to accrue, costs would remain constant. Behavioral programs do not require the purchase of medication and should not increase medical expenditures. Since many variables in cost-effectiveness analysis cannot be pinpointed exactly, feasible ranges of values should be considered.

Two assumptions about future benefits were considered in the sensitivity analysis. One assumption projects the difference between treated and control groups 1 year after the program as one-half of the 0.099 observed difference at 18 months. The difference between treated and control groups will be 0.05 units of well-being. If 50 individuals received this benefit, the additional well-year production under this assumption would be 0.05 units of well being $\times$ 50 patients $\times$ 1.0 year = 2.5 well years. The *total* well year production under this assumption would be 7.33 + 2.50 = 9.83 (see Table 4). Discounting at 5% gives a well-year production figure of 9.13.

A second assumption projects benefits 2 years after the close of the treatment. Under this assumption, we assume that one-half the patients are still available for follow-up, and the treated and control groups differ by one-fourth and observed differences at the 18-month assessment. Multiplying the 0.025 difference between treated and control groups by 25 patients produces 1.25 well years if the improvement lasts 1 year. Adding this 1.25 to the previously calculated 7.33 and 2.5 well-years gives a total well year production of 11.08. The final discounted figure for this assumption equals 10.18 well-years (see Table 4). While these two assumptions treat health status as a constant, in fact it varies naturally. The assumptions we have presented are for illustrative purposes only.

In summary, we have observed an estimated 7.33 well years of benefit in the study, and we might expect an additional 2.5 to 3.75 well years under the two assumptions considered in the sensitivity analysis.

D. Discussion

Patients with COPD may benefit from structured exercise programs. However, compliance to behavioral programs in health tends to be low. Various behavioral interventions for weight control (Foreyt et al., 1981) and for smoking (Leventhal and Cleary, 1980) have not produced impressive results.

The results of the present study suggest that patients in the behavioral treatment groups walked more, displayed greater increases on exercise tolerance, and exhibited better health functioning on Quality of Well-being Scale than the patients in the control groups.

Strategies that include a behavioral component appear to be the most useful for motivating and maintaining compliance to a regular walking program among moderate to severe COPD patients. Patients who adhere to the program and gradually increase their walking over time demonstrate measurable improvement in exercise tolerance. Consistent with other research on pulmonary rehabilitation (Bass et al., 1970; Moser et al., 1980; Petty et al.,

1969; Pierce et al., 1964; Unger et al., 1980) patients in the present study did not improve their pulmonary function as measured by spirometry. However, improvements in exercise performance lead to higher levels of health functioning as measured by the Quality of Well-being Scale. This finding is particularly important since the major purpose of rehabilitation is improvement in the patient's abilities to function independently (Moser et al., 1980).

Self-Efficacy Theory and the Dyspnea-Panic Cycle

Some COPD patients may experience a vicious cycle of fear and dyspnea. Activity may cause shortness of breath which in turn causes panic. The panic results in more dyspnea and the cycle becomes self-perpetuating. Many patients come to think that the situation is beyond their control and may avoid activities because of fear (Dudley, 1981; Mertens et al., 1978). One of our patients described becoming very short of breath while running to escape the rain. He fell and lay on the wet pavement in fear of dying because of his shortness of breath. After this experience he greatly restricted his activity and left home only when absolutely necessary. In other words, he felt unable to cope with dyspnea brought on by activity.

Information may have little impact upon patients affected by the panic-dyspnea cycle. They may understand that panic will complicate the problem but may question their skill in coping with dyspnea. Bandura describes this as a problem in self-efficacy. Self-efficacy is defined as the degree of confidence that a specific behavior can be enacted.

Bandura's self-efficacy theory maintains that behavior is mediated by expectations that particular behaviors can be executed in specifically defined situations. Programs that provide mastery experiences in particular situations will enhance expectations for success in similar situations on future occasions. These expectations in turn serve to mediate future executions of the behavior. Patients in our study were given an individually tailored exercise prescription. In the experimental groups, patients worked out a clearly defined strategy for implementing the walking program. As the focus remained on walking—when, how, where, how long—patients' perceived efficacy for accomplishing exercise improved. A typical answer while filling out the self-efficacy questionnaire at the three-month follow-up was "I know I can walk three blocks because I have done it. I don't know if I can walk five blocks, but I can try."

Past experience serves as a mediating cognitive process (Bandura, 1982), and accomplishing changes in one particular behavior serves to increase expectations that behavior can be executed in the future. At the end of the 3-month training period, patients' expectancies for related exercise behavior, such as climbing stairs and moving furniture, did not change as much. Patients showed least improvement for capacities that were not the focus of training (Kaplan et al., 1984b).

IV. Conclusions and Recommendations

The major objectives of health care should include the extension of the life expectancy and the improvement of quality of life. Preliminary evidence suggests that behavioral programs (as adjuncts to medical treatment) for COPD patients may enhance life quality and provide a relative improvement in health status. The cost-effectiveness of these programs has been evaluated and shown to be comparable with other widely advocated health care services (Toevs et al., 1984). We believe that the mechanism for this improvement is an enhanced sense of self-efficacy (Bandura, 1982) gained through the performance of coping behaviors. Principles of social learning and reinforcement are probably required in order to achieve the enactment and maintenance of these behaviors (Atkins et al., 1984; Kaplan et al., 1984b).

Several alternative behavioral methods are available and it is sometimes difficult to select them. We found an initial benefit from a cognitive-behavioral approach. However, differences between different methods were small and tended to be undetectable by the 6-month follow-up. If asked to recommend a single method, we would choose cognitive-behavior modification. In all analyses, the cognitive-behavioral group was rank ordered first. In addition, cognitive-behavior modification is well understood by older adults and may be better tolerated than a strictly behavioral approach (Thompson and Gallagher, 1980).

There is still a shortage of data on the efficacy of expensive behavioral and rehabilitation programs for COPD patients. We are currently conducting a randomized clinical trial to compare a comprehensive COPD rehabilitation program with didactic education. The evaluation will include a detailed assessment of the costs, risks, and benefits of behavioral rehabilitation.

V. Appendix: Treatment Groups

A. Behavior Modification

The strategies used to help patients in this group (N = 15) follow a regular walking program were based on behavior modification principles. Specifically, the subset of behavior modification principles aimed at developing self-control were utilized. Early in the second session, the patient's daily schedule was outlined, and the patient was asked to identify highly probable behaviors in his or her daily life. Each was then asked to make the self-administration of these reinforces contingent upon daily walking. In addition, patients signed a behavioral contract specifying the time for their daily walk and the reinforcer that would be used for its achievement. The experimenter went for a 5 min sample walk with the patient to identify the proper pace and distance. Then the experimenter provided instructions in self-reinforcement following the walk. For example, some patients made morning coffee contingent upon completing their walk. After the sample walk, the experimenter would have coffee with the patient.

During the third and fourth sessions, the patients were taught progressive muscle relaxation. Anxiety is commonly experienced by patients with COPD and may exacerbate dyspnea or shortness of breath, which in turn may make a patient more anxious. Many COPD patients do not feel they have any control over this vicious cycle. Progressive muscle relaxation was used to help patients gain control over anxiety (Dudley et al., 1980a,b). Breathing exercises were also used in accordance with standard pulmonary rehabilitation procedures. The experimenters stressed appropriate diaphragmatic breathing, purse-lip breathing, and 2:1 exhalation/inhalation ratio during the relaxation sessions (Moser et al., 1980).

B. Cognitive Modification

Recent research has demonstrated the importance of cognitive change in maintaining behavior over time. This other type of strategy that was developed to increase and maintain walking among COPD patients is called cognitive modification (Ellis, 1962; Mahoney and Mahoney, 1976). According to this strategy, individuals are trained to become aware of their own negative and maladaptive thoughts, feelings, and behaviors, and to replace them with more positive cognitions. The assumption underlying this approach is that walking or exercising may be influenced by what the patient says to him or herself during walking. Since exercise is uncomfortable for many COPD patients, they may be actually talking themselves out of walking. Patients who were randomly assigned to receive cognitive modification (N = 16) were first encouraged to monitor their own self-statements, paying particular attention to negative self-statements that might interfere with walking (i.e., "I can't walk very far without getting short of breath, so what's the use?"). They were then trained to substitute negative self statements with more appropriate positive and goal-oriented self statements (i.e., "This walking is uncomfortable, but I can handle it. Soon I will be able to walk farther").

As in the behavior modification strategy, the experimenter went for a 5-min walk with each patient to familiarize him or her with the approximate pace and distance that had been prescribed. In addition, the experimenter pointed out 1/4, 1/2, and 3/4 of the total distance and modeled the appropriate self-cognition (i.e., "Gee, I've already walked 1/4 of the way, that wasn't so bad; half-way there, that didn't take long").

While the cognitive approach is aimed at changing negative self-statements that could interfere with maintaining the walking regimen over time, it is a didactic approach. Patients are not given the specific instructions on how to fit walking into their daily schedule nor are they given any instructions in relaxation. A number of research studies suggest that specific instructions on how to carry out a proposed action should maximize adherence. Thus, a third approach that involved a merger of the cognitive and behavioral techniques was also included.

C. Cognitive-Behavior Modification

The cognitive-behavior modification strategy combined the cognitive, insight-oriented therapy with standard behavior modification and self-control techniques. As in the cognitive modification group, patients who were randomly assigned to this group (N = 16) were encouraged to monitor their own self-statements and they were trained to substitute negative self-statements with more appropriate positive and goal-oriented self-statements. Since contact hours were equivalent across all groups it was necessary to reduce the amount of time spent on cognitive activities in order to make time for the behavioral component. A literal combination of the cognitive and behavioral packages would have taken twice as much time, thus confounding treatment and contact time.

On the behavioral side, the package included relaxation and breathing techniques (two sessions), such as 2:1 expiration-inspiration ratios, diaphragmatic, and pursed lip breathing. Patients were encouraged to practice the relaxation and breathing techniques daily. Since compliance with a regular walking regimen requires self-control, some of the behavioral self-control techniques were also included in the package.

The behavioral components for improving self-control included the specification of regular daily activities and contingency-management techniques for self-administration of reinforcers. The writing and signing of a behavioral contract was not included in this package in order to make time for the cognitive modification component.

As described in the previous two strategies, the experimenter went for a 5-min walk with each patient to familiarize him or her with the walking prescription. As in the other groups, the experimenter pointed out 1/4, 1/2, and 3/4 of the total distance and appropriate self-cognitions were suggested to the patient.

D. Attention Control

The three strategies outlined previously all require personal contact time with each patient. Many researchers have argued that merely spending time with or attending to a patient will lead to increases in compliance (Evans et al., 1970; Hall et al., 1974; Haynes, 1976; Mann and Janis, 1968; Meyer and Henderson, 1974). An attention control group was included in this study (N = 15) to evaluate the effect of attention alone. Patients who were randomly assigned to this group were given information about the importance of stressful life events, personality characteristics, family support, and previous health history on chronic lung disease. As in the other groups, the experimenter met with the patient for five separate hourly meetings in the patient's home. The experimenter also collected walking log information from the previous week or weeks, and administered the self-efficacy measure. The remainder of each session was spent on various paper and pencil tasks. The data from these tasks were used to generate discussion with the patient. The paper and pencil scales included a Social Support Inventory, the Trail Making Test, part B, the Minnesota Multiphasic Personality Inventory, and the Social Readjustment Rating Scale (Rahe, 1972).

E. No-Treatment Control

The no-treatment control group (N = 13) was exercise tested at the first session, given an exercise prescription and a walking log, and advised to implement the walking program. The experimenters were available to these patients for advice via the telephone contact. At the end of 3 months, these patients were invited back to the clinic for a reassessment.

Acknowledgment

This work was supported by grants K04 HL 00809, R01 HL 25109, and R01 HL 34732 from the National Institutes of Health, Heart, Lung, and Blood Institute.

References

Allison, J. A., Sanicos, R., and Anderson, S. D. (1981). Evaluation of exercise training in patients with chronic airway obstruction. *Physical Therapy* **61**:1273-1277.

American Thoracic Society (1981). Pulmonary rehabilitation. *Chest* **80**:475-500.

Anderson, J. P., and Bush, J. W. (1983). *Respondent and Proxy Instruments for Classifying Function Status of Quality of Well-Being.* Unpublished manuscript, University of California, Dan Diego.

Anthonisen, N. R. (1983). Long-term oxygen therapy. *Ann. Intern. Med.* **99**:519-527.

Astin, T. W. (1976). Cigarette smoking and chronic bronchitis. *Br. Med. J.* **2**:1261.

Atkins, C. J., Kaplan, R. M., Timms, R. M., Rinsch, S., and Lofback, K. (1984). Behavioral programs for exercise compliance in COPD. *J. Consult. Clin. Psychol.* **52**:591-603.

Bandura, A. (1982). Self-efficacy mechanisms in human agency. *Am. Psychol.* **37**:122-147.

Bass, H., Whitcomb, J. F., and Forman, R. (1970). Exercise training: therapy for patients with chronic obstructive pulmonary disease. *Chest* **57**:116-120.

Becker, M. H., and Maimen, L. A. (1975). Sociobehavioral determinants of compliance with medical care recommendations. *Med. Care* **13**:10-24.

Bell, C. W., and Jensen, R. H. (1977). Physical conditioning. In *Pulmonary Rehabilitation Home Programs.* Edited by R. H. Jensen and L. Kass. Omaha, University of Nebraska Medical Center.

Blackwell, B. (1973). Drug therapy: patient compliance. *N. Engl. J. Med.* **289**:249-252.

Brashear, R. E. (1980). Chronic obstructive pulmonary disease. In *Current Pulmonology,* Vol. 1. Edited by D. H. Simmons. Boston, Houghton-Mifflin.

Brody, D. (1980). An analysis of patient recall of their therapeutic regimens. *J. Chron. Dis.* **33**:57-63.

California Department of Health Services (1982). *Report to the 1982 California Legislature on Chronic Obstructive Lung Disease Project.* State of California, Health and Welfare Agency.

Carmody, T., Senner, J., Malinow, M., and Matarazzo, G. (1980). Physical exercise rehabilitation: long-term dropout rate in cardiac patients. *J. Behav. Med.* **3**:163-168.

Christensen, D. B. (1978). Drug taking compliance: a review and synthesis. *Health Services Res.* **13**:171-187.

Christie, D. (1968). Physical training in COPD. *Br. Med. J.* **2**:1950-1951.

Cockcroft, A. E., Saunders, M. J., and Berry, B. (1981). Randomized controlled trial of rehabilitation in chronic respiratory disease. *Thorax* **36**: 200.

Davis, M. S. (1968). Variations in patients' compliance with doctors' advice: an empirical analysis of patterns of communication. *Am. J. Public Health* **58**:274-288.

Dudley, D. L. (1981). Coping with chronic COPD: therapeutic options. *Geriatrics* **36**:69-75.

Dudley, D., Glaser, E. M., Jorgenson, B. N., and Logan, D. L. (1980a). Psychosocial concomitants to rehabilitation in chronic obstructive pulmonary disease. Part 1: Psychosocial and psychological considerations. *Chest* **77**:413-420.

Dudley, D. L., Glaser, E. M., Jorgenson, B. N., and Logan, D. L. (1980b). Psychosocial concomitants in chronic obstructive pulmonary disease. Part 2: Psychosocial treatment. *Chest* **77**:544-551.

Ellis, A. (1962). *Reason and Emotions in Psychotherapy.* New York, Lyle Stuart.

Epstein, K. A., Schneiderman, L. J., Bush, J. W., and Zuttner, A. (1981). The "abnormal" screening serum thyroxine (T4): analysis of physician response outcome, cost and health effectiveness. *J. Chron. Dis.* **34**:175-190.

Evans, R. I., Rozelle, R. M., Lasater, T. M., Dembroski, J. J., and Allen, B. P. (1970). Fear arousal persuation, and actual versus implied behavioral change. *J. Person. Soc. Psychol.* **16**:220-227.

Fishman, D. B., and Petty, T. L. (1971). Physical, symptomatic and psychological improvements in patients receiving comprehensive care for chronic airway obstruction. *J. Chron. Dis.* **24**:775-785.

Fix, A. J., Daughton, D., and Kass, I. (1981). Behavioral sciences in pulmonary rehabilitation. *Appl. Techniques Behav. Med.* 263-294.

Fordyce, D. (1983). *Prevention of chronicity in low back pain.* Paper presented at the 91st annual meeting of the American Psychological Association, Anaheim, CA.

Foreyt, J. P., Goodrick, G. K., and Gotto, M. (1981). Limitations of behavioral treatment of obesity: review and analysis. *J. Behav. Med.* **4**:159-173.

Gillum, R. F., and Barsky, A. J. (1974). Diagnosis and management of patient noncompliance. *J.A.M.A.* **228**:1563-1567.

Hall, S. M., Hall, R. G., Nandon, R. W., and Borden, B. L. (1974). Permanence of two self-managed treatments of overweight in inversity and community populations. *J. Consult. Clin. Psychol.* **42**:781-876.

Haynes, R. B., (1976). Strategies for improving compliance: a methodologic analysis and review. In *Compliance with Therapeutic Regimens.* Edited by D. L. Sackett and R. B. Haynes. Baltimore, Johns Hopkins University Press.

Higgins, I. T. T. (1958). Tobacco smoking, respiratory symptoms, and ventilatory capacity: studies in random samples of the population. *Br. Med. J.* **2**:325-329.

Hoepful-Harris, J. A. (1980). Rehabilitation of the cardiac patient: improving compliance with an exercise program. *Am. J. Nursing* **3**:449-451.

Kaplan, R. M. (1982). Human preference measurement in health decisions and the evaluation of long-term care. In *Values and Long-Term Care.* Edited by R. L. Kane and R. A. Kane. Lexington, MA, D. C. Heath.

Kaplan, R. M., and Bush, J. W. (1982). Health related quality of life measurement for evaluation research and policy analysis. *Health Psychol.* **1**: 61-80.

Kaplan, R. M., Bush, J. W., and Berry, C. C. (1976). Health status: types of validity for an index of well-being. *Health Services Res.* **11**:478-507.

Kaplan, R. M., Bush, J. W., and Berry, C. C. (1978). The reliability, stability, and generalizability of a health status index. *Am. Stat. Assoc. Proc. Soc. Stat. Sect.* **26**:415-418.

Kaplan, R. M., Bush, J. W., and Berry, C. C. (1979). Health status index: category rating versus magnitude estimation for measuring levels of well-being. *Med. Care* **42**:365-369.

Kaplan, R. M., and Ernst, J. (1983). Do category rating scales produce biased preference weights for a health index? *Med. Care* **21**:193-207.

Kaplan, R. M., Atkins, C. J., and Timms, R. M. (1984). Validity of a quality of well-being scale as an outcome measure in chronic obstructive pulmonary disease. *J. Chron. Dis.* **37**:85-95.

Kaplan, R. M., Ries, A., and Atkins, C. J. (1985). Behavioral issues in the management of chronic obstructive pulmonary disease. *Ann. Behav. Med.* **7**:5-10.

Kaplan, R. M., Atkins, C. J., and Reinsch, S. (1984b). Specific efficacy expectations mediate exercise compliance in patients with COPD. *Health Psychol.* **3**:223-242.

Katz, I. R. (1982). Is there a hypoxic affective syndrome? *Psychosomatics* **23**:846-853.

Kentala, E. (1972). Physical fitness and feasibility of physical rehabilitation after myocardial infarction in men of working age. *Ann. Clin. Res.* **4**: 1-84.

Lebowitz, N. D. (1982). Multivariate analysis of smoking and other risk factors for obstructive lung diseases and related symptoms. *J. Chron. Dis.* **35**:751-758.

Lenfant, C. (1982). Lung research: government and community. *Am. Rev. Respir. Dis.* **126**:753-757.

Lertzman, M. M., and Cherniack, R. M. (1976). Rehabilitation of patients with chronic obstructive pulmonary disease. *Am. Rev. Respir. Dis.* **114**: 1145-1164.

Leventhal, H., and Cleary, P. D. (1980). The smoking problem: a review of the research and theory in behavioral risk modification. *Psychol. Bull.* **88**:370-405.

Lichtenstein, E. (1982). The smoking problem: a behavioral perspective. *J. Consult. Clin. Psychol.* **50**:804-819.

Mahoney, M. (1974). *Cognition and Behavior Modification.* Cambridge, MA, Ballinger.

Mahoney, M., and Mahoney, K. (1976). *Permanent Weight Control.* New York, W. W. Norton & Co., Inc.

Mann, L., and Janis, I. L. (1968). A follow-up study on the long-term effects of emotional role-playing. *J. Personality Soc. Psychol.* **8**:339-342.

Marston, M. (1970). Compliance with medical regimens: a review of the literature. *Research* **19**:312-325.

McSweeny, A. J., Grant, I., Heaton, R. K., Adams, K. M., and Timms, R. M. (1982). Life quality of patients with chronic obstructive pulmonary disease. *Arch. Intern. Med.* **142**:473-478.

Meichenbaum, D. (1977). *Cognitive Behavior Modification.* New York, Plenum.

Mertens, D. J., Shephard, R. J., and Kavanagh, T. (1978). Long-term exercise therapy for chronic obstructive lung disease. *Respiration* **35**:96-107.

Meyer, A. J., and Henderson, J. B. (1974). Multiple risk factor reduction in the prevention of cardiovascular disease. *Prev. Med.* **3**:225-236.

Moser, D. M., Archibald, C., Hansen, P., Ellis, B., and Whelan, D. (1980). *Better Living and Breathing: A Manual for Patients,* 2nd ed. St. Louis, C. V. Mosby.

Moser, K., Bokinsky, G., Savage, R., Archibald, C., and Hansen, P. (1980). Results of a comprehensive rehabilitation program: physiologic and functional effects on patients with chronic obstructive pulmonary disease. *Arch. Intern. Med.* **140**:1596-1601.

National Institutes of Health (1981). *Chronic Obstructive Pulmonary Disease.* NIH Publication No. 81-2020. Bethesda, Maryland, U.S. Department of Health and Human Services.

National Institutes of Health (1983). *Report of Workshop on Lung Disease and Behavior.* Bethesda, Maryland, U.S. Department of Health and Human Services.

Nocturnal Oxygen Therapy Trial Group (1980). Continuous or nocturnal oxygen therapy in hypoxemic chronic obstructive lung disease: a clinical trial. *Ann. Intern. Med.* **93**:391-398.

Oldridge, N., Wicks, J., Hanley, C., Sutton, J., and Jones, N. (1978). Noncompliance in an exercise rehabilitation program for men who have suffered a myocardial infarction. *Can. Med. Assoc. J.* **118**:376-381.

Pederson, L. L. (1982). Compliance with physician advice to quit smoking: a review of the literature. *Prev. Med.* **11**:71-84.

Petty, T. L. (1977). Pulmonary rehabilitation. *Respir. Care* **22**:68-79.

Petty, T. L. (1978). *Chronic Lung Disease: A Practical Office Approach to Early Diagnosis,* 2nd ed. New York, Beon Laboratories.

Petty, T. L. (1985). Pulmonary rehabilitation. In *Chronic Obstructive Pulmonary Disease,* 2nd ed. Edited by T. L. Petty. New York, Marcel Dekker, pp. 339-354.

Petty, T. L., and Cherniak, R. M. (1981). Comprehensive care of COPD. *Clin. Notes Respir. Dis.* **20**:3-12.

Petty, T. L., Nett, L. M., Finigan, M. M., Brink, G. A., and Corsello, P. R. (1969). A comprehensive care program for chronic airway obstruction. *Ann. Intern. Med.* **70**:1109-1120.

Pierce, A. K., Paez, P. N., and Miller, W. F. (1965). Exercise training with the aid of a portable oxygen supply in patient with emphysema. *Am. Rev. Respir. Dis.* **91**:653-659.

Pierce, A. K., Taylor, H. F., Archer, R. K., and Miller, W. R. (1964). Responses to exercise training in patients with emphysema. *Arch. Intern. Med.* **78**:113-120.

Pulmonary Rehabilitation Study Group (1979). Community resources for rehabilitation of patients with chronic obstructive pulmonary diseases and cor pulmonale. *Circulation* **49**:A1-A20.

Rahe, R. H. (1972). Subjects recent life changes and their near-future illness reports. *Ann. Clin. Res.* **4**:250-265.

Ravenholt, R. T. (1985). Tobacco's impact on twentiety-century mortality patterns. *Am. J. Prev. Med.* **1**:4-17.

Sackett, D. L. (1976). The magnitude of compliance and noncompliance. In *Compliance with Therapeutic Regimens.* Edited by D. L. Sackett and R. B. Haynes. Baltimore, Johns Hopkins University Press.

Sawicki, F. (1972). Chronic non-specific respiratory diseases. *Epidemiol. Rev.* **26**:229-250.

Sobel, B. J., and Emirgil, C. (1977). The first second-timed vital capacity and the course of obstructive lung disease. *Chest* **72**:81-90.

Stimson, G. V. (1974). Obeying doctors' orders: a review from the other side. *Soc. Sci. Med.* **8**:97-104.

Stone, G. C. (1979). Patient compliance and the role of the expert. *J. Soc. Issues* **35**:34-59.

Thompson, L., and Gallagher, D. (1981). *Psychotherapy for Depression in the Elderly.* Final report of NIH Grant R01, MH32157, Bethesda, Maryland.

Timms, R. B. (1982). Sexual dysfunction and chronic obstructive pulmonary disease. *Chest* **81**:398-700.

Toevs, C. D., Kaplan, R. M., and Atkins, C. J. (1984). The cost and effects of behavioral programs in chronic obstructive pulmonary disease. *Med. Care* **22**:1088-1100.

Unger, K., Moser, K., and Hansen, P. (1980). Selection of an exercise program for patients with chronic obstructive pulmonary disease. *Heart Lung* **9**:68-76.

U.S. Department of Health and Human Services (1984). *Health Consequences of Smoking for Chronic Obstructive Lung Disease: A Report of the Surgeon General* (DHHS Pub. No. PHS 84-50205), U.S. Government Printing Office, Washington, D.C.

U.S. Government Task Force (1977). *Respiratory Diseases: Task Force Report on Prevention, Control, and Education* (DHEW Publication No. NIH 77-1248). Washington, D.C., U.S. Government Printing Office.

U.S. Government Task Force (1979). *Epidemiology of Respiratory Diseases: Task Force Report on State of Knowledge, Problems, and Needs* (NIH Publication No. 81-2019). Washington, D.C., National Institute of Health.

Van Der Lende, R. (1969). *Epidemiology of Chronic Non-Specific Lung Disease.* Assen, Netherlands, Van Gorcum.

Weinstein, M. C. (1980). Estrogen use in post-menopausal women—costs, risks, and benefits. *N. Engl. J. Med.* **303**:308-316

Weinstein, M. C., and Feinber, H. (1980). *Clinical Decision Analysis.* Philadelphia, W. B. Saunders.

West, J. B. (1977). *Pulmonary Pathophysiology: The Essentials.* Baltimore, Williams & Wilkins.

Wilhelmson, L., Sanne, H., Elmfeldt, D., Grimby, G., Tibblin, G., and Wendel, H. (1975). A controlled trial of physical training after myocardial infarction. *Prev. Med.* **4**:491-508

Windsor, R. A., Green, L. W., and Roseman, J. M. (1980). Health promotion and maintenance for patients with chronic obstructive pulmonary disease: a review. *J. Chron. Dis.* **33**:5-12.

8

Behavioral Prevention of COPD: Smoking Control

JUDITH FLAXMAN

Illinois School of Professional Psychology
Chicago, Illinois

I. INTRODUCTION

Physicians are in an excellent position to be a major force in preventive medicine by encouraging patients, particularly those with chronic obstructive pulmonary disease (COPD) still in a nonsymptomatic phase, to quit smoking. Physicians seem to be persuaded of the health benefits of quitting smoking themselves; they smoke at a rate lower than the general population and that has decreased over time: from 30% in 1967 to 21% in 1975 (Pechacek and Danaher, 1979). Although Sachs (1984a) has provided compelling evidence of the cost-effectiveness of simple medical advice as a smoking cessation technique, many physicians are not trained in giving prescriptions as complex as the recommendation to quit smoking and, as a result, they sometimes give this recommendation in an ineffective way. This chapter will attempt to provide information about smoking and guidelines for effectively making the recommendation to quit smoking.

This chapter will review the relationship between smoking and COPD,

and current trends in smoking. It will present a model for understanding
cigarette smoking and describe techniques for quitting smoking. It will present an approach to the optimal delivery of the recommendation to quit
smoking in an office practice, discuss when a referral is appropriate, and what
referral resources to recommend.

II. COPD and Smoking

Cigarette smoking is known to be associated with chronic bronchitis, centrilobular emphysema, increased sputum production, decreased ciliary activity,
reduced stability of alveoli by surfactant alteration, depressed alveolar macro-
phage function, bronchial epithelial changes, and mucous gland enlargement
(Brashear and Rhodes, 1978). Such conditions combine to cause disease of
the small airways, which is considered to be the "silent predecessor" to COPD.
Early detection is of significant value because if smoking stops and treatment
begins, the disease process may be reversible and pulmonary function can improve (Hodgkin, 1979).

Because the pulmonary system has a large reserve capacity, significant
changes in function generally occur before symptoms of respiratory disease
are apparent. For this reason, routine spirometry tests are essential for patients who smoke. Hodgkin (1979) recommends that office spirometry take
its place along with the electrocardiograph as a commonly used diagnostic tool
for patients at risk, that is, smokers age 40 and over. Hodgkin suggests that
office spirometer tests be performed at each physical examination to determine whether decreases in forced expiratory flow over the mid-50% of the
vital capacity (previously called the maximum midexpiratory flow rate)—the
measure currently thought to be the best indicator of disease of the small airways—have occurred at a more rapid rate than expected based on the patient's
age. If smoking is stopped early enough, forced expiratory flow is likely to return to normal, thus reducing the risk of COPD (Brashear and Rhodes, 1978).
An approach to using spirometer findings to help patients quit smoking will
be described below.

III. Current Trends in Cigarette Smoking

Since the release of the first Surgeon General's Report on Smoking and Health
in 1964 there has been a steady decline in the proportion of smokers at almost
all age levels (Pechacek and Danaher, 1979). The most dramatic decline has

occurred among men: 52.4% of adult men smoked in 1964 while only 36% were smoking in 1969 (Hunt and Matarazzo, 1982). Among adult women, 34% were smokers in 1966 and that percentage dropped to 29% in 1979. In addition, surveys show that one-third of current smokers do not like smoking (Hunt and Matarazzo, 1982) and 90% of them have tried to quit smoking or indicate that they would like to do so (Pechacek and Danaher, 1979).

Among men, quit rates increase with age, perhaps associated with the increased development of physical symptoms with age. Quit rates are lower for men with more personal turmoil in their lives: those who are divorced or separated, seeking advancement in their jobs, or facing job loss. It has also been reported that blue collar workers in stable job situations often spontaneously reduce or stop smoking during middle age, at a time when their level of life stress is low (Leventhal and Cleary, 1980).

Among women, smoking cessation patterns are not as clear. More affluent women and those in white collar jobs are achieving smoking rates closer to comparable groups of men. Since fewer women than men are quitting smoking there has actually been an increase in the number of female smokers since the late 1960s (Pechacek and Danaher, 1979). Changes in women's participation in various traditionally male rites may be one explanation for this trend. Another possibility is that low tar and nicotine cigarettes are having the unfortunate side effect of easing more women into smoking, perhaps serving as the pharmacologic equivalent of the preadolescent training bra (Hunt and Matarazzo, 1982).

Among teenagers, smoking rates have declined. Between 1968 and 1974 smoking among teenage girls rose from 8% to 15%, while smoking remained stable at 15% among teenage boys. By 1979, however, teenagers' smoking rates had decreased to 11% for boys and 13% for girls.

IV. Patient Compliance

Before considering the special characteristics of cigarette smoking, it is useful to consider the recommendation to quit smoking as one of any number of prescriptions a physician may give to a patient. Numerous failures to quit smoking can be considered along with failures to follow other prescriptions. Stone (1979) reports than only an estimated one-half to one-third of all patients fully follow the treatments prescribed for them. Epstein and Cluss (1982) cite a range of 33-94% compliance rates for long-term preventive regimens, with a mean of 57% compliance. For other long-term regimens they report 41-59% compliance, with a mean compliance rate of 54%.

Levels of compliance vary as a function of the problem, the complexity of the regimen, and the patient population. Quitting smoking is a complex prescription to follow. The patient population more likely to follow it is, in fact, the patient population more likely to adhere to any sort of medical advice: older, better educated and of higher socioeconomic status (Stone, 1979). An approach to overcoming the problem of poor compliance will be discussed at the end of this chapter.

V. A Model for Understanding Cigarette Smoking

A. Introduction

Demographic surveys can tell us who is most likely to quit smoking: older, higher socioeconomic status men with little personal turmoil in their lives. They cannot tell us what process the smoker goes through, however. Psychological research on behavior, emotions, attitudes, and personality as well as pharmacologic research on addictions have all been brought to bear on this difficult problem.

On January 11, 1964, with the publication of the report of the Surgeon General's Advisory Committee on Smoking and Health, smoking "officially graduated from a dirty, messy, unhealthy habit" to a major health hazard (Hunt and Matarazzo, 1982). The most dramatic smoking cessation rate occurred in the year following the publication of this document. Individuals who successfully quit smoking in 1964 had become aware for the first time of a real threat to their health. Living with such a threat when they could eliminate it was so antithetical to their value systems that they were able effectively to exert sufficient willpower to quit smoking (Premack, 1970): they were able to respond to smoking stimuli and to the experience of craving a cigarette with determination and possibly even with a feeling of pride in the action they were taking.

Consistent with the high rate of smoking cessation in 1964, it has been found that successful quitting in response to a health risk is more likely to occur if the risk develops suddenly. More individuals quit smoking after the traumatic experience of a myocardial infarction than after a diagnosis of pulmonary disease (Lichtenstein and Danaher, 1979). Presumably with a slowly developing risk, smoking cessation is put off and continued smoking is rationalized so well that successful quitting becomes less and less likely. Even in the case of myocardial infarctions, however, one study found that the likelihood of quitting was directly related to the severity of the infarction as measured by the average peak CPK level (Baile et al., 1982), with a return to smoking rate of 38% and the first cigarette smoked, on the average, 2.2 days after the occurrence of the infarction. In half of the cases the first cigarette was smoked on the day that patients were transferred out of the coronary care unit.

In general the "relapse" curve shows that the average participant in the average treatment program has a 15-20% chance of remaining abstinent, with more effective programs yielding abstinence rates of 30-40% (Lichtenstein, 1982). A landmark survey of 87 treatment studies (Hunt and Matarazzo, 1970) found that the number of recidivists increases sharply in the first 6 months after a program ends and drops off to plateau gradually by the end of 1 year. This negatively accelerated recidivism curve is also characteristic of alcoholics, heroin addicts, and participants in physical exercise rehabilitation programs (Hunt and Matarazzo, 1982). Although the 15-20% success rate is not an impressive one, it should be noted that the people who seek help in quitting smoking are largely the most difficult cases: those who have been unsuccessful at quitting on their own (Schachter, 1982). Higher success rates can be expected and are found among the millions of individuals who make up the 95% of former smokers who have successfully quit smoking on their own (Lichtenstein, 1982).

Investigations of personality differences between smokers and nonsmokers or between successful quitters and failures have not been very useful (Hunt and Matarazzo, 1982). Successes and failures can be differentiated by failures' tendency to rely on smoking to reduce negative affect (Pomerleau et al., 1978) and successes' increased likelihood of having family members who have quit smoking (Graham and Gibson, 1971). A newer line of investigation (Shiffman, 1982, 1984) has looked at the actions of successes and failures and found that successful quitters were more active in their smoking cessation attempts than were those who failed.

Successes were more likely than failures to substitute alternative behavior for smoking (such as eating, drinking or engaging in distracting activity) or to talk to themselves in useful ways (e.g., reminding themselves of the non-health-related negative consequences of smoking). The specific action taken seemed less important than the readiness to act when cravings were experienced. This finding is consistent with results obtained by Flaxman (1979), who found that self-control techniques used were not correlated with reasons for smoking, but were related to the strength of the smoking habit.

B. Factors in Quitting Smoking

A picture of why it is difficult to quit smoking must include several factors: (1) habit: smoking is a strongly overlearned, positively reinforced habit associated with numerous aspects of daily life; (2) withdrawal: smoking cessation leads to physiological and psychological withdrawal reactions to deprivation of nicotine; and (3) the delayed relapse crisis: even after the physiological withdrawal has ceased a long-term vulnerability to conditioned cravings for cigarettes remains.

Habit

Smokers are most aware of the reinforcing aspects of smoking early in their careers as smokers. Although chronic smokers often report that they do not really enjoy their habit, smoking serves as a powerful immediate reinforcer. Nicotine from an inhaled cigarette reaches the brain in 7 sec. The unpleasant consequences of smoking are much delayed in comparison and have much less influence over continuing smoking behavior (Pomerleau, 1980).

The pervasiveness of the smoking habit can be seen in the variety of reasons people give for smoking. Smokers generally are aware that their smoking meets several of the following six descriptions:

1. Positive affect smoking: cigarettes are used to intensify relaxation and other pleasant sensations, such as after a meal or with alcohol.

2. Negative affect smoking: cigarettes are used to reduce or avoid unpleasant emotions such as anger, anxiety or depression.

3. Stimulation smoking: cigarettes are used to increase alertness and improve one's functioning at a demanding task.

4. Sensory-motor smoking: cigarettes are valued for the ritualized motions involved or the feeling of the smoke in one's lungs.

5. Habit or forgetful smoking: cigarettes are smoked without awareness.

6. Addictive smoking: cigarettes are smoked in order to avoid the unpleasant craving sensation caused by a drop in blood plasma nicotine levels.

The more often any of these patterns is repeated, the more value smoking takes on as a reinforcer and the more it becomes a habitual way of responding. The inevitability of the habit becoming ingrained in this way should be apparent, particularly if we look at the number of situations and mood states associated with smoking and the number of puffs per cigarette over numerous cigarettes per day for years; for a one pack per day smoker this is estimated as more than 70,000 puffs per year (Pomerleau, 1980). Food is the only other substance as readily available as cigarettes. Perhaps this helps explain why former heroin addicts often find that it is easier to get rid of their hard drug habit, which occurs a limited number of times per day, under carefully controlled conditions (of a sort), than to quit smoking (Brecher, 1972).

The emphasis placed here on the tenacity of the smoking habit is not meant to imply that quitting is impossible. We decide which cues to respond to, among many in our environment. A signal to smoke can be ignored, or it can be followed by jogging, eating, calling a friend, or by exerting "will-power" and experiencing a sense of accomplishment for not smoking.

Withdrawal

Of the many substances that people have tried to smoke, tobacco is one of the few that has gained lasting popularity (Domino, 1973). A large part of the reason for this popularity is, presumably, nicotine. The role of nicotine in smoking, however, has not been conclusively established. The World Health Organization has stopped short of considering smoking an addiction, referring to it as an habituation instead (U.S. Public Health Service, 1964).

Smokers have been shown to adjust their smoking sensitively to regulate the amount of nicotine in their blood. They increase their smoking when their plasma nicotine levels drop. Under stress they smoke more heavily, at least in part to compensate for the more rapid drop in plasma nicotine levels that occurs. Unless motivated to cut down their dosage, smokers also tend to compensate for the lower nicotine load delivered by low tar and nicotine cigarettes by puffing harder, more rapidly, or smoking a larger portion of each cigarette.

One prominent psychologist, Stanley Schachter, concludes, in no uncertain terms, that chronic smokers are addicted to smoking. Schachter (1982) describes the situation by saying "the smoker's mind is in the bladder," referring to the rapid elimination of nicotine via urinary excretion during times of stress. This thinking has led to the development of a diet regimen aimed at slowing down the excretion of nicotine in order to reduce withdrawal symptoms (Solomon, 1981).

Whether nicotine is the principal reinforcer for smoking continues to be the subject of controversy, however. Few studies separate out tar and nicotine to test each one independently (Pomerleau, 1980) and the regulation of nicotine levels that occurs is not as tight as the model requires. This situation may change, however, as newly developed, more sophisticated measures of nicotine levels in the body begin to have their impact on research (Pomerleau, 1980). The nicotine regulation model also fails to account for the common phenomenon of successful quitting, followed by recidivism occurring weeks, months, or even years later. Since plasma nicotine levels fall to zero a few days after smoking cessation, something other than nicotine regulation must explain the existence of a 1-year "danger period" during which time exsmokers are at high risk of returning to smoking.

Despite the controversy over whether nicotine is truly an addicting agent, it is clear that concurrent with smoking becoming a strong, conditioned reinforcer, the nonsmoking state becomes increasingly aversive (Solomon, 1981). The habitual smoker who is frantically searching for a cigarette or (a more recent phenomenon) for a place in which smoking is permitted, is a well-known character. With time, in fact, the smoker is more strongly driven by a desire to avoid the discomfort associated with deprivation than by the desire to experience the pleasure associated with smoking.

A wide variety of withdrawal symptoms have been reported. These include hostility and aggressiveness, in monkeys and in humans (Hutchinson and Emley, 1973), irritability, restlessness, sleep disturbances, bowel disturbances, anxiety, and impairment of concentration. Physiological changes that have been observed include decreases in heart rate and systolic blood pressure, declines in body temperature, increase in low-frequency alpha brain waves, and drops in epinephrine and norepinephrine levels (Leventhal and Cleary, 1980).

Withdrawal symptoms differ from one individual to another, however, and they may even differ from time to time in the same person. The fact that withdrawal symptoms are malleable was demonstrated by a group of student nurses who served as subjects for a research project. They were asked to quit smoking for a day, ostensibly for the sake of a study on heart rate (Barefoot and Girodo, 1972). Those who were given a placebo pill said to cause irritability, nervousness, and hunger reported fewer withdrawal symptoms than a control group given a placebo for which no side effects were specified.

The Delayed Relapse Crisis

If a smoker manages to maintain motivation and successfully withstand withdrawal symptoms to abstain from smoking for a month or more, the risk of returning to smoking still remains, as the recidivism curve described earlier demonstrates.

Research has just begun to focus on what is referred to as the delayed relapse crisis. This crisis can be understood as based on the associations between smoking and other situations. If the associations are not broken, environmental stimuli may trigger the sensation of craving months after an exsmoker has quit (Pomerleau, 1980). Retrospective surveys of smokers find that they report relapse to be most likely to occur in situations involving negative affect (e.g., anxiety, anger, and depression; Shiffman, 1982). This phenomenon may be due to smokers' expectations that the cigarette will provide relief in a crisis and to the belief that once they have smoked a single cigarette they have failed and might as well continue smoking (Marlatt and Gordon, 1979). In summary, it seems that the persistence of smoking is due, in part, to the habitual smokers' physiological drive to regulate nicotine and avoid cravings, and, in part, to the powerful habit that develops when smoking occurs in numerous situations. The habitual aspects of smoking create a conditioned craving that can occur even when it has been some time since an individual has smoked. This makes the problem a surprisingly persistent one.

VI. Treatment

A. Pharmacologic Approaches

Nicotine mimetics such as lobeline sulfate (marketed as Bantron or Nicoban) have not been found to be particularly effective (Lichtenstein and Danaher, 1979). Nicotine chewing gum (marketed as Nicorette) has recently been approved as a prescription drug in the United States. When used as the primary treatment it has provided weak results (Lichtenstein, 1982). In the context of a program of behavioral counseling, however, it can be a useful adjunct, perhaps doubling the success rate, particularly for the very heavy smoker (Blum, 1984; Sachs, 1984a). The placebo effect of such a substance as an aid to overcoming withdrawal symptoms can be of particular value. Sachs (1984a) provides specific guidelines for the use of nicotine chewing gum in smoking cessation. Because the effectiveness of nicotine chewing gum depends greatly on its proper use in the context of a behavioral modification program, Sach's article should be reviewed before an attempt is made to use this medication.

B. Altered States of Consciousness

Numerous case reports of success with hypnosis exist but no controlled studies have verified these success rates. The best known hypnotic approaches involve having the smoker repeat short health messages such as "My body is a machine; I live in my body; I must take care of my body; I must not smoke" (Leventhal and Cleary, 1980). Theoretically, this can help create a powerful motivational set that will allow the patient successfully to resist temptations to smoke.

Sensory deprivation may work similarly: Suedfeld (1982) initiates treatment by keeping smokers in dark, sound-reducing chambers for 24 hr. He sees this approach as serving to "unfreeze" or destabilize attitudes and allow change to begin. He has demonstrated some success, particularly when sensory deprivation is combined with behavioral counseling.

C. Smoking Clinics

Both proprietary and nonprofit programs are widely available for helping smokers quit. These programs generally involve a motivational component that consists of education and "scare tactic" demonstrations, a group support component, and behavioral strategies for quitting. The American Cancer Society program is fairly typical. Six group meetings are held over a 3-week period. One evaluation of this program (Evans and Lane, 1980) found an average abstinence rate of 25% 1-2 years after treatment. This success rate may be inflated, however, since it is based on survey responses from only 62% of those who attended the clinics. Unsuccessful quitters might be less likely to respond to such a survey. The Seventh Day Adventists' "5 Day Plan" and the program run by the American Lung Association are similar. In addition many hospital outpatient departments have recently begun to run quit smoking clinics on a regular basis.

The best known proprietary program for quitting smoking is Smok-Enders. SmokEnders provides support over a longer period of time than most nonprofit clinics and uses a 3-week nicotine-fading procedure before requiring abstinence. One evaluation of SmokEnders found a 70% success rate at the end of treatment and 39% success after 4 years. These figures are impressive but again they do not represent the whole sample and, in addition, are not corroborated by objective measures of smoking status. Sachs (1984b) provides additional discussion of the SmokEnders program as well as several similar but less well known programs.

Multicomponent behavioral programs for smoking cessation provide the most promising approaches currently available. There are several excellent manuals describing such programs in a self-help format (Pomerleau and Pomerleau, 1977; Danaher and Lichtenstein, 1978). A typical sequence of events in such a program generally begins with a self-monitoring phase, which serves to make smoking less automatic and to increase smokers' knowledge about their behavior.

After the self-monitoring phase some individuals will choose to quit abruptly (i.e., "cold turkey"), but others will prefer to reduce their smoking gradually to approximately 12 cigarettes per day, and then quit completely on a carefully selected target date. The gradual approach allows some degree of habit-breaking and skill-building to develop while smoking is still occurring. A completely gradual approach to quitting is not feasible, however

(Flaxman, 1978). Any cigarette smoking at all appears to prolong the withdrawal syndrome and make abstinence more difficult to achieve.

If the gradual approach is followed a stimulus control or nicotine fading phase of treatment will be aimed at beginning to break some of the associations between smoking and various daily activities. At the same time, smoking is made less pleasurable by having the smoker switch to progressively lower tar and nicotine cigarettes over a 3 week period (Foxx and Brown, 1979) or by putting cigarettes in an inconvenient location or progressively restricting situations in which smoking is allowed (e.g., no smoking first thing in the morning for 3-4 days, followed by no smoking at meetings and no smoking first thing in the morning for 3-4 days, etc).

A skill-building component of either the abrupt or the gradual program is aimed at teaching the smoker alternative methods for managing affect, such as muscle relaxation or regular exercise to decrease stress, or assertiveness as an alternative to anger. When such treatment is administered by a behavioral counselor the skills taught are tailored to the individual.

An aversive component may be included in a behavioral program for smoking cessation. Rapid smoking to satiation is a technique that has had promising results (Lichenstein et al., 1973; Schmahl et al., 1972). It involves rapidly smoking (a puff every 6 sec) as many cigarettes as possible, to a maximum of 3, during regularly scheduled sessions on several consecutive days. Smoking does not occur at any other time and patients have the option of scheduling emergency sessions if necessary. The potential medical risk and the question of whether this technique induces nicotine poisoning (Horan et al., 1977) have lessened its popularity. An alternative, which can be recommended, involves focused, normal paced aversive smoking (Danaher and Lichtenstein, 1978). A puff on a cigarette is taken every 30 sec and as many cigarettes as one can tolerate are smoked in a session, while one focuses attention on the unpleasant aspects of smoking.

A reinforcement component is generally quite important in behavioral programs. It should be recognized that the reinforcement provided by regular contact with a trusted, supportive authority figure is a crucial ingredient in virtually all smoking cessation programs (Marston and McFall, 1971). Encouragement by the physician and other health professionals can be very reinforcing and may involve no more than a brief (literal or figurative) pat on the back. Other sources of reinforcement should be developed as well, with plans for self-reinforcement established in advance. The money saved by not smoking can be used to purchase a meaningful gift for oneself in celebration of 1 week of abstinence, 1 month, and so on (Fisher et al., 1982).

A relapse prevention component to smoking cessation programs is a new approach, involving analysis of high-risk situations, making plans for coping with them, and practicing trial runs in high-risk situations (for example, a party where alcohol is served and other smokers are present can be staged before a real party is encountered).

D. Smoking Cessation in Office Practice

Organized efforts to help people quit smoking, such as clinics, behavioral treatment programs, and hypnosis are estimated to reach only 5% of the smoking population (Lichtenstein, 1982). It has been suggested that simple smoking cessation messages delivered by medical practitioners can be of comparable or even greater effectiveness (Leventhal and Cleary, 1980; Sachs, 1984a), particularly given the physician's prestige and appropriateness as an authority on the subject and the continuing nature of the physician's relationship with the patient (Lichtenstein and Danaher, 1979). This suggestion is made despite the fact that existing studies show varying success rates, ranging from 9 to 33%, using physician intervention (Leventhal and Cleary, 1980). These studies have used rather weak physician interventions, however, involving only pamphlets and advice, with a discussion lasting, at most, 7 min. In addition, even if simple medical advice is not the most powerful intervention available, it is quite cost-effective. One study suggests that if all physicians in the United States took 60 sec with each of their smoking patients to advise them to quit in a straightforward, unambiguous but noncritical manner, more than 3.5 million smokers would quit who otherwise would continue to smoke (Sachs, 1984a).

In an office practice, physicians and their office staff can do several simple things to encourage smoking cessation among their patients. They can serve as nonsmoking models and a no-smoking rule can be enforced in the office. Over time indirect social pressure of this sort may do a great deal to change smoking habits (Leventhal and Cleary, 1980).

Physicians can conduct routine spirometer tests to monitor patients' lung functioning. As suggested earlier, this is particularly important for smokers over the age of 40. When such tests are used as an early warning of increased risk of COPD, they may provide exactly the "unfreezing" of attitudes toward smoking that some theories of attitude change believe to be required (e.g., Suedfeld, 1982). Although the impact of office spirometer testing on smoking cessation has not been determined empirically, slowly developing pulmonary symptoms, such as cough and sputum production, can be minimized or denied by the patient in a way that test results cannot.

In deciding what to say to patients, consideration should be given to research suggesting that success with public health messages is greatest when a discussion of the seriousness of the problem is coupled with a plan for action (Leventhal and Cleary, 1980). In recommending that patients quit smoking based on spirometer findings it is important that physicians make patients aware of both the risk and the possibility of effectively reducing that risk. Patients need to be sufficiently motivated by the seriousness of the situation to make a change, but not so frightened that they protect themselves by defensively avoiding the problem through denial. If their anxiety is too high they are likely to avoid both the threatening situation and the health information. Like a skilled athletic coach, the physician must motivate the patient by increasing the level of anxiety enough but not too much.

After the recommendation to quit smoking is made, the physician or a nurse should consider with the patient the pros and cons of this action. Ideally, this should be an open consideration of the role smoking plays in the patient's life and the psychological cost of quitting. The advantage of taking time to consider the pros and cons openly is that the decision then becomes the patient's own and will be adhered to much better than if it was coerced.

Several topics should be covered in such a discussion.

The Health Consequences of Continuing to Smoke

Mortality ratios for smokers increase with amount smoked, duration of smoking, age at beginning, depth of inhalation, and tar and nicotine content of cigarettes smoked (Hunt and Matarazzo, 1982). Although some pulmonary damage may have already been done, quitting smoking will prevent further damage and, in some cases, even reverse the damage. Even if the damage is no longer reversible quitting smoking will at least relieve some of the burden on the lungs and allow for better functioning (Hodgkin, 1979). In this regard, it is never too late to quit.

The Benefits of Quitting

Mortality ratios for former smokers decrease as a function of years of discontinuance of smoking (Califano, 1979), money is saved by quitting, nonsmokers lose fewer days of work, self-esteem is gained.

Previous Experience with Quitting and Estimated Likelihood of Success

Willpower is not an all-or-none thing. It is something you *do,* not something you have (Fisher et al., 1982). The fact that patients have not been sufficiently

motivated to quit smoking before does not mean that they are morally deficient, weak-willed, or any other of the names they call themselves. Good
decision-making based on solid information and social support can make this
attempt to quit different from previous ones. The variations in reaction to
withdrawal, even in the same person from one time to another, can be pointed
out. The crucial role that motivation has in determining how difficult it is to
quit can be stressed.

Alternative Goals and Their Feasibility

Although they carry some health risk, cigar and pipe smoking are less dangerous than cigarette smoking (Califano, 1979). Cutting down on the number is
helpful as well, as long as the smoker does not compensate for the reduced tar
and nicotine by inhaling more deeply or smoking a larger portion of each cigarette. It may be more difficult, however, to maintain a low level of smoking
than to quit entirely. The associations that create cravings are continually
being partially reinforced and such partial reinforcement is exactly the sort
of schedule of reinforcement that creates the most persistent behavior, similar to that seen in response to slot machines or video games (Loftus and Loftus,
1983). Attempting to cut down but not quit is not advisable, but could be
viewed as a step in the direction of abstinence in a sequential treatment program.

The Impact the Patient's Smoking Has on Significant Others

Pros and cons must be considered here. For example, although smokers may
be poor models for their children, the short-term irritability that accompanies
withdrawal may be seen as an unacceptable threat to important relationships.
Smoking may be an important ingredient in camaraderie with smoking friends
and these friends may try to sabotage smokers' attempts to quit.

Once the decision to quit has been made the health professional and the
patient should develop a specific plan of action. A frank discussion should be
held about whether patients can quit on their own or whether more support is
needed than the physician's office and friends and relatives can provide. If patients have failed to quit numerous times, are poorly adjusted, very nicotine-
dependent, or often use cigarettes to help themselves deal with anxiety, anger,
or depression, a referral to a proprietary clinic such as SmokEnders or to a behavior therapist is in order. If patients are quite motivated, have not given
smoking cessation a serious try before, and are generally determined, effective
individuals, they may very well be successful on their own with periodic support and encouragement from the physician's office.

If the patient is not being referred elsewhere for help, immediate quitting versus a gradual approach and target date quitting should be decided upon. Once this decision is made a self-help manual can be loaned, given, sold or recommended to the patient. Two good manuals are *Become an Ex-Smoker* by Brian Danaher and Edward Lichtenstein and *Break the Smoking Habit: A Behavioral Program for Giving Up Cigarettes* by Ovide F. Pomerleau and Cynthia S. Pomerleau. The American Lung Association (1981a,b) also offers a pair of self-help manuals. The first, *Freedom from Smoking in 21 Days* provides a program for quitting, whereas the second, *A Lifetime of Freedom From Smoking,* concerns maintenance of cessation. In addition, nicotine chewing gum and an alkaline diet to permit slower excretion of nicotine (described in *Stop Smoking Lose Weight* by Neil Solomon) may be prescribed.

Follow-up phone contacts and visits should be scheduled. The first and third days of abstinence and the first 4 weeks are particularly important times. Appointments for repeat lung function tests should be scheduled regularly beginning 6 months-1 year after the smoker quits, in order to provide tangible evidence of improved lung functioning.

At each follow-up contact motivation should be discussed, high-risk situations should be identified, and active coping strategies (what to remind yourself of and what to do) should be developed. The patient should be warned of the risk involved in negative affect situations and the fallacy of turning to a cigarette to feel better rather than facing the real problem to be dealt with. Also, the tendency to give up because you have had one cigarette should be addressed. An agreement can be made to have patients call the office for help if they are extremely tempted to have a cigarette or do, in fact, have one.

A phone call for help or an outright failure should be dealt with as an opportunity for new learning that can make the next attempt a success. Failure does not mean that the patient should give up. A failure may be an important warning signal indicating that more help is needed or that some aspect of the problem has been ignored and a new strategy must be developed to deal with it. A referral to a clinic or behavior therapist may be in order. If follow-up finds the patient abstinent but battling the urge to smoke, continued success is unlikely. Before the inevitable failure occurs, in this case, a referral is needed to help the patient to find alternative ways to deal with needs previously satisfied by cigarettes.

A successful quitter should be congratulated, given the results of spirometer testing, encouraged to help others quit, and to continue to enjoy the tangible benefits of quitting smoking: better lung functioning, better sense of taste and smell, and perhaps saving someone else's life by serving as a positive model.

VII. Summary

Although 90% of the smokers in the United States indicate an interest in quitting smoking, the problem is a complex and tenacious one. Smokers experience a physiological drive to regulate nicotine; they have a powerful habit; and, even after quitting they experience conditioned cravings for a cigarette, particularly in negative affect situations. Nevertheless, numerous individuals have quit, particularly in the medical profession.

While organized smoking-cessation programs only reach an estimated 5% of the smoking population, physicians regularly see many smokers on a routine basis. The physician is thus in an excellent position to speak as an authority and encourage quitting. The physician can attack smokers' rationalizations about smoking not having any ill effects on them with both information and hard facts provided by a spirometer test. At the same time it is important that the physician raise expectations that quitting smoking is possible and that it is not too late to benefit from quitting.

After delivering a message designed to stress both the importance of quitting smoking and its feasibility, the physician or other health professional can help the smoker develop a plan for quitting smoking. A treatment manual and continued support by the physician and his or her office staff can be provided or a referral to a behavioral counselor, proprietary program, or nonprofit quit smoking clinic can be made. Whatever plan is developed must take into account the tenacity of the smoking problem and the 1-year "danger period" during which recidivism is most likely to occur. A plan of action that recognizes the mechanisms involved in smoking and the effort needed to quit can lead to encouraging success rates when physicians give one of the most complex prescriptions possible: "Quit smoking."

References

American Lung Association (1981a). *Freedom from Smoking in 21 Days.* New York, American Lung Association.

American Lung Association (1981b). *A Lifetime of Freedom from Smoking.* New York, American Lung Association.

Baile, W. F., Jr., Bigelow, G. E., Gottlieb, S. H., Stitzer, M. L., and Sacktor, J. D. (1982). Rapid resumption of cigarette smoking following myocardial infarction: inverse relation to MI severity. *Addictive Behav.* 7:373-380.

Barefoot, J. C., and Girodo, M. (1972). The misattribution of smoking cessation symptoms. *Can. J. Behav. Sci.* **4**:358-363.

Blum, A. (1984). Nicotine chewing gum and the medicalization of smoking. *Ann. Intern. Med.* **101**:121-123.

Brashear, R. E., and Rhodes, M. L. (1978). *Chronic Obstructive Lung Disease.* St. Louis, C. V. Mosby.

Brecher, E. M. (1972). *Licit and Illicit Drugs.* Mt. Vernon, NY, Consumers Union.

Califano, J. A., Jr. (1979). *Smoking and Health: A Report of the Surgeon General.* Washington, D.C., U.S. Government Printing Office, Stock Number 017-000-02180-0.

Danaher, B. G., and Lichtenstein, E. (1978). *Become an Ex-Smoker.* Englewood Cliffs, NJ, Prentice-Hall.

Domino, E. F. (1973). Neuropsychopharmacology of nicotine and tobacco smoking. In *Smoking Behavior: Motives and Incentives.* Edited by W. L. Dunn, Jr. New York, John Wiley, pp. 5-32.

Epstein, L. H., and Cluss, P. A. (1982). A behavioral medicine perspective on adherence to long-term medical regimens. *J. Consult. Clin. Psychol.* **50**:950-971.

Evans, R. I., and Lane, D. S. (1980). Long-term outcome of smoking cessation workshops. *Am. J. Public Health* **70**:725-727.

Fisher, E. B., Jr., Levenkron, J. C., Lowe, M. R., Loro, A. D., Jr., and Green, L. (1982). Self-initiated self-control in risk reduction. In *Adherence, Compliance and Generalization in Behavioral Medicine.* Edited by R. B. Stuart. New York, Brunner/Mazel, pp. 169-191.

Flaxman, J. (1978). Quitting smoking now or later: Gradual, abrupt, immediate and delayed quitting. *Behav. Ther.* **9**:260-270.

Flaxman, J. (1979). Affect-management and habit mechanisms in the modification of smoking behavior. *Addict. Behav.* **4**:39-46.

Foxx, R. M., and Brown, R. A. (1979). Nicotine fading and self-monitoring for cigarette abstinence or controlled smoking. *J. Appl. Behav. Anal.* **12**:111-125.

Graham, S., and Gibson, R. W. (1971). Cessation of patterned behavior: withdrawal from smoking. *Soc. Sci. Med.* **5**:319-337.

Hodgkin, J. E. (1979). *Chronic Obstructive Pulmonary Disease.* Park Ridge, IL., American College of Chest Physicians.

Horan, J. J., Linberg, S. E., and Hackett, G. (1977). Nicotine poisoning and rapid smoking. *J. Consult. Clin. Psychol.* **45**:344-347.

Hunt, W. A., and Matarazzo, J. D. (1970). Habit mechanisms in smoking. In

Learning Mechanisms in Smoking. Edited by W. A. Hunt. Chicago, Aldine, pp. 65-106.

Hunt, W. A., and Matarazzo, J. D. (1982). Changing smoking behavior: a critique. In *Handbook of Psychology and Health,* Vol. I, *Clinical Psychology and Behavioral Medicine: Overlapping Disciplines.* Edited by R. J. Gatchel, A. Baum, and J. E. Singer. Hillsdale, NJ, Lawrence Erlbaum Assoc., Inc.

Hutchinson, R. R., and Emley, G. S. (1973). Effects of nicotine on avoidance, conditioned suppression and aggression response measures in animals and man. In *Smoking Behavior: Motives and Incentives.* Edited by W. L. Dunn, Jr. New York, John Wiley, pp. 171-196.

Leventhal, H., and Cleary, P. D. (1980). The smoking problem: a review of the research and theory in behavioral risk modification. *Psychol. Bull.* **88**:370-405.

Lichtenstein, E. (1982). The smoking problem: a behavioral perspective. *J. Consult. Clin. Psychol.* **50**:804-819.

Lichtenstein, E., and Danaher, B. G. (1979). What can the physician do to assist the patient to stop smoking? In *Chronic Obstructive Lung Disease.* Edited by R. E. Brashear and M. L. Rhodes. St. Louis, C. V. Mosby, pp. 227-241.

Lichtenstein, E., Harris, D. E., Birchler, G. R., Wahl, J. M., and Schmahl, D. P. (1973). Comparison of rapid smoking, warm, smoky air, and attention placebo in the modification of smoking behavior. *J. Consult. Clin. Psychol.* **40**:92-98.

Loftus, G. R., and Loftus, E. F. (1983). *Mind at Play: The Psychology of Video Games.* New York, Basic Books.

Marlatt, G. A., and Gordon, J. R. (1980). Determinants of relapse: implications for the maintenance of behavior change. In *Behavioral Medicine: Changing Health Lifestyles.* Edited by P. O. Davidson and S. M. Davidson. New York, Brunner/Mazel.

Marston, A. R., and McFall, R. M. (1971). Comparison of behavior modification approaches to smoking reduction. *J. Consult. Clin. Psychol.* **36**:153-162.

Pechacek, T. F., and Danaher, B. G. (1979). How and why people quit smoking: a cognitive-behavioral analysis. In *Cognitive-Behavioral Interventions: Theory, Research, and Procedures.* Edited by P. C. Kendall and S. D. Hollon. New York, Academic Press.

Pomerleau, O. F. (1980). Why people smoke: current psychobiological models. In *Behavioral Medicine: Changing Health Lifestyles.* Edited by P. O. Davidson and S. M. Davidson. New York, Brunner/Mazel, pp. 94-115.

Pomerleau, O. F., Adkins, D., and Pertschuk, M. (1978). Predictors of outcome and recidivism in smoking cessation treatment. *Addict. Behav.* **3**:65-70.

Pomerleau, O. F., and Pomerleau, C. S. (1977). *Break the Smoking Habit: A Behavioral Program for Giving Up Cigarettes.* Champaign, IL, Research Press Co.

Premack, D. (1970). Mechanisms of self-control. In *Learning Mechanisms in Smoking.* Edited by W. A. Hunt. Chicago, Aldine, pp. 107-123.

Sachs, D. P. L. (1984a). Office strategies to help your patients stop smoking. *J. Respir. Dis.* **5**(2):35-48.

Sachs, D. P. L. (1984b). Smoking cessation: what are your referral options? *J. Respir. Dis.* **5**(3):49-57.

Schachter, S. (1982). Recidivism and self-cure of smoking and obesity. *Am. Psychol.* **37**:436-444.

Schmahl, D. P., Lichtenstein, E., and Harris, D. E. (1972). Successful treatment of habitual smokers with warm, smoky air and rapid smoking. *J. Consult. Clin. Psychol.* **38**:105-111.

Shiffman, S. (1982). Relapse following smoking cessation: a situational analysis. *J. Consult. Clin. Psychol.* **50**:71-86.

Shiffman, S. (1984). Coping with temptations to smoke. *J. Consult. Clin. Psychol.* **52**:261-267.

Solomon, N. (1981). *Stop Smoking Lose Weight.* New York, Putnam's.

Stone, G. C. (1979). Patient compliance and the role of the expert. *J. Soc. Issues* **35**:34-57.

Suedfeld, P. (1982). Environmental factors influencing maintenance of lifestyle change. In *Adherence, Compliance and Generalization in Behavioral Medicine.* Edited by R. B. Stuart. New York, Brunner/ Mazel, pp. 125-144.

U.S. Public Health Service. (1964). *Smoking and Health.* Report of the Advisory Committee to the Surgeon General of the Public Health Service. Washington, D.C., U.S. Dept. of HEW, PHS Pub. 1103.

9

Psychobiological Evaluation and Treatment of COPD

DONALD L. DUDLEY

Washington Institute of Neurosciences
and University of Washington
Seattle, Washington

JUDITH SITZMAN

Massachusetts General Hospital
Boston, Massachusetts
and Comprehensive Psychiatric Centers
Santa Rosa, California

I. Introduction

The treatment of psychobiological aspects of chronic obstructive pulmonary disease (COPD) is best considered in the light of factors that influence the development of disease and the continuation of disability and insufficiency. Disability is the decrease in the patient's productivity and comfort and insufficiency is the loss of organ function. We find it instructive to differentiate between acute and chronic disease in discussions of COPD and its treatment.

A. Acute Treatment Model

The acute treatment model takes into consideration the self-limiting aspects of many disease processes. The patient is ill for a period of days, weeks, or, at the most, months, and then returns to an acceptable level of physiological and psychological functioning. The physician is congratulated on the "cure," and the patient has an increasing respect for the physician.

Acute treatment is best accomplished with an efficient, competent manner that is reassuring and supportive and that decreases the dramatic, excited nature of an emergency. A relaxed, unhurried approach to the patient conveys a sense of concern and facilitates interaction. The importance of the patient should be increased and the importance of medical equipment decreased. Highly verbal patients can tolerate longer interviews, while very anxious or physically weak, debilitated patients require brief interactions.

Reassurance and support in the form of information regarding the condition should be given early in the course of treatment and should be shared with important family members. If the patient has a stable pulmonary embolus, a statement such as, "You have a blockage of a small vessel in your lung that is clearing and will now heal like a broken arm or leg," is important. It is helpful to provide the patient with an easily understood reference from everyday life. Patients hospitalized for diagnostic tests should be informed by the physician of the purpose and nature of each test, when it will be scheduled, where it will take place, and generally what he or she may experience during and after the procedure. For example, patients undergoing routine pulmonary function tests often feel more comfortable knowing they will not experience pain and will simply be breathing in and out of a mouthpiece. It may be important to have a close family member with the patient during the acute phases of treatment.

The patient, family, and staff should be assured that the patient deserves all the help that can be provided. However, it is important to decrease dependency early in treatment. What is desirable during an acute emergency (passive cooperation) becomes undesirable during the rehabilitation phase. The patient and family should have the feeling that they need to help the staff. This will avoid passivity, depression, and fright when faced with the need for emotional and physical activity as the patient returns to productive life.

In selected patients, once the acute emergency is over, angina pectoris, hypertension, dyspnea, or congestive heart failure may only respond to treatment of psychiatric problems with appropriate psychoactive medications. Above all, it is important to treat in a nonaversive setting. Treatment instructions should not be coupled with threats of dire consequences for noncompliance. They should be coupled with positive consequences. This avoids treatment being directly related to negative feelings or fright and thus increases the probability of compliance.

B. Chronic Treatment Model

The chronic treatment model takes into consideration the long-term effects of continued organ insufficiency and bodily disability. The patient is continuously ill and may never return to an acceptable level of physiological and psychiatric functioning. The physician is confronted with a patient and family who have learned that modern medicine will not cure the condition. They may be disillusioned, angry, depressed, or frightened. They need to be congratulated on their ability to deal with the problem and assured that there will be someone to take care of them regardless of how bad things get. The physician often finds that the patient and family feel cheated by life and are not capable of expressing appreciation, regardless of the physician's interest and dedication. This is obviously a difficult social situation in which to practice medicine.

It is useful to arrange the treatment plan around positive attainable rewards and goals. The reward may be added attention by the physician, increased attention by the family, material objects, and so on. The goal may be increased independence, increased exercise tolerance, and so on. With this approach, the emphasis is not on eliminating the disease, but on gradually increasing understanding and ability to deal with the disease and the surrounding environment. To accomplish this task, it may be necessary to use the usual clinical treatment method plus education, group psychotherapy, psychoactive medications, or any other useful method of increasing the patient's and significant others' ability to cope with life.

C. Discussion

In the acute disease situation, the patient and doctor are seen as rewarding each other. In the chronic disease situation, both doctor and patient are faced with their own relative impotence; the patient is often seen as weak, lacking drive and spirit, or both; the doctor may be seen as lacking clinical competence. Since the patient never gets well, there is often little reason for the patient and family to reward the doctor with the positive feedback needed to be able to deal with chronic disease. For many physicians this is sufficient reason not to deal with such patients. In addition, friends encourage the patient to "see my doctor—his patients get well," and thereby actually undermine treatment. Patients with chronic respiratory disease often try a number of doctors before realizing that no one is going to cure them and that they must learn to live with the disorder and the the doctors.

II. Psychosocial and Psychophysiological Issues in COPD: Environment and the Patient

The interaction between environment and disease can be illustrated in a number of ways: (Dudley et al., 1969a; Dudley and Welke, 1977).

achievement. Those items were included because they clustered before disease onset in the same manner noted for socially undesirable items such as divorce, death of a close friend, and being fired from work. Change, rather than desirability or undesirability, was the characteristic of life events that contributed to their association with psychological adjustment and hence disease. Using the same techniques that allowed the quantification of psychosocial events in life change units, disease was measured in "seriousness of illness units" (Wyler et al., 1970, 1971). In all, 126 diseases were quantified. These ranged from number 1 (dandruff) with a value of 21, to number 126 (leukemia) with a value of 1,080. Using this system, the diseases commonly encountered by the clinical pulmonary specialist spanned the entire spectrum of diseases.

The quantification of disease in this manner has two uses for the clinician. The first is some appreciation of people's perception of the seriousness of a given disease and thereby the amount of time, effort, and dedication the patient expects to be given. An asthmatic, for example, may give asthma a value of 1,000, while the family gives it a value of 413. It may be difficult to treat the patient until there is agreement in the family regarding the seriousness of the disease and the amount of their lives it should justifiably control. The second is related to the relationship between life change as measured in life change units and the seriousness of the disease developed. There is a positive relationship between life change units and seriousness of illness units. Thus, people who have 1,000 life change units are more likely to develop a disease such as a blood clot in the lung or heart failure, and those with 100 life change units are more likely to develop the common cold or hay fever. Not only is the probability of getting sick increased with life change, but the probability of getting a serious disease or dying is also increased.

D. Use of Psychosocial Assets

With the advent of the Schedule of Recent Experience for quantification of psychosocial input, measurements of the ability to deal with this input became essential. In this regard a person's overall ability to deal with the environment can be called "psychosocial assets." There are three categories of psychosocial assets:

Category 1: Social Support

> Being in a setting in which one receives love.

> Being in a setting in which one is esteemed.

> Being in a mutually defensive system (if attacked, those around you will come to your aid).

Category 2: Coping Ability

The patient's ability to change environments to meet needs.

Category 3: Adaptive Ability

The patient's ability to adapt to existing environments.

A patient who rates strongly in all of these areas is considered to have high psychosocial assets. Currently the only single test that takes all of the above factors into consideration is the Berle Index. In general, patients who score above the 80th percentile on this test get well, control their disease without a great deal of difficulty, and seldom get sick. Patients who score below the 60th percentile tend to do poorly. It is usually not possible to predict health status if the score is between the 61st and 79th percentiles.

The essential explanation for why life change induces illness is that life change requires one to adapt to or cope with a stressful life event. The adaptation requires use of the body and its organ systems. A few individuals display a near fathomless ability to muster coping behaviors with coping mechanisms to deal with life changes. These people probably never get sick. A few people rely only on one or two coping behaviors and are sick all the time. Most of us fall somewhere between in the number of coping behaviors we utilize.

Coping behaviors include emotional responses (anger, sorrow, elation), personal habits (eating, smoking, physical activity, sex), and unconscious habits (nail biting, sighing, finger drumming). Attention to one's job and hobbies are coping behaviors, as is time spent with one's family.

Initial interviews with patients should involve a comprehensive psychological screening. Quantitative measurements may include the Schedule of Recent Experience, the Berle Index, and a self-rating scale for depression. Interviews should cover the patient's perception of his illness and how it has affected his relationship with significant others and his occupational and recreational activities. How a patient adjusts to an illness depends on inner resources, outside support systems, and adequate finances and housing. Since significant relationships may be affected by the patient's illness, it is important to interview spouses or people that the patient identifies as close to her. Understanding the nature of these relationships, and the significant others' perception and reaction to the patient's illness guides staff in defining problem areas and setting realistic treatment goals.

E. Social Indicators of Disease

Layman and physicians alike tend to confuse the symptoms of disease with the disease itself, but they are not the same. A patient can be terribly sick and have no disease. The explanation for this paradox is that culturally we interpret being sick or ill as experiencing a loss of comfort, productivity, or both. A patient may have hypertension, a disease with no loss of comfort or productivity. During a smog alert he or she may wheeze, feel miserably ill, uncomfortable, and unproductive while having no disease. The schizophrenic may be very comfortable but wholly unproductive. In order to live with disease and sickness, it is essential to understand that the disease and being sick are not the same thing. On the other hand, it also complicates the interaction of the disease with our culture, since people with recognizable disease entities who do not fit the cultural definition of illness may be seen as malingerers and be treated with hostility. This is true with many chronic diseases.

Another cultural problem is related to the laboratory diagnosis of diseases. It is easy for a patient to understand that he is ill if he has severe leg pain and his leg is bent at an unusual angle. It is obviously broken. But what if she feels well, comfortable, and productive, yet has an electrocardiogram that indicates heart disease, has a chest x-ray that indicates pulmonary carcinoma, or gross ventilatory testing indicating chronic obstructive pulmonary disease. Subsequently, she is told that a devastating disease is present for which she must take the doctor's word and submit to treatment that may be well beyond her understanding. In these circumstances "well" patients are subjected to medical and surgical procedures that may radically change their lives. Few patients adjust easily to this. They need to "feel sick" if something is physically wrong and in this kind of setting many people begin to act sick simply to communicate the severity of their disease. Developing a carcinoma is a frightening and life-threatening situation, but others will not understand this unless one acts sick. Without this cultural expression of illness, the carcinoma patient must face a potentially devastating situation alone. Few of us choose to do that.

Another clinical situation can be equally distressing. The patient may find himself with a symptom of disease but no sign of disease, for example, early COPD with dyspnea but no "significant" reduction in pulmonary function variables. Examination after examination is performed without positive findings. There is simply "no reason" for the dyspnea. What can the patient do? Should he grin and bear it while awaiting the occurrence of some sign that will make the symptom socially acceptable? Should that happen, the patient can be "appropriately ill." If it does not happen, the patient may find himself in a position where people will not believe that he experiences dyspnea or they will suggest that the dyspnea is "all in your head." In this situation it is helpful to remember that all symptoms are "in the head."

Unfortunately, dyspnea without an appropriate sign may lead to alienation from the physician or an increasing reliance on less traditional or even phony treatment. When this occurs it is essential that the physician be understanding and tolerant. The patient may need to try different and even unorthodox treatments, and needs a physician who will stand by her and care for any serious trouble resulting from the dyspnea or the treatments. Situations in which incurable symptoms are encountered should be met maturely and the limitations of treatment spelled out. The physician and patient can then be comfortable with each other and arrange the best possible clinical management.

Pain and Dyspnea Compared

Pain is a symptom that all agree is closely associated with needing medical attention. Pain is always analyzed as uncomfortable and dangerous. Still, no matter how articulate the patient or sophisticated the diagnostician, the only test of pain's severity is the patient's report. Avoidance of pain has played a profound role in our evolution. Since prehistoric times, we have searched for ways to deal with pain and pain-producing situations. So instilled in us is pain as a danger signal that its presence in even small and innocent amounts triggers massive physiological reactions throughout our nervous system. Despite the massive problem of chronic pain, physicians and patients feel comfortable with pain. The pathways are known, treatment modalities have been described, and it is a traditional symptom.

Dyspnea, like pain, is a common presenting symptom. Unlike pain, it is not a generalized danger signal. It specifically alerts the physician to the cardiopulmonary system and as a symptom is localized to that system. Like pain, its identification is based on the subjective judgment of the patient and is generally not definable in terms of blood gas or ventilatory abnormalities.

Patients vary in their descriptions of dyspnea, but the general complaint is of uncomfortable sensations arising in the chest or airways that are interpreted as interfering with normal breathing. The patient feels smothered, breathless, and that not enough air is available. Some patients experience severe dyspnea with little or no structural change in the cardiopulmonary systems, while others experience mild or no dyspnea with severe structural change. Dyspnea is sometimes experienced by normal, healthy people during strenuous exercise and periods of emotions.

When people prone to dyspnea attacks are studied in detail, dyspnea is found to be associated with both activating and nonactivating emotions. With nonactivating emotions such as depression, dyspnea is associated with decreased ventilation or hypoventilation. With action-oriented emotions such as anger or anxiety, dyspnea occurs in association with hyperpnea or hyperventilation. Thus, emotionally triggered dyspnea is associated with both increased and decreased ventilation.

Since healthy people and cardiopulmonary patients both experience dyspnea, and either a relative increase or decrease in ventilation may act as a trigger, it can be a confusing symptom. The best explanation for this is that dyspnea can be learned. It can depend upon past conditioning experiences. Events such as breath holding or excessive crying during childhood, congestive heart failure, allergic reactions, and bronchial infections apparently lead to physiological reactions that are associated with emotion and in which dyspnea occurs. In other words, people who suffer dyspnea attacks may be sensitized or conditioned to respond to emotionally induced changes in their carciopulmonary system with dyspnea. They experience a kind of psychobiological drowning, a respiratory short circuit. Other people are unaware of these changes and do not suffer the dyspnea symptoms. Also, as with so many other illness symptoms, emotional reactions to dyspnea attacks often trigger more and worse dyspnea attacks because of the same conditioning.

Since dyspnea is associated with danger in only two organ systems, unlike pain it is not recognized as a general danger signal. Hence, a patient with dyspnea is more likely to be called a malingerer. People tend not to understand the reason for the inability to work or play, thereby producing difficult social relations unless the dyspnea becomes severe enough to be interpreted by others as being painful.

In summary, there are three important differences between dyspnea and pain: (1) dyspnea is not a generalized danger signal; (2) there are no specific nerve pathways that have been demonstrated reliably to produce dyspnea (i.e., dyspnea must be learned or there must be cardiac or pulmonary disease present to initiate it), and (3) dyspnea is closely associated with physical and emotional activity.

The patient with dyspnea should remain physically active unless there is a medical problem that prohibits it. As patients with dyspnea exercise to toleration, they learn that the dyspnea is not life-threatening. The more they exercise, the more control is learned and the less threatening the symptom becomes. The patient is "deconditioned" or "desensitized."

There are many other symptoms that patients with pulmonary disease may exhibit, such as fatigue, anxiety, and depression. It is important that each symptom be understood by the patient in terms of its effect on emotion and behavior, and that the patient learn to quantify the symptoms and the degree of "cultural impairment." For any given symptom, 100 can stand for the most the patient has ever experienced and 0 for the absence of the symptom. The patient can then report a definite number as representing the current symptom level. In addition, the patient can specify the amount of the symptom that is tolerable, and attaining this can be one of the goals of treatment. Such psychophysical judgments regarding subjective phenomena are clinically accurate.

Psychophysical Assessment

These measurements provide an indication of how sick the patient thinks he is. They are important in quantifying this for the physician. Most patients who use this method find that they are *not as sick as they thought they were* and are reassured. In addition, it gives the physician an indication of what the patient's treatment goals are. If they have been reached there may be no reason to pursue aggressive treatment, since the physician may be met with passive resistance. On the other hand, a patient may insist on a 100% return to function while the physician knows that only 50% is possible, even with very aggressive treatment. This patient may need assistance in readjusting his goals downward, while another patient whose goals are too low may need to adjust goals upward.

Nonverbal Communication (Dudley and Welke, 1977)

It is always constructive to understand what the situation means to the patient. This can lessen tension for both the patient and physician. The physician can ease potentially stressful circumstances by understanding what is being communicated. Since, in any person-to-person transaction, as much as 50% of what is communicated is nonverbal, some knowledge of this nonverbal behavior is essential if the physician is going to deal with patients in a systematic and reasonable manner.

All of us recognize certain nonverbal cues. When meeting people, we automatically notice their facial expressions, their body posture, and whether their speech is rapid or slow. We notice if they are tense or relaxed. Few of us, however, do this in a systematic manner or use the information to benefit the interpersonal transaction.

The Telltale Handshake

When first meeting someone, the physician should notice how far away the person stands and the temperature of the hand when the physician shakes it.

Hand temperature and body distance are important indicators of emotional depression in our culture.

Hand temperature tends to be cool or cold during three emotional states: anger, anxiety, and depression. Hand temperature increases to warm or hot during periods of resentment and during periods of comfort and contentment. By shaking the patient's hand the clinician can obtain a general idea of his or her emotional state.

In some situations it is appropriate to have cold hands, for example, before a traumatic procedure. If the patient's hands are warm and the face is flushed, the physician might consider the presence of resentment and the possibility of legal and interpersonal difficulties with the patient should anything go wrong. On the other hand, cold hands could mean that the patient is angry rather than anxious over the procedure, thereby leading to possible problems.

Facial Expression and Physical Appearance
(Ekman et al., 1971; Knapp, 1972)

Nonverbal communication is an inseparable part of the communication process. Under some circumstances it may contradict, modify, or elaborate on verbal messages. Frequently, it regulates the flow of communication between people. For example, a head nod, eye movement, or shift in position may signal someone to speak or stop speaking.

Since we are concerned about how people react to their illness, it is important to understand the patient's emotional state. Facial expressions may often reflect one or several emotions. Rapidly changing facial expressions may reflect repressed affective states. These may be fleeting and not noted during an interview. Facial expressions may also conflict with verbal messages. A typical example is that of a patient who smiles when telling someone he's upset. His words say, "I'm angry." His smile says, "Not really," or "I'm not serious." The smile may serve to reduce the tension or anxiety experienced when expressing anger. When nonverbal and verbal messages are incongruent, therapeutic communication between staff and patient is disrupted. It is important during interviews to acknowledge and clarify, when possible, incongruent messages.

What we think of ourselves, our self-image, may also be communicated through our physical appearance. Clothes may convey such personal attributes as sex, age, nationality, socioeconomic status, identification with a specific group, occupation, mood, interests, and values. For example, depressed people often perceive themselves as unattractive and their dress may reflect their attitude.

Body Space (Dudley and Welke, 1977)

The distance at which someone stands while talking with others is another index of emotional condition. In American society we normally hold people a "handshake" distance away, or the distance needed to reach out and shake someone's hand. Most people feel uncomfortable when anyone either gets closer than handshake distance or further away during normal conversation. Thus, the handshake distance, or about 3 feet, is the optimal distance for good communication. If the physician knows a patient is feeling depressed or dependent, however, moving in and, standing or sitting, touching the patient 1 or 2 feet away is best, because a depressed or dependent person is acutely aware of a space immediately around his or her body but does not pay much attention to things that occur beyond that distance (reduced body space). However, if the practitioner notices that someone is shy, uncomfortable, hostile, or suspicious, it will be easier to communicate while standing or sitting 4-6 feet away (expanded body space). Suspicious people have a body space that exceeds 4 feet. When someone approaches closer than 4-5 feet, they feel the way one normally does when someone comes closer than 3 feet and literally talks into one's face. To maintain good communication it may sometimes be necessary to establish a distance that is not comfortable for the physician but is for the other person.

Being An Aversive Stimulus

These kinds of observations are helpful in dealing with patients, but they only scratch the surface of nonverbal clues. A primary issue the physician must learn to deal with is related to becoming an aversive stimulus. For example, a patient may get dyspneic each time he or she is anxious. If the physician's manner makes the patient feel uncomfortable and anxious, the patient may well get dyspneic. Imagine that this happens on weekly or monthly visits over a period of a year. The physician becomes an aversive stimulus. Simply looking at or thinking about the physician may produce dyspnea. This patient can then easily become a real problem in terms of management and from a medical standpoint. The physician must learn to be a positive element in the patient's life, one whose presence must be associated with comfort and help. Otherwise, the patient's well-being and compliance with treatment are sacrificed.

The physician should avoid seeing the patient only in crisis situations or during exacerbations of the illness. Schedule the patient for occasional meetings in which progress is reviewed and additional information that has been added to the understanding of the disease is transmitted to the patient. Often it is appropriate for the physician to write the patient a letter explaining the latest laboratory findings and expressing continued interest in the patient's safety and well-being. In all events, avoid becoming an aversive stimulus.

F. Loss and Depression

Losses may be sudden or gradual. Some are predictable; others unpredictable. Chronically ill respiratory patients experience varied losses. Their positive feelings associated with health are often replaced by fatigue, dyspnea, and reduced exercise tolerance. Knowing that their illness is irreversible may create feelings of hopelessness and fears of losing control. When their illness progresses, positive self-attitudes often diminish. Independence and pride are lost as patients are forced to retire, change their recreational activities, and rely on others for assistance in performing household tasks or in meeting personal needs such as dressing or bathing. Feelings of inadequacy may result when social roles change.

A major part of our self-image is our body image: the perceptions, attitudes, and feelings we have toward our body. Alterations in our body image may be a major source of frustration and stress. Body image changes occur in respiratory patients when they begin to notice and feel uncomfortable about their barrel chest resulting from hyperinflation, or ankle swelling due to congestive failure. People who value trimness react to the weight gain and facial changes accompanying long-term steroid therapy. Continuous use of home oxygen not only affects one's social situation but can create feelings of unattractiveness.

People react to the same stressor in various ways. Minor emergency responses include fantasy, swearing, weeping, laughing, talking it out, and walking it off. Under major stress the ego is more taxed, and people may resort to extended use of repression, depression, excessive fantasy, somatic reactions, and detachment from reality.

Reactions to loss are called bereavement states: the thoughts, feelings, and actions that are consequences of the loss. Generally, such states are limited in intensity and duration. However, some are maladaptive, lasting for years. The most adaptive response to loss is the grief and mourning process. Families of dying patients may be deprived of their relationship unless medical personnel intervene to prevent their withdrawal. Less adaptive responses to loss include delayed or absent grief, depression, hypochondriasis, acting-out behavior, or neurotic and psychotic states.

Depression appears to be a common problem in chronically ill respiratory patients. This may be because of the accumulation of losses they experience as a result of their illness. Health personnel need to recognize cues of depression so that appropriate treatment is instituted early. When uncertainty exists about the presence of depression, its severity or management, psychiatric consultation is necessary.

The behavior of depressed people has been described as falling into 4 categories: physical, emotional, cognitive, and motivational. Physical symptoms often experienced by depressed people are decreased appetite, difficulty sleeping, and increased fatigue. Since respiratory patients usually experience fatigue as a result of the increased work of breathing, and sometimes experience difficulty in falling asleep because they are taking bronchodilators, physical symptoms of depression may be masked.

Feelings of hopelessness and helplessness characterize the emotional state of depressed people. Some patients experience fluctuating mood, while the severely depressed express more persistent feelings of hopelessness. Crying spells may be frequent or absent. The sense of humor is usually decreased. Relationships suffer as patients experience less consern and affection of those close to them. Diminished interaction occurs as they focus more on themselves than others. Sexual activity may be limited. Therefore, it is imperative to understand spouses' or significant others' reactions, discuss the patient's depression with them, and suggest how they may be of support to the patient.

The cognitive state is marked by indecisiveness and low self-esteem. Having perfectionist standards, many depressed people engage in self-criticism and overreact to errors. These patients are drawn to activities that are less demanding and involve less responsibility. They prefer passivity to activity, dependence to independence. Suicidal ideation may take various forms, such as obsessive thoughts, daydreams, and passive or active wishes.

Several brief screening measures may be used to evaluate patients for depression. The Beck Depression Inventory (Beck et al., 1961) and Zung Self-Rating Scale (Zung, 1965) and DSM-III-R-derived scales are particularly recommended. Management of the depressed patient involves the alleviation of guilt and suffering, stimulation and hope, and the protection from self-injury. This is accomplished through psychotherapy and, in some cases, the use of antidepressant medication. Some patients who refuse referrals to mental health facilities may be willing to meet with social workers or nurses prepared to do supportive counseling. Office visits can also have a counseling value.

Patient interviews should be considered in a serious, concerned manner. Since spontaneity of speech is decreased, the professional must be more active in the interview. Humor should be avoided. Commenting on the patient's mood may elicit various emotional reactions that can be acknowledged and discussed. For example, some patients may deny they are depressed but acknowledge they are discouraged. In this instance, a discussion about their discouragement is more helpful than telling them they are depressed. Daily routines should be investigated, as structure is often absent and may need to be part of the treatment plan. Inquiring about any suicidal wishes or thoughts shows concern and conveys the message that suicide is not a taboo topic.

G. Muddling Through

In our culture, muddling through is expected for us. Those among us who are terrified of flying in airplanes, or frightened of swimming, or intimidated by crowds are expected from early childhood to "grow up" and "bite the bullet" to "get a grip" on ourselves. Since our society admires these feats of overcoming anxiety and fear, most of us do "tough it out," and the subsequent jolts to organ systems we recognize as discomfort, sometimes severe discomfort. But we try and we somehow hang on.

Despite popular opinion, why should anyone who reacts with severe stress to public speaking force himself to accept public speaking invitations? To be sure, in a job in which public speaking is expected, one might seek professional counseling to help overcome the problem. But to "tough out" such events on a regular basis, whether part of the job or not, is nothing more than a sure way to get sick. If one can learn to stop reacting with stress to public speaking, that is one thing. It is certainly worth some effort to do so. However, if one cannot overcome the phobia, one should avoid public speaking. Continuing to engage in an activity that is overtly and continuously distressing makes as much sense as forsaking sleep or giving up food.

This does not mean one should avoid everything that might lead to uneasiness. Often the anticipation of an event will cause some discomfort or even considerable discomfort. Inevitably, a sprinter feels ill at ease before the gun goes off for an important track race. It is natural for actors to have opening-night butterflies before the curtain rises. But when the curtain rises, they can go on like the professionals they are. When the gun fires, the sprinter takes off with practiced fluid strides. There is, however, a considerable difference between some nervousness preceding a great performance and clutching the seat for the duration of a 2-hour airplane flight, or feeling panic in crowded rooms, or experiencing terror in entering an elevator. In essence, these kinds of stress reactions represent your effort to communicate non-verbally with yourself. You are saying to yourself, "I shouldn't be here because this is not good for me." For a number of patients, avoiding life events that trigger discomfort is good business. There is no reason for everyone to "muddle through," particularly if their heart and lungs are failing them.

III. Psychosocial and Psychophysiological Treatment

A. Intensive Care Unit

Management of patients with severe COPD requiring treatment in the intensive care unit is difficult at best. There is recognition by the patient and staff that the unit is bringing only temporary relief. Patients' lives may or may not be extended, but they will not become more functional even if treatment is "successful." In this setting it is difficult for either the patient or the medical team to maintain an optimistic, hopeful outlook. The grim reality of the situation makes it difficult to maintain staff morale and can lead to perfunctory and dehumanized treatment of the patient. The treatment of these patients during the intensive care unit stay can be greatly facilitated by understanding the patient's psychosocial and psychophysiological situation as outlined in this chapter.

The path that leads to the intensive care unit may be a long one of graually increasing disability, and the patient may arrive with an acutely failing pulmonary system superimposed upon his chronically disabled state. His level of pulmonary function is usually such that it marginally sustains him while he is resting quietly. Any change in metabolic demand will lead to rapid onset of symptoms. One way that metabolic demand, and thereby symptoms, are increased is by placing the patient in a situation in which he is unable to avoid emotional stress. Patients who are severely ill with a pulmonary crisis are rarely able to tolerate emotional stresses of even a routine nature.

Most or all of these problems with emotional stress may change when the patient is placed on assisted breathing. If completely successful, for the first time in years the patient is receiving a sufficient amount of oxygen to supply his metabolic needs totally. The patient is then able to allow herself to participate in emotional expression that was denied previously because of pending respiratory embarrassment secondary to the physiological results of emotional change. There is little doubt that this type of experience will lead to dependence on the machinery required to assist breathing. The dependence often is not related to the patient's lack of drive or determination to breathe on her own but rather to the reluctance to give up feeling emotionally normal or near normal.

The intensive care unit staff is presented with a person who will in all probability not reward it by becoming symptom-free and who will continue to complain of discomfort after the staff has done its best. For reasons noted above, these patients often lack warmth and the capacity to relate; thus they will frequently seem to lack emotional involvement with the staff no matter how hard it works. It takes a highly motivated staff to absorb the emotional punishment of caring for these patients when the rewarding admiration of a grateful patient is absent. The staff seldom feels adequately rewarded for its hard work and dedication to patient care and is often left with only the satisfaction that its clinical expertise has given the patient additional time to live.

Acutely ill patients suffer from some sleep deprivation, sensory overstimulation, and isolation. Death may be an imminent concern. Besides investigating the patient's immediate concerns, the staff can reduce stress through:

1. Orienting patients to their environment and daily activities

2. Planning activities to minimize fatigue and the work of breathing

3. Maintaining an attitude of competency in the patient's presence

4. Controlling the environment for traffic and noise

5. Utilizing resources for patient and staff support

Too frequently families are neglected in the acute care setting. Families should be familiarized with the physical surroundings, visiting hours, and informed when they can receive progress reports. For example, spouses may be told that flexible visiting hours will be allowed while the patient is critical but that the usual schedule for visiting will be reinforced once his or her condition stabilizes. Guidelines for family involvement in patient care should be clarified by the nursing staff.

Often patients become increasingly independent as the crisis begins to resolve. However, some patients show increased dependency in the recovery phase or in the ambulatory care setting when it is time for them to begin doing more for themselves. This helpless-dependent position may be reflected in a patient's unwillingness to cooperate with a treatment program. He may express feelings of helplessness and resentment. Staff may also be manipulated against each other by such a patient. His dependent attitude may also be manifested in the clinging nature of his relationships and in his lack of initiative in seeking instructions.

Too often patients alienate others by their self-preoccupation. Staff members become irritated and frustrated and may unintentionally ignore the patient or express their frustration and resentment. Rather than avoid the patient, a consistent treatment approach should be agreed upon. Reflecting on the patient's behavior during an interview may reveal particular fears and anxieties related to her illness, treatment program, or hospital discharge that can be discussed and sometimes alleviated. When a patient's anxiety is decreased, her dependent behavior may decrease. Management also includes clarifying the amount of time spent in interviews, introducing patients to other resource staff in a given setting, and reinforcing independent behavior. Maintaining a nonjudgmental attitude is essential, since these patients are often highly sensitive to criticism and unable to express anger, since they fear rejection by others.

B. Group Psychotherapy

Reports in the literature have indicated the salutary effects of group treatment on both patient status and staff-patient relations. However, patients with COPD present a complex therapeutic problem. The patients most likely to need this type of therapy are the same ones who would need it if they did not have COPD. The intimate interdependence between the emotional state of the patient and pulmonary function creates special problems. Emotional states of action-orientation such an anger and anxiety increase respiratory and metabolic activity. Conversely, emotional states of action-inhibition such as depression or apathy decrease respiratory and metabolic activity. In normal subjects or minimally diseased persons such shifts in affect and behavior with the concomitant shifts in pulmonary function may be uncomfortable and result in dyspnea, but there is adequate physiological reserve for the person to maintain pulmonary compensation. However, the patient with severe COPD has a very narrow range within which he can maintain pulmonary balance. A rapid shift to either action-activation or action-inhibition may set the stage for production of pulmonary embarrassment (Dudley and Pattison, 1969; Pattison et al., 1971).

Patients who need group psychotherapy have a history of precarious psychosocial balance that left them ill prepared for the stress of severe debilitating disease and its concomitant need for continuous medical care and intermittent hospitalization. Their inability to deal with emotions was further compromised by the precarious pulmonary balance. When faced with emotional conflicts they may be unable to deal with the affect involved without precipitating pulmonary decompensation and disabling symptoms.

Patients who have reasonable interpersonal and social resources and some physiological reserve have the capacity to respond to the frustrations of their illness without upsetting their pulmonary balance. These types of patients are able to participate in group discussions involving insight-oriented therapy and profit from them.

Observations of the relationship between physiological and psychological factors highlight the importance of structuring group methods to the needs

of the patient population. Physiological limitations and particular psychological defense mechanisms make it impossible for particular patients to participate in a group treatment method that focuses on the exploration of affect
and conflict.

In general, patients with higher psychosocial assets and good pulmonary
function demonstrate successful participation in group treatment. Unsuccessful patients have low psychosocial assets and severe physiological limitations.
These patients' reactions to group treatment are characterized by a guarded
pose and avoidance of emotionally charged or personally related topics. It is
not uncommon to observe them react to emotionally charged topics with
anxiety, anger, depression, dyspnea, and physiological insufficiency. Supportive didactic discussions or activity and social groups that are task-oriented are
usually positive experiences, regardless of the degree of physiological insufficiency.

Relation of Variables Affecting Group Participation

Two hypotheses can be advanced concerning the severe repression, denial, and
isolation that characterize the severely incapacitated COPD patient. The first
suggests that these patients had reasonably adequate coping mechanisms prior
to their disease and that the emotional crippling is an adaptive response to the
severe physiological limitation. In support of this is the fact that most patients had been self-sufficient throughout their lives without known psychiatric symptoms or complaints. However, many also had a history of unsuccessful marital relations, suggesting difficulties in interpersonal relations.

The second hypothesis suggests that these patients had always overutil-
ized the psychological defenses of denial, suppression, repression, and isolation
and that the disease process was superimposed on this pattern of defense. Observations by other workers on the premorbid personality of the tuberculosis
patient lend support to this hypothesis.

In either case the end result is that the only psychological mechanisms
available for handling affect and interpersonal conflict are gross denial, suppression, repression, and isolation. This, of course, becomes a vicious cycle,
for as they face the realistically severe problems associated with an incapacitating disease and chronic treatment, they cannot face their feelings or deal
with the interpersonal conflicts without literally endangering their lives. The
rigid avoidance of affect and conflicts only perpetuates the problems and increases frustration, anger, and despair, which in turn cannot be dealt with by
the patient.

These observations are pertinent to the development and prescription of group methods for the treatment of patients with chronic lung disease as well as other medically disabling diseases. Based on these observations, significant questions should be raised by therapists regarding selection and outcome criteria for group treatment.

Selection criteria for group treatment usually depends on the structure, procedures, and goals of the therapy group. Admission of a patient to a group is also influenced by the theoretical orientation, experience, and professional background of the therapist. Standard psychological diagnostic tests have failed to yield valid predictions as to how patients may behave in group treatment. The relationship between interpersonal behavior, expression of affect, and pathophysiology when selecting medical patients for group treatment may prove an effective predictive method. There is a question of whether or not group treatment should be undertaken with any severely disabled medical patient who may compromise a physiological system temporarily when confronted with the exploration of affect and interpersonal conflict. Usual group methods may not be applicable to these populations, and new group approaches may need to be developed and tested. Further clinical and research evidence is also needed that will support the indications and contraindications for varied group treatment approaches with varying medical populations experiencing varying degrees of disability. Since families are often affected by the patient's illness, under what circumstance should they be included in group treatment? It is often assumed by therapists that families or spouses should be directly involved. Yet it is important to consider what characteristics may contradict their inclusion.

There is also a need to establish successful outcome criteria. Patients may perceive improvement in different ways. For example, respiratory patients who associate expression of affect with dyspnea may learn that expressing emotions does not consistently produce dyspnea. Socially isolated patients may learn what they fear about intimacy, and the group may function as a socialization process for them.

Insight in group treatment may occur on at least four levels. Patients may learn how they are seen by others; some learn what they are doing to and with other people; others learn why they behave in certain ways and why they have not been able to behave differently; and, lastly, some gain an understanding of the cause of their present interpersonal behavior.

Discussion

The use of educational, psychotherapeutic, and medical principles in a unified approach to the treatment of patients with chronic pulmonary disease has a long history in the United States. Joseph Hersey Pratt, a Boston internist, developed the first such treatment method in 1905 for tuberculosis patients. This early program consisted of a combination of group psychotherapy, didactic teaching, and medical treatment. It was referred to as the Thought Control Clinic, and a derivation of it was called the Class Method of Treatment. The results of this early work were impressive, and Pratt and his colleagues extended use of the method to patients with diabetes and cardiac disease. Other groups of researchers extended his work to patients with hypertension and peptic ulcer. Around 1921, as a direct result of Pratt's work, St. Elizabeth's Hospital in Washington, D.C., instituted group therapy for the treatment of chronic schizophrenic patients. Despite the intent of Dr. Pratt and his colleagues and its demonstrated effectiveness, the integrated use of group therapy and teaching in treatment of chronic disease had almost disappeared from the field of internal medicine by the 1940s, with the exception of the tuberculosis sanatoriums. With closure of these institutions in the 1960s and 1970s, the technique disappeared as an organized treatment method in internal medicine.

In the past decade the increasing emphasis on treatment of chronic disease and the acceptance of a chronic disease model have resulted in increased interest in such an integrated approach to patient care. In addition, treatment techniques have in many instances become virtually too much for the patient to handle without special instruction and support. Some hemodialysis programs utilize a programmed test in self-care for patients to overcome some of these difficulties. In other programs patient manuals or textbooks have been developed for use by diabetics and patients with chronic airway disease and arthritis. These all appear to be effective in aiding the patient to adapt better to disease. Work in the Netherlands on the use of group education and group therapy for treatment of asthma and diabetes is of particular importance because of the demonstration of a significant reduction in morbidity. These teachers recommend a treatment program unlike the model followed by most American programs in that the integrative process is done by a skilled internist, and emphasis is not limited to the giving of information. Emphasis is placed on the integration of the patient's degree of incapacity with the pattern of life.

These observations are pertinent for the development and prescription of group methods for the treatment of patients with severe chronic lung disease. Programs conducted on the wards, which include various group treatments, have been developed in many tuberculosis wards. Group treatment has been used successfully with outpatients with tuberculosis, bronchial asthma, and emphysema.

However, authors report that they avoid involving patients who are severely debilitated, who are so seriously ill that death is an imminent possibility, or who are severely immobilized by physical illness. Thus, the usual group methods described do not seem directly applicable to the most severely ill patient population. The few exceptions have been group work with patients such as those in poliomyelitis respiratory wards.

Yet in even the less physically handicapped patients, group leaders report that they have found it necessary to modify discussion groups and joint group social and vocational activities. Further, they report that group techniques that focus on immediate exploration of affect and interpersonal conflict have not been successful with patients with moderate to severe lung disease, nor with debilitated aged patients.

In this light it is pertinent to report 2 group methods that seem to be uniformly successful. Most patients and staff who were involved concluded that these two group activities did have a salutory effect.

The first is a discussion group conducted by a physician and a well-trained paramedical person. It is important that the physician and the family be directly involved. Pertinent aspects of pulmonary and cardiac physiology and pathology are reviewed and effects of chronic lung disease on patterns of life activity are described. All information is provided to the group in a neutral manner, and the talks are didactic with time for questions and discussion. There is no forced emotional intervention. The second is a physical therapy or rehabilitation group. This should be prescribed treatment in which six to eight patients (and families, if appropriate) assemble to exercise, practice breathing, or share experiences with their disease. It is useful to have the sessions conducted by outgoing, energetic people with whom the patients can identify. There is generally joking, sharing of experiences, and friendly competition over the adequacy of their performance. The patients perceive these group experiences as positive because it is their disease and not themselves that is in question. These groups play into their denial mechanisms in part, but also afford some measure of secondhand intervention in patterns of interpersonal relations.

C. Ambulatory Care

Patient and Family Education

The goals of patient and family education are to maintain health, prevent complications, maximize individual growth. Success or failure of educational programs depends on many interrelated factors such as the following:

1. Teaching skills of the educator

2. Patient/family involvement in planning the program

3. Adequacy of program objectives

4. Identification of resources and barriers

5. Effectiveness of the evaluation process

Teaching Skills

Professionals who are successful teachers use teaching-learning principles and strategies that optimize the learning situation. Since the physical environment influences learning, teachers can achieve a suitable atmosphere by regulating room size, ventilation, heat, and light. Respiratory patients in particular are sensitive to crowded rooms and ventilation changes. Learning is also enhanced by clarifying guidelines on attendance and participation and selecting material best suited for the learner. If information is presented at too high a level of comprehension, patients become frustrated, while they lose interest and become annoyed when the material presented is too simplified. Increased anxiety can also result when patients' questions are ignored or when too much information is given to a patient too rapidly.

If you wish to create an atmosphere of self-expression and shared problem-solving, small patient groups arranged in circular fashion without a table are more effective than large groups seated in rows of chairs facing the educator. Guided discussion in small groups places increased responsibility on the learners. As a result they become active participants, more aware of their styles of communication and problem-solving skills, and may eventually increase varied interpersonal skills.

When the professional functions as a leader of a discussion group, the learning objectives may be facilitated through various techniques. For example, he or she may use inductive learning to help patients and families understand the principles related to anxiety by asking them to describe anxiety-provoking situations and how they have coped with them. Principles and generalizations may then be drawn from their observations and experiences. Questions may also be used to seek more information, clarify behavior, and compare and contrast situations.

Positive reinforcement strengthens behavior and can be achieved by giving patients feedback about the nature of their performance. When patients present incorrect information, they can be rewarded for their effort while they are informed of correct information. In any learning situation the educator must decide what behavior to reinforce. He or she may wish to reinforce the participation of a withdrawn patient in a discussion group, someone's willingness to tackle a problem, or another's performance of a task. In group situations it is important to recognize the achievements of each other.

Patient and Family Participation

Active participation in the learning process enhances learning and increases autonomy. Patients and families should have some control over the information they receive and when it is presented. Too frequently educational programs are planned for them without assessing their learning needs, their readiness to learn, and how their cultural backgrounds may affect the learning process. Educators must also set realistic expectations. For example, anxious, depressed, or dependent patients may not be able to participate fully in initial planning sessions.

Adequacy of Program Objectives

Perhaps one of the most difficult tasks is that of clearly defining learning objectives. When goals are hazy, it is impossible to select appropriate content and evaluate a program efficiently. Useful objectives are statements that identify the kind of performance desired and demonstrate that someone has achieved the objective; that establish conditions under which the behavior will be expected to occur; and that specify how well the educator wants the learner to do it: the minimal level of acceptable performance.

Identification of Resources and Barriers

Educators need to evaluate the following resources prior to planning any educational program: support within the organization, financial support, time, space, and personnel affected by the decision. Such assessments prevent unnecessary conflicts that may occur at a later date, since they help the educator analyze the factors that may oppose or strengthen an educational program. The use of force-field analysis as a tool for evaluating resources and barriers may be of considerable assistance. Awareness of the constraints and strengths of a program helps educators plan strategies to weaken the opposing forces.

Effectiveness of the Evaluation Process

Evaluation is a continuous process in any educational program. Educators evaluate program objectives, instructional materials, and patients' progress towards achieving the objectives. Generally, evaluation measurements are used to determine the effectiveness in attaining program goals and objectives. Educators need to decide whether clinical observations should be used alone or in conjunction with measurements that are valid and reliable. Evaluation resources may also be limited to clinical settings because of inadequate funds, staff, or time.

In summary, patient education is often considered to be a viable part of any pulmonary rehabilitation program. Clinicians planning these programs may want to consider the following factors that contribute to an improved psychological state and performance in a rehabilitation program.

1. Progressive exercise leading to decreased fear of activity

2. Education in self-care, leading to increased autonomy in control of symptoms

3. Staff attitudes stressing that the patient is worth the effort

4. Setting realistic goals leading to improvement in self-esteem

5. Monthly follow-up to consolidate gains

6. Mutual support from group interaction

7. Factors within patients that lead to strong motivation

IV. Dealing with Psychiatric Disease

A. Introduction

In contrast to the previously discussed psychosocial and psychophysiological problems and their accompanying emotions that afflict many or most patients with severe pulmonary disease, psychiatric disease is probably no more frequent than in patients without pulmonary disease. The distinction between psychophysiological and psychosocial problems and significant psychiatric disease is a critical issue. The treatment of the former can often be by various psychotherapies, behavioral therapies, and social support systems, with medication as adjuncts *when necessary,* while treatment of the latter should initially be primarily with medications. Other types of therapy may be needed in the recovery period, but there likely will be no recovery period without the use of medications.

In general, the psychiatric diseases to be concerned about are the schizophrenias, manic depressive illness (unipolar and bipolar types), major depression, and delirium (acute brain syndromes). Specific pharmacologic treatments are also available for anxiety and depression not classified in the above categories. A review of psychiatric diseases can be obtained from any of the current textbooks of psychiatry.

Patients with combined psychiatric and pulmonary disease are more likely to have serious problems than patients without such combinations. A good way to screen for possible psychiatric disease can be to identify patients with (1) marked pulmonary disease but with no complaints or no response to the reality of the disease at all; (2) those with little pulmonary disease who are incapacitated; (3) patients who overreact and feel little hope for coping with the concomitant problems. This clinical information suggests an increased probability of the patients' having a psychiatric problem but does not necessarily confirm the diagnosis.

In early states of pulmonary disease, changes in psychological activation are often associated with dyspnea only. As the disease progresses in severity, it may reach a point where increases in emotional activation of any type produce elevations in oxygen consumption and carbon dioxide production that cannot readily be compensated for physiologically because of the patient's impaired ventilation. Even minimal changes in alveolar ventilation then become difficult to accommodate. With psychological activation, the patient with an unimpaired muscular system (that is, one who is not paralyzed and thus can contract muscles) is likely to then develop hypoxia and possible hypercarbia. When there is a decrease in psychological activation, there is a drop in the amount of air the patient breathes, but there is no equivalent drop in oxygen need and nutritional requirements of the skeletal muscles. Thus, any and all emotional change may be associated with uncomfortable symptoms because the pulmonary system then tends to deliver less oxygen than is required to meet metabolic demand.

The secondary reaction to dyspnea, wheezing, cough, sputum production, and pain that occurs can be anxiety, fear, and/or depression that in turn serves as another emotional stimulus, further compromising the patient's physiological and emotional state.

It is understandable that these people tend to avoid interpersonal contact because of the psychological stress involved. They thereby decrease psychological stressors. By using denial and repression, they lessen the impact of emotionally loaded events. The psychological defenses used to protect a failing organ system, however, are often regarded by others as socially inappropriate, since the patient may be perceived as rejecting, bland, and unresponsive. The preceding problems can be magnified many times in patients with psychiatric disorders (Dudley et al., 1980a,b,c; Dudley and Pitts-Poarch, 1980; Dudley and Sitzman, 1979).

Table 1 Neuroleptics: Major Tranquilizers[a]

Specific medication	Special properties	Usual daily dosage	Daily dosage in moderate to severe COPD
Phenothiazines Thioridazine HCL (Mellaril)	Similar to chlorpromazine, but it has been reported to produce pigmented retinitis in doses over 800 mg. Mild D-2, highest alpha-1, moderate alpha-2, and high cholinergic receptor blocking	Oral: 50-800 mg	Oral: 5-200 mg
Chlorpromazine (Thorazine)	Older dose forms may contain tartrazine and should be avoided if this medication is used in asthmatics. Current dose forms should be free of tartrazine. Can be very sedating. Associated with the production of antinuclear antibodies. Mild to moderate D-2, high alpha-1, moderate alpha-2, high H-1, and high cholinergic receptor blocking effect	Oral: 500-2000 mg IM: 50-100 mg every 30-60 min until symptoms are under control to a total dose of 200 mg	Oral: 5-200 mg IM: 25 mg every 30-60 min until symptoms are under control to a total dose of 100 mg
Trifluoperazine HCL (Stelazine)	Can be activating. Moderate D-2, low alpha-1, low alpha-2, moderate H-1, and moderate cholinergic receptor blocking effect	Oral: 10-40 mg	Oral: 2-5 mg

Dihydroindolones Molindone HCL (Moban)	Apparent low cardiovascular toxicity. Does not block guanethidine. Mild D-2, low alpha-1, moderate alpha-2, low H-1, and low cholinergic receptor blocking effect. There is little experience with this medication in COPD	Oral: 30-100 mg	Oral: 10-30 mg
Thiothanxenes Thiothixene (Navane)	No tartrazine. Low anticholinergic effect. May have significant antidepressant effect. Decreases sensory input. Can be non-sedating or sedating. Strong D-2, moderate to low alpha-1, moderate alpha-2, high H-1, and low cholinergic receptor blocking effect. (D-2 receptor blocking refers to antipsychotic effect. Higher D-2 blockade is thought to be synonymous with greater antipsychotic effect)	Oral: 5-80 mg IM: 5-20 mg every 30-60 min to a total dose of 80 mg	Oral: 2-20 mg IM: 5 mg every 30-60 min to a total dose of 40 mg
Butyrophenones Haloperidol (Haldol)	1, 5, and 10 mg tablets of haloperidol contain tartrazine. These dose forms should be avoided if this medication is used in patients with asthma. Can be nonsedating; decreases sensory input. Likely to produce movement disorders that can interfere with chest movement. Moderate D-2, moderate alpha-1, low alpha-2, low H-1, and low cholinergic receptor blocking effect	Oral: 2-40 mg IM: 5-10 mg every 30-60 min to a total dose of 40 mg IV: 2 mg every 6-8 hour dose	Oral: 1-10 mg IM: 2-5 mg every 30-60 min to a total dose of 20 mg IV: 2 mg every 6-8 hour

Table 1 (continued)

[a]From Thioridazine to haloperidol, extrapyramidal symptoms increase, and, moving backward, alpha-adrenergic blocking, allergic responses, sedation, atropinelike effects, seizures, and orthostatic hypotension generally increase. For all neuroleptics listed, drowsiness or lack of attention may make operation of machinery dangerous, particularly during initial treatment. Selected patients may need the usual daily dose. Respiratory depression with aggravation or onset of hypoxia and hypercarbia is always a possible complication when the neuroleptics are used in the COPD population.

Neuroleptics in general can alter sexual function and drive. Each medication in this class can produce specific types of problems. For example, thioridazine may contribute to delayed or inhibited ejaculation and chlorpromazine may contribute to a simple reduction in sexual dirve. On the other hand, both may increase sexual drive and performance in specific patients. In addition, sexual dysfunction is so common in patients who need to be treated with neuroleptics that it is often difficult to know what the cause of the change in sexual function is secondary to.

Common side effects	Precautions with	Contraindications
Blurred vision	Seizures	Comatose states
Dysuria	Depression	Central nervous system depression
Constipation	Pregnancy	Bone marrow depression
Nasal congestion	Respiratory disease	Subcortical brain depression
Postural hypotension	Cardiac disease	Seriously impaired liver function
Photosensitivity	Respiratory depression	Hypersensitivity
Drowsiness	May reverse the hypertensive	Uncontrolled epilepsy
Fatigue	action of medications such as	Severe retarded depression
Weight gain	epinephrine, and block the	
Extrapyramidal side effects	antihypertensive effect of	
Respiratory depression	guanethidine	
Potential difficulty handling secretions		
Changes in temperature control		

these tables as a guide, thiothixene is the best D-2 blocker, being almost nine times more effective than haloperidol. Since D-2 receptor blocking is an indication of antipsychotic activity, this agent may be the best antipsychotic on the market. One hundred milligrams of thiothixene is the equivalent of 888 mg haloperidol in D-2 receptor blocking effect, the equivalent of 254 mg of diphenhydramine in H-1 blocking, 0.08 mg of atropine in anticholinergic activity, and the equivalent of 0.8 mg prazosin in alpha-1 blocking.

Similar figures for thioridazine would be 14.0, 13.3, 93, and 18.2, respectively. In other words, by using Tables 5 and 6, one can choose a neuroleptic such as thioridazine that provides a high dose (low D-2) effect that has high anticholinergic and high alpha-1 blocking. If low dose (high D-2 effect), low anticholinergic activity, and relatively low alpha-1 blocking are desired thiothixene could be chosen. These data have been provided by Richelson (1983/83, 1985) and are based on receptor studies done on human brain. The relationships listed are rough guides. Much information of this nature is based on data from rat or other nonhuman brains and the technology varies. The particular set of studies was used because they seemed to parallel clinical experience and the information was translatable in terms of milligrams of standard blocking agents.

Rapid treatment of extrapyramidal reactions is important in maintaining unimpaired respiratory movements. These reactions to neuroleptics can be treated with benztropin mesylate, 1-2 mg, or with diphenhydramine hydrochloride, 50-100 mg intravenously in most cases of respiratory impairment. Oral maintenance therapy can be accomplished with any of the antiparkinsonian medications, such as benztropine mesylate or procyclidine hydrochloride.

Antidepressants

In the treatment of depression, it is helpful to have information on the clinical use of antidepressants that can be used to produce sedation and activation. Since nomifensine has been removed from the market it is hoped that an activating compound such as Fluoxetine and bupropion will be available and that the compound will be compatible with COPD.

Doxepin is the antidepressant of choice in agitated, depressed patients with COPD. In addition to its antidepressant characteristics, it is sufficiently sedating to reduce or eliminate agitation. The sedative effect is apparent in minutes or hours, while the antidepressant effect may take days to weeks to be apparent. As with other antidepressants, it appears to have little or no effect on the respiratory center, and seems to act as a bronchodilator (Knapp et al., 1976; Steen, 1976). It should be noted that doxepin and other psychotropic agents have been found to decrease seizures in patients with seizure disorders. One hundred milligrams of doxepin contains the equivalent of 0.2 mg haloperidol in D-2 blocking, 2.7 mg atropine in anticholinergic effect, 77,500 mg diphenhydramine in H-1 blocking, 0.3 mg prazosin in alpha-1 blocking and 4.0 mg phentolamine in alpha-2 blocking (see Tables 6 and 7).

Fluoxitene or bupropion is probably the antidepressant of choice in retarded, depressed patients, with low drive and motivation. The activating effect can appear in hours and the antidepressant effect in days or weeks. The most common side effects are sleep disturbance, restlessness, and diaphoresis. These medications are under consideration for commercial use and information of a clinical nature awaits their release. They reportedly have little or no anticholinergic effect and are not cardiotoxic. A reliable receptor blocking profile should be available soon.

Doxepin has a relatively low incidence of side effects if used for the appropriate indications. It is generally not advisable to utilize doxepin in the morning or fluoxitene or bupropion at night, because patients will not adapt well to such regimens. To obtain optimal therapeutic effect, advantage should be taken of the initial sedation or activating characteristics by prescribing these agents when sedation or activation will not interfere with the patient's life.

In utilizing antidepressants and neuroleptics, it is important to remember that blood levels may have little relationship to oral dose, and cellular levels may be poorly related to either. Since these compounds may have a therapeutic window, above or below which there will be no positive clinical effects, it is essential to maintain optimal blood levels. This is particularly true for the antidepressants. The desired clinical response can be associated with a specific blood level and then maintained. This is the preferred method of determining dosage in patients with combined psychiatric and pulmonary disease. Since metabolism varies greatly between individuals, major side effects such as cardiotoxicity can be avoided by the measurement of blood levels and appropriate adjustment in dosage.

Although it is important for the clinician to deal with side effects of individual psychoactive agents it is also important to understand that certain medications are converted to known psychoactive agents in the course of their metabolism in the human body. For example, imipramine is broken down to desipramine and amitriptyline is broken down to nortriptyline. The metabolite varies from the parent compound by having different receptor blocking characteristics and different side effects (see Tables 2 and 7). The issue is complicated by the fact that once a steady state is reached (7-10 days) the ratio of desipramine to imipramine is about 2:1 and the ratio of nortriptyline to amitriptyline is about 1.2:1.

Table 2 Heterocyclic Antidepressants[a]

Specific medication	Special properties	Usual daily dosage	Daily dosage in moderate to severe COPD
Tricyclic agents			
Amitriptyline HCL (Elavil)	Information uncertain. May act as a mild bronchodilator and may depress ventilation. Generally not recommended in COPD patients with arrhythmias. Metabolically converted to nortriptyline (Aventyl or Pamelor); thus may begin as sedating and end up in 7-14 days as nonsedating or activating. Low D-2, moderate H-1, high cholinergic, low alpha-1, and moderate serotonin receptor blocking effect	Oral: 50-300 mg	Oral: 10-100 mg
Doxepin HCL (Adapin, Sinequan)	Adapin contains tartrazine and should be avoided in asthmatics. Some preliminary evidence indicates comparatively low bioavailability for Adapin. Low cardiac toxicity; little or no effect on respiratory center; may act as a mild bronchodilator. Particularly effective in treatment of panic attacks associated with depression. Antidepressant of choice for agitated/depressed patients. Acts	Oral: 50-300 mg	Oral: 10-100 mg

Table 2 (continued)

Specific medication	Special properties	Usual daily dosage	Daily dosage in moderate to severe COPD
Tetracyclic amines			
Maprotiline (Ludiomil)	Generally similar to protriptyline and desipramine with the exception that it appears to have the highest incidence of seizures of any antidepressant on the United States market. D-2 blocking unknown, H-1 blocking low to moderate, cholinergic blocking low, alpha-1 blocking low, and unknown serotonin receptor blocking	Oral: 75-225 mg	Oral: 10-100 mg
Triazolopyridines			
Trazodone (Desyrel)	Contains tartrazine in the 50 mg and 150 mg dose forms, which should be avoided in asthmatics. Associated with priapism and impotence subsequent to treatment of the priapism. Generally sedating. Low D-2, low H-1, low cholinergic, low alpha-1, and unknown serotonin receptor blocking	Oral: 150-400 mg	Oral: 50-150 mg
Dibenzoxazepine			
Amoxapine (Asendin)	Useful in psychotic, depressed patients (in roughly the group of patients treated with combinations of antidepressants and neuro-	Oral: 75-400 mg	Oral: 25-100 mg

leptics.) Has some of the side effects of neuroleptics including extrapyramidal symptoms. Generally sedating. High D-2 (for an antidepressant), low H-1, low cholinergic, low alpha-1, and unknown serotonin receptor blocking

Benzodiazepine
(Triazolobenzodiazepine)

Alprazolam (Xanax)	An anxiolytic with what may prove to be reasonable antidepressant characteristics.	Oral: 0.25-4 mg	Oral: 0.125-2 mg

[a]For all antidepressants listed, drowsiness or lack of attention may make operation of machinery dangerous, particularly during initial treatment.

A beneficial side effect of these medications in COPD patients may be mild bronchodilation. Selected patients may need the usual daily dose.

Common side effects	Precautions with	Contraindications
Dry mouth	Urinary retention	Acute myocardial infarction
Potential difficulty handling secretions	Cardiovascular disorders	Hypersensitivity
Blurred vision	Narrow angle glaucoma	Acute schizophrenia
Constipation	Organic brain syndrome	Mania
Nausea	Schizophrenia	Monoamine oxidase inhibitors
Heartburn	Mania	
Hypotension	Convulsive disorders	
Weight gain	Thyroid disease	
	Pregnancy	
	Potentiation of sympatho-mimetic amines	
	Blocking guanethidine	

Lithium

Understanding lithium therapy has been increasingly important as clinical studies continue to demonstrate its effectiveness in controlling mania, depression, or cyclic swings from mania to depression. Mania may be treated initially with a neuroleptic and depression with an antidepressant. However, lithium should be started concomitantly if mood swings are a serious problem. The starting dosage of lithium is generally 150-450 mg/day. This dosage may require modification if the patient is taking theophylline or a diuretic, since theophylline tends to cause an increased excretion of lithium, and most diuretics will decrease excretion of lithium. In addition, lithium excretion may vary with salt intake, which should thereby be kept stable during lithium administration. A fasting morning level of lithium (9-10 hr after the evening dose) of 0.5-1.0 mEq/liter (or lower) is usually therapeutic in patients with moderate to severe lung disease. It may take 3-10 days to equilibrate a therapeutic blood level. Lithium usually has a 7-10 day lag between the onset of therapy and the therapeutic response. When the maintenance dose is reached, the neuroleptic or antidepressant can often be withdrawn. Note that some COPD patients obtain good therapeutic effects with blood levels less than 0.5 mEq/liter.

Patients should be monitored carefully for signs of toxicity (particularly hyperthermia) and alternative treatment should be planned in advance. Lithium carbonate occasionally produces a severe depression. If this occurs, it is necessary to treat with an antidepressant with or without lithium carbonate.

It should be noted that increasing experience is being gained with the use of carbamazapine, valproic acid, lecithin, and other agents in the treatment of the approximately 25% of patients who cannot tolerate or do not respond to lithium (see Table 3).

Anxiolytic Agents

These psychopharmacologic agents are often overused. They tend to be given in sympathy for the patients' condition and our inability to cure them rather than for specific indications. As with any medication, it is better not to prescribe anxiolytic agents if clinical indications for their administration are unclear. These are potent compounds, and prescribing them indiscriminately (that is, to a patient who may not need them or needs some other type of medication such as an antidepressant or neuroleptic) can be antitherapeutic and even dangerous in the COPD patient. Without a positive diagnosis, it is likely that the only effect will be sedation and potentiation of depression

Table 3 Manic-Depressive Agents

Specific medication	Special properties	Usual daily dosage	Daily dosage in moderate to severe COPD
Lithium carbonate[a] (Eskalith, Lithane)	Reduces or stops cyclic mood swings. Prophylactic against recurrent mania or depression. Often takes 7-14 days for therapeutic effect to be seen. Give with psychiatric supervision. 20% or more of the population with manic-depressive disease do not respond or have unacceptable side effects and other agents need to be utilized. Can produce diabetes insipidus.	Oral: 900-1800 mg/day until blood level of 0.8-1.2 mEq/L is attained; may have to be reduced to 1/2 to 2/3 of starting dosage for maintenance	Oral: Same dosage; aim for serum level of 0.6-1.0 mEq/L (stay on low side)
Carbamazapine (Tegretal)	An iminodibenzyl derivative with a tricyclic structure similar to the tricyclic antidepressants. For treatment of acute episodes, it is particularly efficacious in mania. It has a growing use in bipolar or schizoaffective patients who do not respond to or tolerate lithium. It has also been used in treatment of lithium-induced diabetes insipidus. Usually used as an anti-seizure agent, but has growing applications	Oral:	Oral:

Table 3 (continued)

Specific medication	Special properties	Usual daily dosage	Daily dosage in moderate to severe COPD
	as a psychotropic medication. The feared adverse effect of aplastic anemia is rare, but white blood cell count suppression early in treatment is common. Regular hematologic monitoring is recommended. Common side effects are dizziness, ataxia, and clumsiness. Use only under the supervision of those familiar with the medication.		
Valproic acid (Depakote)	A GABA-ergic drug, strong antiseizure agent. Preliminary studies indicate that this medication may have antimanic characteristics. It should be used only by those familiar with its action and with the failure of other methods of controlling manic depressive disease.	Oral:	Oral:

| Lecithin and Choline | Lecithin in doses between approximately 20 and 40 g has been shown to exert some antimanic activity. Adverse side effects seem to be onset of depression and diarrhea. Choline can produce an unpleasant body smell in about 20% of those who take it and is not recommended for those individuals. | Oral: 20-40 g | Oral: 20-40 g |

[a]Blocks release of T-4; likely to precipitate depression; contraindicated with brain damage or significant cardiovascular or renal disease.

Considerable caution should be used with diuretics since lithium carbonate may be substituted for sodium and toxic levels of lithium rapidly produced, leading to potentially fatal cardiac arrhythmias. Caution should also be used when it is utilized in hot weather and the patient is losing salt.

Contraindicated in comatose states, presence of a large amount of CNS depressants, hypersensitivity, and history of addiction or habituation.

and/or behavioral disorganization that can further aggravate problems with
COPD. Generally these agents should be used to attain short-term goals such
as overcoming an acute stress reaction. The statement that giving them over
long periods of time leads to significant problems with habituation and addiction needs to be studied. In particular, some newly released, not yet released,
and probably some older compounds in this category may carry roughly the
same probability of causing habituation and addiction as digitalis or hydrodi-
uril. If an anxiolytic agent has been administered in high dosage over a period
of months, withdrawal should be carried out by gradual reduction of dosage
rather than abrupt withdrawal. A reasonable schedule is to withdraw at the
rate of 10% of the current dosage each week. In some cases it may be desirable to replace one type of anxiolytic by another rather than to withdraw
the medication and have the patient experience recurrence of the symptoms
it was originally prescribed for. Abrupt withdrawal is not desirable for any
medication, and anxiolytic agents are no exception. Sudden withdrawal will
often result in such symptoms as nervousness, anxiety, tremor, and insomnia.

Commonly used anxiolytic agents include diazepam, chlordiazepoxide,
chlorazepam, alprazolam, triazolam and hydroxyzine (see Table 4).

Anticholinergic Problems

Medications with high anticholinergic properties such as antiparkinsonian
agents, thioridazine, and amitriptyline occasionally lead to an anticholinergic psychosis (delerium). The use of multiple medications increases the probability of the reaction. This will be associated with the signs and symptoms
of atropine ingestion, including mild temperature elevation; flushed, warm
skin; increased heart rate; decreased sweating; mydriasis; and an acute brain
syndrome. It is important that this be recognized early, since increasing the
dosage of the offending agents will increase the severity of the psychosis.
Treatment with intramuscular or intravenous physostigmine (1 mg) is recommended, if necessary, for the patient's well being and/or survival (Burks et
al., 1974; El-Yusef et al., 1973). Reversal is rapid (in minutes). Only physostigmine will cross the blood-brain barrier; neostigmine will simply produce
symptoms of peripheral cholinergic action. Methscopolamine (0.5-1.0 mg
intramuscularly) can be used to block the peripheral effects of physostigmine to help avoid respiratory problems, if necessary.

Summary

Four primary types of medications are useful in the treatment of psychiatric
disease or sustained emotional upsets in patients with COPD:

Table 4 Anxiolytic Agents (Minor Tranquilizers or Sedative Hypnotics)[a]

Specific medication	Special properties	Usual daily dosage	Daily dosage in moderate to severe COPD
Benzodiazepines			
Chlordiazepoxide HCL (Librium)	May be drug of choice in alcohol withdrawal. Poor absorption by intramuscular route	Oral: 10-20 mg IV: for treatment of acute reactions including seizures and delirium tremens: 0.5 mg/kg at rate of 5 mg/min to total dose of 50 mg every 4-6 h	Oral: 10-100 mg IV: one-half the usual dose
Diazepam (Valium)	Good muscle relaxant. Poor absorption by intramuscular route	Oral: 5-50 mg IV: For treatment of acute reactions including seizures and delirium tremens: 0.1 mg/kg at a rate of 1 mg/min to a total dose of 5-10 mg every 4- 6 h	Oral: 5-50 mg IV: one-half the

Table 4 (continued)

Specific medication	Special properties	Usual daily dosage	Daily dosage in moderate to severe COPD
Chlorazepate dipotassium (Tranxene)	Antiseizure agent	Oral: 3.75-45 mg	Oral: 3.75-15 mg
Alprazolam (Xanax)	Often recognized as the medication of choice in panic attacks and similar conditions. Also noted by some to have antidepressant properties (see above)	Oral: 0.25-4.0 mg	Oral: 0.125-2.0 mg
Triazolam (Halcion)	Short half life: approximately 2.5 hr. Usually well-tolerated sleep medication. Can be utilized in low doses as a temporary treatment for anxiety (0.0625-0.125 mg) with low risk of sedation. Has reportedly been given in a dose of 0.125 mg daily for up to a year without producing habituation.	Oral: 0.125-0.5 mg	Oral: 0.0625-0.25 mg

[a]Barbiturates produce unacceptable central nervous system depression, sedation, dependency, and addiction risk and have a low safety margin compared to the medications listed above, with the exception of meprobamate. For all anxiolytics listed, drowsiness or lack of attention may make operation of machinery dangerous, particularly during initial treatment. Selected patients may need the usual daily dose. Respiratory depression with aggravation or onset of hypoxia and hypercarbia is always a possible complication when the anxiolytic agents are used in the COPD population.

In selected patients with high anxiety levels, there may be no effect on respiratory drive, sedation, or habituation and the primary effects may be symptom reducing and life saving.

Common side effects	Precautions with	Contraindications
Drowsiness	Glaucoma	Hypersensitivity
Ataxia	Anticoagulants	Porphyria (do not use meprobamate)
Confusion	Renal impairment	Comatose states
Slurred speech	Respiratory depression	Severe dependency or addiction
Headache	Hepatic impairment	
Dizziness	Pregnancy	
Impaired visual accommodation	Withdraw slowly when used long term to avoid problems such as convulsions	
Dependency	Breast-feeding mothers: medication may be transferred via milk	
Dry mouth	May occasionally produce paradoxical rage, anxiety, or depression	
Potential difficulty handling secretions		

Table 5 Receptor Blocking Properties of Selected Neuroleptics

	D-2 (Haloperidol)	Cholinergic (Atropine)	H-1 (Diphenhydramine)	Alpha-1 (Prazosin)	Alpha-2 (Yohimbine)
Thiothixene	8.88	0.00081	2.5373	0.00827	0.0081
Haloperidol	1.00	0.00010	0.0079	0.01455	0.0004
Chlorpromazine	0.21	0.03333	1.6418	0.03455	0.0021
Thioridazine	0.14	0.1333	0.9254	0.18182	0.0019
Molindone	0.03	0.00001	0.0001	0.00004	0.0026
Haloperidol	1				
Atropine		1			
D-Chlorpheniramine			1		
Prazosin		0.1		1	
Yohimbine		8.0			1

Figures represent the number of mg of the reference blocking agent effect represented by 1 mg of the psychotropic agent. For example: 1 mg of thiothixene = 8.88 mg of haloperidol in terms of D-2 blocking effect, 0.00081 mg of atropine in terms of anticholinergic effect, 2.54 mg of diphenhydramine in terms of H-1 blocking effect, 0.008 mg of prazosin in terms of alpha-1 blocking effect, and 0.008 mg of phentolamine in terms of alpha-2 blocking effect. Receptors are cellular recognition sites for neurotransmitters and neurotransmitter blockers. They are generally membrane-bound proteins on the outside of the cell and have the ability to recognize specific molecular structures. The names of the receptor recognition sites are usually related to the function of the site. For example, D-1 and D-2 are recognition sites for dopamine. The D-2 site seems to be the one that when blocked decreases psychotic activity. Histamine recognition sites are called H-1 and H-2 sites. The antihistamine action of diphenhydramine and d-chlorpheniramine is secondary to their ability to block H-1 cellular recognition sites. Similarly, there are two subclassifications of alpha-adrenergic receptors called alpha-1 and alpha-2 sites, found in both the central and peripheral nervous system. These play important roles in the regulation of blood pressure. Blocking alpha-1 recognition sites lower blood pressure, while blocking alpha-2 recognition sites increases blood pressure.
Source: Richelson, 1985; and Richelson, E., personal communication.

Table 6 Receptor Blocking Characteristics of Four Psychotropic Medications

	D-2 (Haloperidol)	Cholinergic (Atropine)	H-1 (Diphenhydramine)	Alpha-1 (Prazosin)
Thiothixene	888.0	0.08	254	0.8
Haloperidol	100.0	0.01	1	1.5
Doxepin	0.2	2.30	77,500	0.3
Amitriptyline	0.4	10.00	19,250	0.2

Figures represent the approximate number of mg of the reference blocking agent effect represented by 100 mg of psychotropic agent. For example: 100 mg of thiothixene = 888 mg of haloperidol in terms of D-2 blocking, 0.08 mg of atropine in terms of anticholinergic effect, 254 mg of diphenhydramine in terms of H-1 blocking effect, and 0.8 mg of prazosin in terms of alpha-1 blocking effect.
Source: Richelson, 1982/83, 1985; and Richelson, E., personal communication.

1. Neuroleptics, previously called major tranquilizers or antipsychotic agents. They are used in the treatment of diseases such as schizophrenia, mania, acute psychotic reactions, and, in some cases, delirium and dementia.

2. The heterocyclic antidepressants, previously called tricyclic antidepressants, before the introduction of molecular structures that were not tricyclic in origin. They are used in the treatment of depressive disease whether bipolar or unipolar, recurring or single episodes.

3. Medications for the control of swings in mood from depression to mania, from depression to a normal mood or from mania to a normal mood. The only medication in this group recognized in the past was lithium carbonate. Increasing evidence indicates that there is a role for carbamazepine, lecithin, valproic acid, and other compounds.

4. Anxiolytic agents. These medications can be used for control of anxiety in conjunction with the use of any of the above compounds. They vary from medications used to treat panic, seizures, and anxiety, or to induce sleep. They are safe, if not abused. In general, by themselves, they have little effect on major psychiatric problems and, in this group of patients, should be used as an adjunct to the primary neuroleptic, antidepressant, or medication for mood control. They

Table 7 Receptor Blocking Properties of Selected Antidepressants

	H-1 (Diphenhydramine)	Cholinergic (Atropine)	Alpha-1 (Prozosin)	Alpha-2 (Phentolamine)	Serotonin (Methysergide)	D-2 (Haloperidol)
Doxepin	775.0	0.02708	0.00257	0.040	0.067	0.002
Triimipramine	250.0	0.03542	0.00256	0.065	0.049	0.025
Amitriptyline	192.5	0.11458	0.00236	0.050	0.067	0.004
Maprotiline	25.0	0.00416	0.00067	0.005	?	?
Amoxapine	2.8	0.00208	0.00122	0.017	?	0.028
Nortriptyline	3.5	0.01458	0.00098	0.017	0.042	?
Imipramine	2.5	0.02292	0.00067	0.014	0.015	0.002
Protriptyline	0.7	0.08333	0.00050	0.007	0.014	0.002
Trazodone	0.4	0.00001	0.00171	0.087	?	0.001
Desipramine	0.1	0.01042	0.00045	0.006	0.005	0.001
Diphenhydramine	1					
Atropine		1				
Protozin			1			
Phentolamine				1		
Methysergide					1	
Haloperidol						1

Figures represent the approximate number of mg of the reference blocking agent effect represented by 1 mg of the psychotropic agent. These data may vary with differing studies.
Source: Richelson, 1982/83, 1985; and Richelson, E., personal communication.

are most useful in the person who is acutely or chronically emotionally upset.

With the availability of receptor blocking profiles (Tables 5-7) for many of these agents the clinician can look up a particular medication and estimate its amount of specific receptor blocking characteristic. For example, if there is worry about anticholinergic effect it is possible to find out how much of this characteristic the medication has in comparison with atropine, a familiar blocking agent. This is an area of medicine with a number of imponderable questions, but the information is of undoubted use to the clinician.

References

American Psychiatric Association (1987). *Diagnostic and Statistical Manual of Mental Disorders: Third Edition-Revised.* Washington, D.C., The American Psychiatric Association.

Beck, A. T., Ward, C. H., Mendelson, M., Mock, J., and Erbaugh, J. (1961). An inventory for measuring depression. *Arch. Gen. Psychiatry* 4: ɔ61-571.

Burks, J. S., Walter, J. E., and Rumach, B. H. (1974). Tricyclic antidepressant poisoning. *JAMA* 230:1405-1407.

deAraujo, G., Dudley, D. L., and Van Arsdel, P. P., Jr. (1972). Psychosocial assets and severity of chronic asthma. *J. Allergy Immunol.* 50:257-263.

deAraujo, G., Van Arsdel, P. P., Jr., Holmes, T. H., and Dudley, D. L. (1973). Life changes, coping ability and chronic intrinsic asthma. *J. Psychosom. Res.* 17:359-363.

Diagnostic and Statistical Manual of Mental Disorders: Third Edition (DSM-IIIs). American Psychiatric Association (1980). Washington, D.C., The American Psychiatric Association.

Dudley, D. L., and Pattison, E. M. (1969). Group psychotherapy in patients with severe diffuse obstructive pulmonary syndrome. *Am. Rev. Respir. Dis.* 100:575-576.

Dudley, D. L., and Pitts-Poarch, A. R. (1980). Psychophysiologic concepts of respiratory control. *Clin. Chest Med.* 1:131-143.

Dudley, D. L., and Sitzman, J. (1979). Psychosocial and psychophysiologic approach to the patient. *Semin. Respir. Med.* 1:59-83.

Dudley, D. L., and Welka, E. (1977). *How to Survive Being Alive.* New York, Doubleday.

Dudley, D. L., Holmes, T. H., Martin, C. J., and Ripley, H. A. (1964a). Changes in respiration associated with hypnotically induced emotion, pain and exercise. *Psychosom. Med.* 26:46-57.

Dudley, D. L., Martin, C. J., and Holmes, T. H. (1964b). Psychophysiologic studies of pulmonary ventilation. *Psychosom. Med.* **26**:645-660.

Dudley, D. L., Martin, C. J., and Holmes, T. H. (1968). Dyspnea: Psychologic and physiologic observations. *J. Psychosom. Res.* **11**:325-339.

Dudley, D. L., Martin, C. J., Masuda, M., Ripley, H. S., and Holmes, T. H. (1969a). *The Psychophysiology of Respiration in Health and Disease.* New York, Appleton-Century-Crofts.

Dudley, D. L., Verhey, J. W., Masuda, M., Martin, C. J., and Holmes, T. H. (1969b). Long term adjustment, prognosis and death in irreversible diffuse obstructive pulmonary syndromes. *Psychosom. Med.* **91**:310-325.

Dudley, D. L., Aickin, M., and Martin, C. J. (1977). Cigarette smoking in a chest clinic population—psychophysiologic variables. *J. Psychosom. Res.* **21**:367-375.

Dudley, D. L., Glaser, E. M., Jorgenson, B., and Logan, D. L. (1980a). Psychosocial concomitants to rehabilitation in chronic obstructive pulmonary disease. Part I: The psychosocial and psychophysiologic format. *Chest* **77**:413-420.

Dudley, D. L., Glaser, E. M., Jorgenson, B., and Logan, D. L. (1980b). Psychosocial concomitants to rehabilitation in chronic obstructive pulmonary disease. Part II: The psychosocial and psychophysiologic treatment. *Chest* **77**:544-551.

Dudley, D. L., Glaser, E. M., Jorgenson, B., and Logan, D. L. (1980c). Psychosocial concomitants to rehabilitation in chronic obstructive pulmonary disease. Part III: Dealing with psychiatric disease. *Chest* **77**:413-420.

Dudley, D. L., Sitzman, J., and Rugg, M. (1985). Psychiatric aspects of patients with chronic obstructive pulmonary disease. *Adv. Psychosom. Med.* **14**:64-77.

El-Yousef, K. M., Janowsky, D. S., and Davis, H. M. (1973). Reversal of anti-parkinsonian drug toxicity by physostigmine: a controlled study. *Am. J. Psychiatry* **130**:141-145.

Knapp, M. L. (1972). *Nonverbal Communication in Human Interaction.* New York, Holt, Rinehart and Winston, Inc.

Knapp, P. H., Mathe, A. A., and Vachon, L. (1976). Psychosomatic aspects of bronchial asthma. In *Bronchial Asthma-Mechanisms and Therapeutics.* Edited by E. B. Reiss and M. Segal. Boston, Little, Brown.

Pattison, E. M., Rhodes, R. J., and Dudley, D. L. (1971). Response to group treatment in patients with severe chronic lung disease. *Int. J. Group Psychother.* **21**:214-225.

Petrich, J., and Holmes, T. H. (1977). Life change and illness onset. *Med. Clin. North Am.* **61**:825-838.

Richelson, E. (1985). Pharmacology of neuroleptics in use in the United States. *J. Clin. Psychiatry* **46**:8-14.

Richelson, E. (1982/83). Pharmacology of antidepressants in use in the United United States. *J. Clin. Psychiatry* **43**:4-11, **44**:4-9.

Steen, S. N. (1976). The effects of psychotropic drugs on respiration. *Pharmacol. Ther.* **2**:717-741.

Wyler, A. R., Masuda, M., and Holmes, T. H. (1970). The seriousness of illness rating scale reproducibility. *J. Psychosom. Res.* **14**:59-64.

Wyler, A. R., Masuda, M., and Holmes, T. H. (1971). Magnitude of life events and seriousness of illness. *Psychosom. Med.* **33**:115-122.

Zung, W. W. (1965). A self-rating depression scale. *Arch. Gen. Psychiatry* **12**:63-70.

10

Nursing Care of Patients with COPD: A Sociobiological Perspective

MARCIA A. KOPACZ*

Henry Ford Hospital
Detroit, Michigan

I. Introduction

The focus of this chapter is to provide a basis for the nursing care of persons with chronic stable obstructive pulmonary disease (COPD). For purposes of this discussion, the spectrum of diseases included within the classification of COPD includes emphysema, chronic bronchitis and intrinsic adult-onset asthma. An in-depth discussion of the patient care problems associated with COPD and the nursing interventions designed to ameliorate the severity of the symptoms and/or assist the patient and family to cope with the chronic nature of these diseases is provided. A brief review of the pathophysiology of COPD, selected psychosocial factors, nursing diagnosis concepts, and self-care issues is presented.

Present affiliation: Oakland General Hospital, Madison Heights, Michigan

II. Review of Systems Involvement

Patients with COPD are complex in part because the pulmonary physiological
aberrations are multiple and varied among persons with the same diagnosis.
Furthermore, COPD affects more than the lungs. The direct and indirect effects of the pulmonary pathology coupled with the potential iatrogenic effects
of the ensuing treatment regimen result in multiple somatic complaints. These
produce stress not only on the patient's physiological reserves but also on his
or her psychosocial supports and skills. The challenge to nursing is to assist
the patient and his or her family to live within the psychophysiologic limitations of this slowly progressive disease.

A. Respiratory Dysfunction

The cluster of diseases included within the spectrum of chronic obstructive
lung disease are characterized by expiratory airflow obstruction. A detailed
description of the pulmonary pathology is found in Chapter 1. The major
physiological findings are summarized in Table 1. Emphysematous changes
are the least reversible because they involve permanent parenchymal and
alveolar changes. Loss of tractional support from the parenchymal structures results in premature airway closure with expiration. Alveolar destruction reduces the surface area available for gas exchange. These destructive
changes make treatment measures in patients with primarily emphysema
less efficacious than for those with chronic bronchitis or asthma.

Chronic bronchitis causes chronic airway narrowing due to edema and
mucus hypersecretion. Furthermore, the chronic bronchitic with a smoking
history produces mucus that is thicker and more tenacious than that of the
nonsmoker due to actual structural changes in the mucus-producing cells
lining the airways. Chronic productive cough is the hallmark of chronic
bronchitis. Mucociliary clearance is less effective because of (1) loss of elastic recoil of the alveoli, (2) reduced conductance of the upstream airways,
and (3) reduced caliber of the airways due to inflammation and thickened
bronchial mucosa. Chronic mucus retention in turn serves as a focus for bacterial infection that further aggravates the sensation of shortness of breath.

Chronic asthma presents with a picture of intermittent airway plugging
and smooth muscle spasm. Smooth muscle hyperactivity results in intermittent episodes of wheezing and shortness of breath. While there is generally
little relation to ectopy, some factors suggested to precipitate or aggravate
bronchospasm include infection, exercise, smoke, cold air, pollution, overuse of medications, and emotions. In marked contrast to the person with

Table 1 Causes of Airflow Obstruction in COPD

Sources	Emphysema	Chronic bronchitis	Asthma
↓ Tractional support	+++	–	–
Alveolar	+++	–	–
Bronchial atrophy	++	?	–
Bronchial obliteration	+	++	–
Airway edema	–	Chronic +++	Intermittent ++
Mucus hypersecretion with plugging	–	Chronic +++	Intermittent ++
Smooth muscle spasm	–	–	Intermittent +++

either emphysema or chronic bronchitis, the patient with chronic intrinsic asthma may initially feel normal between acute exacerbations. If the disease persists and progresses, the frequency and severity of acute symptoms increase with a reduction in the symptomless periods. This results in a picture of more persistent airway obstruction.

For all three disease types, the most common presentation is that of an overlap syndrome with symptomatic features of two or more disease processes. The most important factor is to determine which are the clinically predominating and/or acutely exacerbated clinical features about which the patient is currently complaining.

Airway obstruction, whatever the mechanism, results in increased work of breathing (WOB) for COPD patients. WOB refers to the amount of energy utilized by the body for the purpose of breathing. In healthy individuals this is approximately 3% of the total energy expenditure. In persons with COPD the work of breathing at rest and with exercise is increased as both inspiration and expiration become more labored requiring more accessory muscle use. Thus, more oxygen and muscle energy are required for even quiet breathing. In times of acute exacerbation it is easy to understand how simple actions such as talking, eating, bathing, and other basic daily tasks may be beyond the capabilities of the patient with COPD.

Dyspnea or shortness of breath (SOB) is a subjective state that cannot be defined in terms of arterial blood gas or pulmonary function test abnor-

malities. The genesis of SOB is poorly understood. The degree of SOB is
generally unrelated to the amount of physical activity performed. The unpre-
dictability of the degree of SOB that COPD patients can experience from
minute to minute causes disruption of routine activities of daily living (ADL)
and an inability to plan for the immediate and the more distant future. A
regimented work routine becomes increasingly difficult to maintain. This
difficulty is a major factor in the establishment of COPD as the second most
frequent cause of Social Security disability grants in the United States.

B. Cardiovascular Dysfunction

An indepth discussion of the major cardiac changes observed in patients with
COPD is beyond the scope of this chapter. A brief synopsis is provided below,
which will serve as a basis for nursing interventions.

Alterations of Cardiac Rhythm

Cardiac arrhythmias of many types are common among COPD patients. The
major causative factors associated with dysrhythmia in COPD include hypoxemia, acidosis/alkalosis, electrolyte imbalance, underlying cardiac disease, pulmonary hypertension, drugs, and ventilators. The mechanism therefore can
be (1) hemodynamic (e.g., loss of vagal restraint secondary to potassium de-
pletion, ventilators, etc.), (2) metabolic (changes in acid/base level of the
blood), or (3) drug-induced (diuretics, antihypertensives, bronchodilators, etc.).
The site of cardiac malfunction with COPD is generally the right ventricle. Chronic hypoxemia results in pulmonary vasoconstriction requiring increased right-sided pressure to circulate the blood through the pulmonary
vasculature. This produces excessive strain on the right ventricle as it attempts
to pump against greater resistance. Acid/base disturbances alter cardiac muscle irritability. Studies have found that atrial arrhythmias are more frequent
among COPD patients than those with coronary artery disease. The incidence
of ventricular dysrhythmia is similar in both groups (Kleiger and Senior, 1974).
Flick and Block (1979) studied nocturnal versus diurinal cardiac arrhythmias among COPD patients and found that 9 of the 10 subjects were desaturated on room air and had chronic arrhythmias. The authors noted that the incidence of PVCs doubled during sleep. In general, arrhythmias, especially ventricular arrhythmias, have been associated with a rather poor prognosis.

Alterations of Pump Function

Chronic hypoxemia, as previously noted, produces pulmonary vasoconstriction that leads to cor pulmonale and congestive heart failure (CHF). Dysrhyth-

Table 2 Clinical Features of Emphysema (Pink Puffers) and Chronic Bronchitis (Blue Bloaters)

Clinical features	Pink puffer	Blue bloater
History of congestive heart failure	Late in course	Frequent
Secondary polycythemia	Absent	Frequent
PO_2 (chronic stable level	WNL	Low
CO_2 (chronic stable level)	WNL	High
Major complaints	↑↑↑ ↓↓↓	Cough, sputum, fluid retention ↑ Dyspnea ↓ Activity tolerance
Clinical course	Progressively ↑ dyspnea ↓ activity tolerance. Alterations of ABGs and onset of CHF near terminal events	Recurrent infection and respiratory failure with gradually worsening ABGs and cardiac function

mias produce additional pump function compromise. Other factors increasing the COPD patient's risk for CHF include acid/base disturbances, underlying cardiac disease, systemic hypertension, and pulmonary embolus.

The onset of the first acute episode of CHF has varying degrees of significance for patients with COPD. The concept of "pink puffers" and "blue bloaters" was developed in part to explain this difference. As described in Table 2, patients with primarily chronic bronchitis, "blue bloaters," generally have documented chronic hypoxemia, hypercarbia, and CHF earlier in the course of their disease than patients with emphysema. The emphysematous patient, the "pink puffer," fights by increasing his or her minute ventilation to maintain near-normal oxygen and carbon dioxide levels. The development of overt CHF is later in the course of his or her disease and has an associated poor prognosis. Burrows in his classic article, "The Course and Prognosis of Chronic Obstructive Lung Disease," found that the most important variables affecting survival at 3 or 5 years when considered in conjunction with FEV 1.0 were resting heart rate, the physician's assessment of severity of disease and the history of edema (Burrows and Earle, 1969).

The onset of cor pulmonale with or without overt CHF in the chronic asthmatic generally signifies an increase in underlying irreversible airways disease. As the disease progresses to its more chronic form the risk for cardiac failure increases due to the same factors affecting cardiac function as in patients with chronic bronchitis and emphysema.

Alterations of Peripheral Vascular Function

Secondary polycythemia (increased red blood cell concentration) is a reflex response of the body to hypoxemia. This can be observed in healthy individuals who live in high altitudes as well as in patients with chronic hypoxemic lung disease. The purpose of this compensatory reflex is to improve oxygen transport by increasing the number of red blood cells and thus hemoglobin attachment sites available for oxygen binding. The resultant increased blood viscosity, however, can impinge on cardiac pump function by increasing the amount of pressure required to circulate the cardiac output. The role of phlebotomy (venous puncture) is unclear. Some investigators have found that periodic venesection can improve cardiac function and activity tolerance. The duration of benefit is uncertain (Chetty et al., 1983).

Pulmonary embolus (PE) has been noted at autopsy in 38-51% of patients with COPD. The frequency of nonfatal PE is unknown because of the difficulty in establishing the diagnosis when COPD is present. Deep vein thrombosis (DVT) of the lower extremities produce 87-90% of the PE (Prescott et al., 1981). The sources of risk among COPD patients for DVT and PE are not well defined. Some investigators attribute it to inactivity and cor pulmonale (Lippmann and Fein, 1981). The role of polycythemia is controversial (Lippmann and Fein, 1981; Prescott et al., 1981; Moser, 1977). Other variables that increase the susceptibility to DVT and ensuing PE among COPD patients include dysrhythmia, injuries of blood vessel walls, and age.

C. Gastrointestinal Dysfunction

Gastrointestinal complaints may be among the most bothersome to the COPD patient. Not only is their ability to participate in work and leisure activities limited, but their capacity to enjoy food and the accompanying socialization is also impaired. Inactivity, drug side effects, fluid, and solid intake can affect bowel function and/or produce gastric distress. Further, the risk for ulcer disease is higher among this population.

Alterations of General Nutrition

COPD patients despite their reduced activity level have relatively high caloric needs because of their increased work of breathing. Adequate cellular function depends on balanced nutritional intake, adequate fluids, and gas exchange. Complaints of early satiety and postprandial shortness of breath are common. These can be the result of a combination of factors. Low-lying diaphragms mechanically compromise the gastric space. It therefore takes less food and/or fluids to produce a sense of satiety. As the stomach fills it presses on the diaphragm further inhibiting its movement, thus causing more shortness of breath. Aerophagia or air swallowing as the patient eats and drinks produces abdominal distention, which additionally compromises both diaphragm function and the ability to ingest adequate calories. Thus the subjective discomfort associated with eating reduces the patient's appetite and ability to enjoy eating.

Additional factors that can negatively affect the nutritional efforts of the patient include economic or environmental stresses, other health problems, past eating habits, and mental attitude. Economic and environmental considerations include the cost and ease of procuring and preparing food. The energy costs of meal preparation and clean-up may be prohibitive for the COPD patient. Lack of social supports or a significant other to assist in the procurement and preparation of food or to make mealtimes a pleasant event can be an important problem. Concomitant health problems can have profound effects on the individual's appetite and/or ability to be independent in this self-care activity. Dental disease, reduced visual acuity, additional dietary restrictions, and musculoskeletal limitations are common.

Alterations of Bowel Function

Healthy bowel function depends on three major factors: fluids, solids, and activity. A balance of all three is necessary; alteration of any one factor can result in bowel dysfunction. In general, COPD patients are at risk for deficits in any or all three areas.

As noted in the general nutrition section, early satiety, postprandial (after eating) SOB, and aerophagia can inhibit fluid and/or solid intake. Breathing patterns result in increased insensible water loss. Generalized reduction of activity levels is almost universal. Medications can produce constipation and/or diarrhea. Therefore, complaints of bowel dysfunction among COPD patients are frequent. Determination of the predominant contributing factors is essential for treatment success.

Alterations of Gut Integrity

The incidence of peptic ulcer disease in patients with COPD is estimated
to range between 15 and 37%. Monson (1970) found the risk for comorbidity
of COPD with duodenal ulcers to be significantly higher than for other chronic
disease combinations. The mechanism for these associations is unclear. Genetic
predisposition has been found to be significant in two subgroups, patients with
alpha 1 antitrypsin deficiency and the ABH antigen nonsecretors. It is theo-
rized that these patients have less enzyme activity to protect the epithelial
tissue in the lungs and portions of the gut (Cohen et al., 1980). Other epidemiologic factors that increase the risk for ulcers in COPD patients include age,
smoking history, sex, concomitant cardiovascular disease, and multiple drug
therapy.

The comorbidity of peptic ulcer disease with COPD has grave significance with regards to mortality. Bonnevie (1977) reported higher death rates
among persons with COPD and ulcer disease than in patient populations with
other combinations of chronic disease. In ambulatory and hospitalized patients, investigators have noted a death rate five times higher than predicted
if COPD and peptic ulcer disease coexist (Sleisenger and Fordtran, 1983).

D. Musculoskeletal Dysfunction

Shortness of breath on exertion (SOBOE) or complaints of easy fatigability
are often the first symptoms reported. The diminution in activity tolerance
is so gradual and insidious that, by the time professional help is sought, significant airways disease is present. Inefficient respiratory muscle function contributes significantly to these symptoms. Nocturnal leg cramps are another
frequent complaint of COPD patients.

Alterations of Respiratory Muscle Function

As we discussed in the section on pulmonary function, COPD patients typically have an altered breathing pattern related to inefficient use of the respiratory muscles. The lungs are expanded and contracted two ways. The downward and upward movement of the diaphragm rhythmically increases and decreases the longitudinal length of the chest cavity. In health, diaphragmatic
movement produces 75% of the air volume change during quiet inspiration.
The other major inspiratory muscle group is the external intercostals. The
primary expiratory muscles are the internal intercostals and the abdominals.
Expiration, in contrast to inspiration, is primarily a passive event requiring
negligible amounts of muscle work. Accessory muscles of respiration include

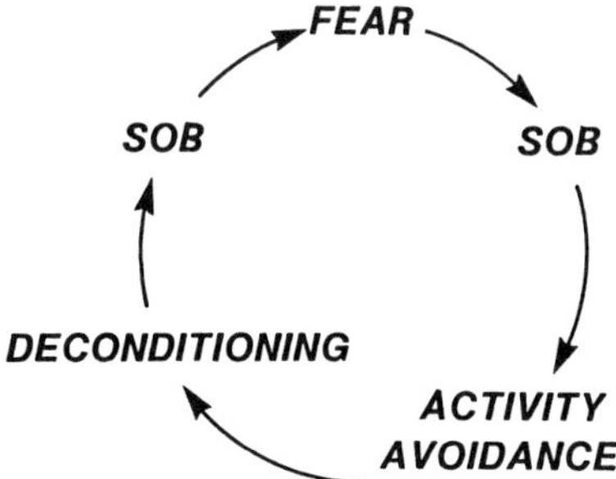

Figure 1. Deconditioning cycle.

the sternocleidomastoids, scapulae elevators, anterior and posterior serrati, scalene, and the erectus muscles of the spine.

COPD patients with significant amounts of air trapping have enlarged lungs that mechanically reduce diaphragm movement and efficiency. Increased accessory muscle use is an almost reflexive response to SOB. The patient attempts to move greater volumes of air, but unfortunately, any increments in volume are exceeded by the marked increase in energy costs associated with the breathing pattern.

Impaired Activity Tolerance

SOB is a frightening and uncomfortable sensation. Patients learn anecdotally that by avoiding certain activities they can minimize their discomfort. This starts the cycle of activity avoidance with ensuing muscle deconditioning as illustrated in Figure 1. The fear of SOB, almost universal among COPD patients, can be more debilitating than the decline in measured pulmonary function or gas exchange capabilities. In an effort to prevent the onset of acute SOB, there is a general reduction in activity. Inactivity causes muscular deconditioning. Deconditioned muscles have higher oxygen requirements than conditioned ones. The COPD patient with impaired gas exchange has great difficulty meeting the additional demands of activity. Haas and Cardon (1969) reported that with selected exercises, COPD patients took longer to reach an oxygen steady state, the ensuing oxygen debt was larger, and recovery slower than in a matched control group. Thus routine ADL becomes inordinately difficult and unpleasant. The avoidance response results in a smaller and smaller life space for the patient. Life holds few pleasures; the only positive reward is less shortness of breath. This cycle is very difficult to break. It can be interrupted only by concerted action usually involving strong patient motivation and professional guidance.

Motor Muscle Dysfunction

Deconditioning not only reduces the efficiency of the motor muscle groups
but also produces alterations in comfort. Nocturnal leg cramps are a recurrent
complaint of the COPD patient. Primary causative factors include disuse,
muscle tendon shortening, and electrolyte imbalance.

E. Neuropsychological Dysfunction

Until recently there has been a relative dearth of knowledge regarding the long-
term effects of COPD on neuropsychological function. This subject is reviewed
in detail in the chapter by Prigatano and Grant.

Alterations in Brain Function

Grant et al. (1980) studies the effects of chronic hypoxemia on patients with
moderate to severe COPD. The findings suggest that these patients have reduced
abstracting ability and diminution of complex perceptual motor integrative abilities. Deficits in the more simple motor skills and attention span were also
noted while language and memory were largely intact.

Alterations of Sleep/Wake Cycle

Sleep/wake cycle disturbances have been reported by patients and/or their families (McSweeny et al., 1982). The cause of this complaint is unclear. Contributing factors may include reduced activity levels, anxiety, medications, and
frequent daytime napping producing nocturnal wakefulness.

F. Psychosocial Dysfunction

The complex interplay of psychosocial factors and the physiological changes
associated with COPD has resulted in increased research and interest in the behavioral aspect of these diseases. An in-depth discussion of relevant psychosocial issues can be found in chapter by McSweeny. A brief overview follows.

Behavioral Dysfunction

Dirks and his colleagues (1977, 1978a,b) have developed a wealth of information regarding asthmatics using the Minnesota Multiphasic Personality inventory (MMPI) and the Asthma Symptom Checklist (ASC). The MMPI panic-
fear scale measures a stable character trait unaffected by the disease or treatment. The ASC measures a state response affected by the duration, plus sever-

ity of the disease and the ensuing treatment regimen. The MMPI suggests that asthmatics are generally more fearful, dependent, emotionally labile, and experience more feelings of helplessness than norms. Three ranges of the panic-fear trait have been identified. Patients with a high score on the panic-fear scale of the MMPI exhibit "symptom exaggeration" and helplessness, which result in the use of more medications, longer hospital stays, and higher rehospitalization rates. Patients who score in the moderate range maintain an attitude of "symptom vigilance" that fosters prompt treatment of symptoms and adherence to the therapeutic regimen. At the other extreme, those who have low MMPI panic-fear scores utilized a "symptom minimization" approach to their disease and treatment. Undertreatment secondary to symptom denial may ensue. Rehospitalization is frequent because of symptom neglect. Dirks suggests that treatment focus should be different for each group. Patients with high panic-fear scores need to be assisted to develop coping mechanisms that promote feelings of independence and personal control. Those who use symptom minimization as their primary coping technique need assistance in accepting adherence to their therapeutic regimen as an independent strategy. Individuals in the moderate range need to be encouraged in their efforts to maintain appropriate levels of symptom vigilance and compliance with the treatment plan. Interestingly, additional relationships between patients' MMPI scores, the use of steroids, and the physician's judgment of illness severity have been noted. Those patients with high scores on the MMPI panic-fear scales were judged to be most ill and received more prednisone than the other two groups (Dirks et al., (1978a,b).

The ASC is hypothesized to measure "signal anxiety," which is described as a personal warning identifying impending danger and the need for protective measures. Dirks and his colleagues suggested that patients can be taught to use signal anxiety responses to generate purposeful constructive plans and adaptive measures (Dirks et al., 1978).

Dr. Dudley describes his research on the psychophysiology of COPD in his chapter. His theoretical approach is based on the assumption that physiological changes have psychosocial inputs and results. The theory that the more psychosocial assets an individual possesses the better he or she will be able to cope with the limitations of chronic disease and rehospitalization has been supported by many investigators (Pearlin and Schooler, 1978; Post and Collins, 1981-1982; Dudley et al., 1980a,b). Dudley delineates three categories of psychosocial assets, suggesting that individuals with broader experiences may be better able to cope with situational changes because they

have more available options (Dudley and Pitts-Poarch, 1980). Isolation, denial, and regression were found to be the classic defense mechanisms of the
COPD patient. These withdrawal strategies produce an "emotional straight
jacket," which results in an existence in a "constricted living space" as the
patient tries to avoid the SOB associated with either positive or negative
states of emotional arousal (Dudley et al., 1980a,b).

The recently completed Nocturnal Oxygen Therapy Trial (NOTT) results support many of the findings of Dirks and Dudley. The chapter by
McSweeny presents a cogent description of these trial results. Specifically,
McSweeny and his colleagues again found depression to be the major emotional disturbance. The lack of reported anger supports Dudley's theory
of emotional arousal avoidance. Age, socioeconomic status, and neuropsychological function affected life quality more than objective measures of disease
severity. McSweeny describes four dimensions of life quality: emotional
functioning, social role functioning, behavioral functioning, and the ability
to enjoy hobbies and recreation. The NOTT results provide some preliminary
quantitative and qualitative data regarding the effect of COPD on these life
quality dimensions. A 40-50% reduction in pleasurable activities was reported.
Difficulties with home management activities and reductions in social interaction were the primary social-role deficits. Problems with ambulation, alterations
of sleep/rest cycle, and interference with recreational pastime were also reported (McSweeny et al., 1980, 1982).

Post and Collins (1981-1982) propose that the cause and maladaptive behavior may be related to the patient's inability to mourn his or her losses successfully. A major obstacle confronted by the COPD patient is the continuing
decline in function, which requires continual readjustment to losses. Successful adaption of the patient's expectations and goals is extremely difficult. They
suggest that interventions should focus on (1) facilitating acceptance of loss
and restructuring life goals; (2) interrupting the cycle of alienation and social
withdrawal; and (3) increasing the patient's sense of control.

An infrequently studied aspect of emotional role functioning is sexual
activity. Fletcher and Martin (1982) studied sexual dysfunction in men and
found that it worsened as pulmonary function declined and that COPD may
be associated with male impotence. Additional contributing factors to sexual
dysfunction include information deficits, medications, poor physical or mental
health (Stockdale-Woolley, 1983), internalization of society's pressures, anxiety, boredom, fatigue, and fear (Stanford, 1977).

Vocational Activity Dysfunction

A job has many implications symbolically and practically. It is often "a measure of the individual's perceived worth" and thus affects his or her self-esteem and self-image. The economic effects of unemployment or underemployment can be devastating. Financial stress, superimposed on an individual or family network already strained by the physical and emotional burdens imposed by COPD, can be overwhelming. Role shifts within the family are a frequent result adding more psychosocial stress. Research in the area of vocational rehabilitation for COPD patients has been limited. Dyksterhuis's (1972) research suggests that the vocational rehabilitation potential is greatest when the patient is first confronted with a need to change his or her life-style. Patients generally respond better to vocational rehabilitation efforts if they are still marginally employed rather than unemployed. Dyksterhuis further suggested that vocational rehabilitation efforts that can be incorporated into on-the-job training programs may be more effective in initiating career renewal efforts. Objective measures identified as contraindications for inclusion in vocational rehabilitation programs were a pulmonary artery perfusion scan classification of 4±, an FEV 1.0 less than 50%, or the presence of moderate to marked right heart failure (Dyksterhuis, 1972).

Kass et al. (1975) support and add to these findings. They found the independent variables most highly correlated with vocational rehabilitation success potential in addition to an FEV 1.0 greater than 50% were an FEF 25-75 greater than 27% and MVV greater than 40%. Additional research by Kass and his colleagues suggest that IQ scores coupled with FEV 1.0 have a 90% degree of accuracy in predicting vocational rehabilitation success (Daughton et al., 1979). Most investigators concur that the success rate is greater among patients who (1) are still working, (2) well enough to keep working, and (3) have an economic incentive to keep working.

Compliant Behavior Dysfunction

Introduction

Compliant or noncompliant patient behaviors represent a major focus of research in all areas of health care. Compliance or adherence are expressions used to describe the extent to which individuals follow the recommendations of health professionals. As the focus of long-term treatment shifts from hospital-based to community-based care, there is a concomitant increase in the patient's responsibility in self-management. Thus, compliance becomes an even more important issue. A brief synopsis of selected research on patient compliance follows.

Selected Review of the Literature

Though little compliance research has actually been conducted using COPD patients, studies in other areas have potential implications. Many factors have been suggested as potential determinants of compliance. These include demographic variables, sociobehavioral characteristics, situational factors in the patient's life, the nature of the illness, treatment regimen characteristics, and the quality of interaction between the patient and health care provider (Haynes, 1976). Results have been conflicting regarding the relative importance of these factors. There is general agreement that demographic factors are the least reliable predictors and that there is no specific personality type associated with noncompliance (Blackwell, 1973). Kinsman and co-workers (1980) found that asthmatic patients who were noncompliant with as needed (PRN) medications did differ in some psychological dimensions relating to personality. Factors found to be more predictive are the nature of the illness and treatment regimen (Stone, 1979; Charney, 1972) and the complexity and degree of behavior change required by the treatment regimen (Hulka et al., 1976; Davis and Eichhorn, 1963; McAlister et al., (1976). Preliminary research findings regarding the relationship between the patient's beliefs, attitudes, and compliance have been promising. Marston (1970) reported patient attitudes as one of the major determinants of compliance. There is also evidence suggesting that patients who perceive themselves as having an "internal focus of control" are more likely to seek information about health status (Wallston et al., 1976), follow advice for self-care (Kirscht and Rosenstock, 1979), and increase behavioral commitment and adherence (Collins and Hoyt, 1972; Rodin and Janis, 1979; Lazarus, 1966; Seligman, 1975). As indicated in the psychosocial section, social support is viewed as enhancing self-esteem and motivation for well-being (Rogers, 1968; Caplan and Killilea, 1976; Friedman and DiMatteo, 1979). The deleterious impact of social isolation has been described (Neeley and Patrick, 1968) and other investigations have linked social isolation to noncompliance among patients with tuberculosis (Kasel, 1975) and other chronic illnesses (Baekland and Lundwall, 1975). Help and approval from significant others has been shown to enhance compliance (Donabedian and Rosenfeld, 1964; Caplan et al., 1976). Barstow (1975, 1979) studied coping strategies of emphysema patients and found that the single most important influence on the patient's adjustment was the presence of a supportive "significant other."

Evidence from numerous research studies supports the theory that the quality of interaction between the patient and health care provider is the most salient determinant of compliance (DiMatteo, 1979; Mazzulo et al., 1974; Hulka et al., 1976). Kasel (1975) stressed the need for discussions of "mutual expectations" rather than mere exchange of information and facts. Information given alone has not been shown to increase compliance (Tagliacozzo et al., 1974; Bille, 1977; Sackett et al., 1977). A key element in provider-patient interaction seems to be the provider's ability to comprehend and provide feedback. Stone (1979) defined the provider's responsibilities as: (1) fully assessing the individual patient's situation, (2) anticipating difficulties following recommendations, and (3) communicating information in a way that will maximize its effectiveness. Hallburg outlines guidelines for teaching aged adults that emphasize the need for mutuality and the establishment of a supportive learning environment (Hallburg, 1976). Thus, research to date indicates that the factors most associated with compliance include (1) presence of overt symptoms, (2) beliefs about threat to health and efficacy of action, (3) knowledge regarding therapeutic recommendations and their purpose, (4) social support and family stability, and (5) positive interactions with health care providers.

Intervention strategy research has focused on two general areas: the effects of patient attitudes and beliefs on behavior, and the interactions that have an impact on beliefs and behaviors. Most agree, as noted above, that information given alone may increase knowledge but not necessarily affect behavior. Research indicates that strategies to mobilize patient support systems through use of a health care provider in a "significant other" role may be more successful (Caplan et al., 1976). Among the behavioral strategies, various types of reminder systems have been successful in assisting patients to keep clinic appointments and adhere to the medical regimen (Finnerty et al., 1973; Gillum and Barsky, 1974; Gates and Colburn, 1976). Other interventions that show promise are self-monitoring, tailoring, contracting, and graduated regimens.

III. Nursing Management of Patients with COPD

A. Overview

From the preceding review, it is apparent that the nursing care of patients with COPD is complex, demanding, and can be at times overwhelming and frustrating. COPD is a chronic progressively debilitating disease that leads inexorably, despite the patient's or professional's best efforts, to disability and death.

While COPD primarily affects the lungs, the secondary effects on other body systems can be equally incapacitating. Thus the goal of nursing care is to assist the patient in maintaining the highest level of self-care function allowed by his or her social and physiological resources. Implicit in this philosophy is an understanding that both the patient and his family will need counseling, instruction, support, and assistance as the patient's ability to be independent wanes.

B. Generic Application of Orem's Self-Care Model in the Long-Term Management of COPD Patients

The goals of long-term care with the COPD patient include prevention of disease progression, control of symptoms, prevention of secondary complications, and minimization of the gap between actual and potential function. A general framework for the long-term management of COPD patients has been repeatedly identified (Lertzman and Cherniak, 1976; Hass and Cardon, 1969; Davido, 1980; Petty and Cherniak, 1981; Petty, 1970, 1974, 1976; Petty et al., 1974; Wynne and Block, 1973; Lustig et al., 1972).

The cornerstones in the management of these patients are education and self-care. Specific educational areas include pathophysiology of COPD, medication therapy, breathing retraining, exercise reconditioning, pulmonary hygiene techniques, and self-monitoring regarding the effects of the disease and its treatment. Treatment modalities are described in the chapter by Petty. The regimen of COPD patients is complex, not only because of the number of medications and treatments measures prescribed but also because of the amount of behavior change required.

Orem (1980) defines self-care as those activities that an individual initiates and performs in maintaining life, health, and well-being. The aged, disabled, and ill may require partial or complete assistance with self-care management. Based on this definition, she identified five broad areas of nursing interventions: (1) acting or doing for, (2) guiding, (3) teaching, (4) supporting, and (5) providing a developmental environment. This discussion will focus on application of the latter four intervention categories to the care of COPD patients.

There is considerable overlap of activities within Orem's four areas of nursing care. She defines guiding as a method of assisting individuals to make choices or pursue a course of action that requires direction or supervision. Techniques involved in this guidance process include suggestions, instructions, direction, or supervision. One example of a guiding intervention is training patients to know when and how to use breathing techniques in various daily situations.

Supportive interventions focus on sustaining the patient's efforts and preventing failure or avoidance of unpleasant situations or decisions. They can involve both physical and psychological support. For example, a nurse may ambulate a patient, producing SOB. She then verbally encourages and physically guides him or her to use breathing retraining techniques to regain control of breathing. This helps to foster confidence in the patient and promote a sense of personal control over his or her symptoms. Thus, the nurse's physical presence, words of encouragement, and physical contact demonstrate three different types of supportive measures.

As defined by Orem, teaching is a method of assisting an individual who needs instruction to develop knowledge or specific skills. Instruction regarding the performance of actual breathing techniques exemplifies this nursing intervention category.

Nursing actions are required that foster a developmental environment in which individuals can form or change attitudes or values, creatively use their abilities, and adjust their self-concept. This type of millieu is conducive to the success of other intervention strategies. Both physical and psychosocial conditions must be considered when one is selecting actions aimed at promoting a developmental environment. The verbal and nonverbal communication skills of the nurse are essential components of millieu development.

COPD patients and their families not only need to learn specific psychomotor skills such as diaphragmatic breathing but must also develop fairly sophisticated problem-solving skills such as when to start using antibiotics and how to adapt breathing techniques to various daily activities. Nurses therefore must utilize guiding, teaching and supporting nursing interventions to foster a developmental environment.

Table 3 relates the strategies derived from the review of literature to the management of COPD patients. This table is by no means exhaustive; it attempts to provide the reader with a readily applicable model using multiple theories and research findings. The first column lists the standard treatment measures used in the long-term care of COPD patients. Columns 2, 3, 4, and 5 identify specific nursing actions that can be classified within Orem's four intervention categories.

Just as no one treatment component has been conclusively proven to be superior to the others, so there is no one correct nursing intervention. The more nursing options available, the greater the potential for success. The reader

Table 3 Nursing Intervention Categories Applied to Components of COPD Long-Term Management Plan

Treatment components in the long-term management of COPD patients	Teaching strategies	Guiding strategies	Supporting strategies	Developmental environmental strategies
Breathing Retraining Pursed lip breathing Diaphragm breathing Relaxation Positioning *Exercise Reconditioning* *ADL Modification* Energy conservation Work simplification Postural drainage Percussion Coughing	Explain rationale for and demonstrate specific techniques Return demonstrations by patient and family Encourage verbal feedback Reminder systems Keep language simple Content concrete Apply new information to patient's personal experiences	Counseling re: Modification of measures to personal life style Ways to use information Evaluation of treatment intervention When to seek PRN/ER assistance Provide opportunities for role playing Telephone assistance Emergency situations	Positive reinforcement Desensitization to SOB Frequent repetition of information with concrete application Mutual evaluation of technique performance and efficacy of results Recognition of and reward for therapeutic actions Encourage and acknowledge patient/family's efforts re: self-care	Mutual definition of: Roles Therapeutic goals Evaluation of Treatment regimen Treatment options Include family when possible Focus on impact of disease on emotions and coping abilities Encourage open communication

General Measures	Keep teaching time short with opportunity for frequent reinforcement and clarification	Application of information to vocational, home, and recreational situations	Assist patient/family in viewing adherence to total regimen as positive and independent	+ Reinforcement
Patient/family education re:	Pace instruction	Assist patient in identifying referral sources as needed	Assist patient/family in viewing referral as positive	Provide (adequate)
Pathophysiology of COPD	Minimize disruptions			Space
Signs/symptoms CHF/URI				Time
General health measures				Personnel
O_2				Patient aides
Long-Term Monitoring				Promote staff enthusiasm and interest in patient/ family
Compliance to regimen				
Medications				
Exercise regimen				
Pulmonary hygiene				
Breathing retraining				
Counseling needs				
Referrals				

should consult the other chapters in this volume for discussions of additional intervention strategies.

Breathing retraining, ADL modification, and pulmonary hygiene techniques require intellectual understanding of their rationale and use as well as psychomotor skills to implement them. One goal of these interventions is to increase the individual's sense of personal control over symptoms. The purpose of general education measures is to provide information that will assist in the development of the patient's problem solving skills including appropriate modification of the treatment regimen and assistance seeking when necessary. Long-term monitoring skills assist the patient in evaluating the effects of the disease and its treatment on daily life. All these measures attempt to augment the patient's independence in the performance of self-care activities and to promote self-confidence.

Intervention should be planned to maximize success potential. The nurse needs to define with the patient "success criteria." Nursing interventions can be aimed at different "levels of success." For instance, when pulmonary hygiene presents a therapeutic challenge to the patient and nurse, intervention can be presented and success evaluated at four levels. This evaluation includes assessment of the patient's ability to (1) *identify* the rationale for the procedure, (2) *perform* a return demonstration of the technique, (3) *modify* the instruction to his or her personal life style, and (4) *utilize* techniques independently. Mutually developed objective criteria can be clearly delineated and used by both the patient and the nurse to evaluate intervention success.

Important underlying principles relating to teaching strategies include language simplicity, repetitive frequent instruction, concrete application of information to the patient's personal situation, provision of opportunities for return demonstrations, and use of techniques such as reflection to ascertain the patient's retention and personal application of information. The reader is again referred to Hallburg's teaching guidelines (1976).

Guiding strategies shift the focus from nurse-initiated instruction to patient-initiated clarification or adaption of instruction. The nurse's role is to assist the patient in making decisions regarding alternatives in his or her health care regimen. Careful assessment of what patients are really asking is essential. For instance, a patient may ask, "Do I have to make a bed that way?" The real question may be, "I never made a bed before, do I have to now?" or "That's too threatening a modification for me now, isn't there some other way?" Therapeutic listening and counseling are the basis for many of the guiding strategies.

Supporting strategies (outlined in column 4 of Table 3) attempt to sustain the patient's efforts at self-care. As mentioned earlier, these patients are depressed, debilitated, and withdrawn; their physical and emotional status are not conductive to high motivation or perseverance. Frequent positive reinforcement of the patient's and family's efforts acknowledges the value of their efforts, confirms the individual's importance, and enhances self-esteem. Mutual reassessment of treatment measures, the patient and family's goals, and anticipatory counseling are supportive strategies. Furthermore, interventions that increase the patient's sense of personal control stimulates self-confidence, perseverance, and adherence to the treatment regimen. Desensitization to SOB is one technique. Desensitization involves deliberate inducement of a problematic symptom (e.g., SOB) and then allows the patient, under supervision, to use strategies (e.g., breathing retraining techniques) to ameliorate the symptom's severity.

Strategies fostering a developmental environment (column 5 of Table 3) include mutual goal setting and problem identification, nurse-patient role definitions, and use of the nurse as a "significant other." Discussions of "mutual expectations" regarding roles and goals as noted previously have been found to enhance compliance. Mutual evaluation of the impact of the disease and its treatment measures further supports compliance, reinforces the patient's active rather than reactive role as a member of the health care team, and promotes a sense of personal control. Nurses' education and communication skills augment their ability to function as a "significant other" for COPD patients and potentiate the supportive aspects of the health care system. The involvement of family members and friends activates the patient's personal support network, which in turn increases the frequency of compliant behaviors. The physical factors identified in column 5 of Table 3 are self-explanatory.

C. Integration of Nursing Diagnosis, Causative Factors, and Nursing Intervention Strategies to Promote Self-Care of COPD Patients

Overview

The nursing diagnosis concept provides a framework linking the psychosocial-physiological basis of patient care problems with intervention strategies. As defined by the nursing section of the American Thoracic Society (1981), a nursing diagnosis describes actual or potential health problems that nurses are capable of identifying and licensed to treat. A patient with the medical diagnosis of COPD frequently presents with multiple nursing diagnoses.

Table 4 presents a suggested taxonomy of the major nursing diagnoses, possible causative factors, and nursing interventions. The individuality of each patient demands frequent modification of all three to personalize nursing

Nursing Diagnosis Approach to the Nursing Care of COPD Patients

Nursing diagnosis	Causative factors	Nursing interventions
spiratory dysfunction		
Alteration of breathing pattern	A. Alveolar destruction	A. Breathing retraining techniques
	↓ Tractional support	Pulmonary hygiene techniques
	↑ Accessory muscle use	Desensitization to SOB
	↓ Mechanical efficiency of diaphragm	Counseling
	Airway edema	Patient/family education
	Mucus plugging	Medications
	↓ Mucociliary transport	Signs/symptoms CHF/URI
	Ineffective cough	Fluids
	Acute URI	
	Acute CHF	
	Fear	
Impaired airway clearance	B. Impaired mucociliary transport	B. Pulmonary hygiene techniques
	Airway edema	Fluids
	Mucus plugging	Discontinue smoking
	Ineffective cough	Patient/family education
	Dehydration	Signs/symptoms URI
	Smoking	
	Acute URI	

C. Risk for respiratory infection

C. Impaired mucociliary transport
  Airway edema
  Mucus plugging
  Ineffective cough
  Dehydration
  Poor nutrition
  Chronic debilitation

C. Immunizations
  Modification of ADL patterns
  Pulmonary hygiene techniques
  Fluids
  Patient/family instruction
    Signs/symptoms URI
    Actions to take
    General health measures

II. Cardiovascular dysfunction
  A. Alterations of pump function

A. Chronic hypoxemia
  Dysrhythmia
  Acid/base disturbances
  Pulmonary embolus
  Systemic hypertension
  Cardiac disease
  Polycythemia

A. Patient/family education
  O_2
  Medications
  Diet/fluid modifications
  ADL modification
  Monitoring
    Medications
    Acid/base status
    Cardiac function

Table 4 (continued)

Nursing diagnosis	Causative factors	Nursing interventions
B. Alterations of cardiac rhythm	B. Chronic hypoxemia Acid/base disturbance Pulmonary hypertension Drugs	B. Patient/family instruction O_2 Medications Monitoring Acid/base status Cardiac function
C. Alterations of peripheral vascular integrity	C. Inactivity Cor pulmonale Dysrhythmia Vessel wall injury Age	C. ↑ Activity Patient/family instruction Vessel wall protection Risk factors
III. Gastrointestinal dysfunction A. Alterations of nutrition	A. Aerophagia ↓ Gastric space SOB Diet restrictions	A. Pursed lip breathing ↑ Activity ↑ Socialization Small, frequent feedings

	Economics	Patient/family instruction
	Impaired home management skills	Diet
	Concomitant health problems	Energy conservation
	↓ Socialization	Work simplification
	↓ Activity	Monitor
	Medications	Medications
		General health
B. Alterations of bowel function	B. ↓ Bulk intake	B. Patient/family instruction
	↓ Fluid intake	Diet/fluid modification
	↓ Activity	Bowel function
	Medications	Safe use laxatives
		Monitor
		Medications
		Bowel function
C. Alterations of gut integrity	C. Enzyme deficiency	C. Discontinue smoking
	Smoking	Patient/family instruction
	Medications	Medications
	Cardiovascular disease	Diet
	Age/Sex	

Table 4 (continued)

Nursing diagnosis	Causative factors	Nursing interventions
		Monitor
		Medications
		Effects of concomitant disease
		Signs/symptoms of ulcer
IV. Musculoskeletal dysfunction		
A. Impaired activity tolerance	A. Deconditioning	A. Breathing retraining
	SOB	Reconditioning program
	Fear	Desensitization to SOB
	Impaired O_2 transport	Energy conservation
	↑ O_2 debt with exercise	Work simplification
	Prolonged recovery time	
	Inadequate nutrition	
B. Alterations of comfort	B. Inactivity	B. Leg/foot stretching exercises
	Muscle tendon shortening	↑ Activity
	Electrolyte imbalance	Monitor electrolyte status

V. Neuropsychological dysfunction

A. Impaired abstracting ability	A. Chronic hypoxemia	A. Monitor O_2 therapy
	Hypercarbia	Encourage socialization
	↓ Socialization	Encourage maintenance of routine
		Instructional strategies
		Terminology: simple
		Nontechnical
		Information: concrete
		Practical
		Relate to patient's experiences
		Frequent repetitive use
		Adjunctive patient aids
B. Alterations in sleep/wake cycle	B. Lack of routine	B. ↑ Activity
	Anxiety	Encourage maintenance of routine
	Inactivity	Monitor
	SOB	Signs/symptoms CHF/URI
	Acute CHF/URI	± Use of medications

Table 4 (continued)

Nursing diagnosis	Causative factors	Nursing interventions
VI. Psychosocial dysfunction		
A. Individual maladaptive coping patterns	A. Fear Past coping styles ↓ Social supports Environmental stresses ↓ Self-image Informational deficits Communication pattern	A. Individual counseling Desensitization to SOB Breathing retraining Expanding social support network Work simplification Energy conservation Patient education Disease and treatment Mutual goal setting Mutual role definition
B. Ineffective family coping patterns	B. Family's past coping style Fear Environmental stresses Communication patterns Information deficits Misconceptions	B. Family counseling Environmental stress modification Family education Disease and treatment Mutual goal setting Mutual role clarification

C. Impaired social role functioning	C. Employment/role stresses ↓ Activity tolerance Environmental stresses Informational deficits	C. Exercise reconditioning program Employment counseling Energy conservation Work simplification
D. Impaired emotional functioning	D. Fear SOB ↓ Activity tolerance Coping style Informational deficits Misconceptions	D. Desensitization to SOB Breathing retraining General counseling Sex counseling Disease and treatment Clarification of misconceptions
E. Noncompliance with therapeutic regimen	E. Informational deficits Health attitudes Coping styles Environmental limitations Physical limitations Social supports Motivation Unrealistic goal setting	E. Patient/family education Counseling Identify appropriate environmental manipulations Assist in therapeutic problem-solving skill development Community referral

care. Nursing care is a dynamic rather than static process. The table is organized by systems rather than priority to enhance clarity of discussion. The
first column identifies nursing diagnostic categories, the second column possible
causative factors, and the third shows specific nursing interventions that have,
as a goal, enhancement of the patient's ability to participate in self-care. The
nursing interventions specifically apply the general principles underlying Orem's
self-care model to the COPD patient. They include examples of teaching, guiding, and supporting interventions to promote a developmental milieu within
which the patient and his or her family can enhance their self-care skills.

Accurate identification of the diagnosis and contributing factors is essential for effective planning and implementation of nursing care. Treatment failure frequently occurs because of an incorrect diagnosis and/or assessment of
causative factors. Many additional creative nursing strategies must be developed
and evaluated to increase the armamentarium of nursing interventions available
to the practitioner.

Systematic Application of the Nurse's Taxonomy

Respiratory Dysfunction

Respiratory dysfunction problems can be grouped within three broad nursing
diagnostic categories: alterations of breathing patterns, impaired airway clearance, and increased risk for recurrent respiratory infections.

Currently available treatment modalities have no effect on the loss of
tractional support or tissue destruction associated with emphysematous changes.
Nursing interventions, as noted in column 3, must therefore focus on the reversible components of the pulmonary pathology. Breathing retraining is the cor-
nerstone of nonpharmacologic treatment. The techniques encompassed by this
term are pursed lip breathing, diaphragmatic breathing, positioning, and relaxation. The specific procedure for performing these and their efficacy in symptom relief are described in the chapter by Petty. Nursing strategies include instruction regarding indications for and use of the modalities as well as physical
guidance regarding actual performance. Breathing retraining interventions are
directed toward improving the efficiency of the diaphragm, reducing accessory
muscle use, and increasing the patient's sense of personal control over his or
her symptoms.

Pulmonary hygiene techniques include postural drainage, percussion,
fluids, coughing, and cessation of smoking. These strategies are thought to improve airway clearance, reduce mucus plugging, and reduce the frequency of
or augment the treatment of respiratory infections.

Both of these categories of pulmonary dysfunction require relatively high levels of effective and affective patient behavior changes. The generic teaching, guiding, supporting, and environmental strategies outlined in Table 3 must be implemented if the goal of improved pulmonary function is to be achieved.

Cardiovascular Dysfunction

As noted in the systems review section, COPD patients are at risk of developing three types of cardiovascular complications. These include alterations of pump function, cardiac rhythm, and peripheral vascular integrity.

Chronic hypoxemia is the major causative factor in the pathogenesis of the first two complications. The indications for and use of oxygen therapy are well described in the chapter by Petty. The decision to implement oxygen therapy is medical. The education of the patient and family is most frequently a nursing intervention. Table 5 outlines the clinical indications for long-term use of oxygen, the instructional process and goals developed by the Respiratory Home Care Service of the Division of Pulmonary and Critical Care Medicine at the Henry Ford Hospital, and based in part on the American Thoracic Society position statement of 1977. Instruction begins with assessment of patients' perceptions of indications for and use of home oxygen. Focus then shifts to information giving, clarification of misconceptions, alleviation of inappropriate fears, and modification of oxygen delivery systems to meet individual situational needs. Individual needs to be considered when selecting an oxygen delivery system are the cost of the oxygen system, the need for ambulatory source within or outside the home, and available social supports. An often neglected aspect of oxygen therapy instruction is therapeutic goal setting. SOB is not an acceptable behavioral criterion for the patient to use to determine oxygen use. Telling a patient to use oxygen when he feels short of breath is analogous to instructing a patient to take an anticoagulant when his blood feels thick. A precise oxygen dose determination should be done. Duration of use generally falls into one of three categories: continuous (at least 18-20 hr/day) for the chronically hypoxemic, nocturnal for sleep desaturation, and with exercise for those with only exercise desaturation. Continuous use is the most common therapeutic oxygen prescription for COPD patients.

Maintenance of a developmental environment is essential if adherence to an oxygen program is to be achieved. The patient and his or her family must feel safe to discuss recurrent or episodic concerns regarding oxygen therapy. Social concerns frequently expressed regarding oxygen include body

Table 5 Oxygen Therapy Guidelines[a]

Clinical indications for long-term use

    Any patient with a PO_2 while "clinically stable" on room air $\leqslant 55$ mmHg

    Patient with 60 mmHg $\geqslant PO_2 \geqslant 55$ mmHg with at least *one* of the following additional clinical findings:

        Exercise-induced hypoxemia ($PO_2 \leqslant 55$ mmHg)

        Nocturnal hypoxemia ($PO_2 \leqslant 55$ mmHg)

        Secondary polycythemia

        EKG or clinical evidence of cor pulmonale

Instructional goals

    Enhance patient adherence

    Prevent iatrogenic complications

    Promote safe use of equipment

Instructional process

    Explain indications for and use of home oxygen

    Explain flow rate and use of flow meter for presecribed system

    Care of oxygen humidifier

    Care of and use of portable unit if appropriate

    Safety precautions

        Remove oxygen if smoking, using stove, etc

        Avoid use of oil-based lotions/ointments on face or nose

---

[a]Developed for use by the Respiratory Home Care Service of the Division of Pulmonary and Critical Care Medicine, Henry Ford Hospital, Detroit, Michigan.

image changes associated with using and wearing the equipment, safety concerns regarding fires, and isolation fears related to limitations in activity.

Additional treatment measures used for pump and rhythm disturbances include instruction and monitoring of medication regimen, diet and fluid modification, ADL adaptions, and monitoring of fluid and electrolyte imbalance. ADL modification will be discussed in more detail below.

The primary alterations of peripheral vascular integrity are deep vein thrombosis and pulmonary embolus. They are related to the secondary effects of COPD, cardiac compromise, inactivity, and increased fragility of blood vessel wall. Nursing strategies are those of teaching and supporting. Patients should be encouraged to ambulate and and increase their participation in ADL. The success of the recommendation depends to a great deal on the patient's ability to utilize breathing retraining techniques to control his or her symptoms. Vessel wall protection includes general measures such as avoiding temperature extremes, restrictive garments or positioning, and bruising. Smoking cessation helps to improve respiratory and cardiovascular function as well as promote gut integrity.

Gastrointestinal Dysfunction

Alterations of nutritional state, bowel function and gut integrity are the most frequent of GI complaints. Pursed lip breathing can specifically aid in the reduction of aerophagia. By inhaling through the nose and exhaling through pursed lips, the patient can minimize air swallowing. Antacids aid in reducing gas and maintaining gut integrity. Increasing activity stimulates the appetite and bowels. Instruction regarding the monitoring of diet and medication is another aspect.

Musculoskeletal Dysfunction

Of the two identified problems in this area, impaired activity tolerance is the most debilitating. Leg cramps can be treated effectively with calf stretch exercises, increased activity, and maintenance of serum potassium level within normal range. Improving activity tolerance is much more complex. The interventions identified in Table 4 require high levels of patient motivation and dedication. Furthermore, psychomotor skills utilized in the performance of breathing retraining and exercise reconditioning are complex. Patients and their families must be assisted in setting realistic short and long-term goals related to activity.

Energy conservation and work simplification techniques used with COPD patients have been adapted from those used by cardiac patients. The goal with cardiac patients is prevention of chest pain and decreased cardiac work; with COPD patients it is the prevention or control of SOB. Table 6 defines the concepts of energy conservation and work simplification and identifies the indications for and use of these interventions.

Neuropsychological Dysfunction

Impaired abstracting ability must be a major consideration when planning any nursing intervention. Terminology should be simple and nontechnical. Presen-

Table 6 Work Simplification/Energy Conservation[a]

Work simplification

Definition: Task analysis promoting utilization of adaptions to accomplish an ADL task while consuming the least amount of personal energy necessary

Indications

Patient's disability/limitations prevent or inhibit completion of ADL tasks

Available modifications either in methods or equipment offer potential for increasing patient's participation in ADL

Teaching intervention methods

Verbal instruction

Task performance

Combination

Techniques

Plan ahead

Organize activity/work area

Task analysis

Identification of proper body positioning

Proper selection of tools/equipment

Identification of proper location/positioning/utilization of tools/ equipment

Energy conservation

Definition: Application of the general principles of posture, body mechanics, and work simplification techniques to ADL thus minimizing the patient's energy costs and maximizing his or her ability to participate in vocational/avocational pursuits

Indications

Patient's ability/limitations inhibit/prevent performance of routine ADL

Patient verbally identifies and/or demonstrates lack of knowledge or inability to apply basic principles to ADL

Teaching intervention methods

Verbal instruction

Table 6 (continued)

Task performance

Combination

Techniques

Identification of actual/potential problem areas

Identification of proper body mechanics during selected activities

Identification of appropriate work simplification techniques for selected activities

[a]Developed for use in the Henry Ford and Sinai Hospitals Pulmonary Rehabilitation Programs.

tation of information should have concrete application to the patient's personal experiences. Various types of patient aids (booklets, medication cards, etc.) provide visual reminders of treatment regimen. Oxygen therapy for the chronically hypoxemic is indicated.

From a behavioral perspective, maintenance of regular activity routine and increased socialization provide intellectual and emotional stimulation. They also assist in the reestablishment or maintenance of a normal sleep-awake cycle. Acute exacerbations of CHF and respiratory infection symptoms frequently are noticed initially because of sleep disturbances. Judicious monitoring of prescribed and over-the-counter drugs is indicated because of the myriad potential side effects.

Psychosocial Dysfunction

Maintenance of a developmental environment with emphasis on communication and interpersonal skills is the basis for nursing care interventions directed toward improved psychosocial function. Doctors Kaplan and McSweeny discuss in detail behavioral and psychosocial interventions with COPD patients in their chapters in this book.

The five nursing diagnostic categories identified as types of psychosocial dysfunction are individual maladaptive coping patterns, ineffective family coping patterns, impaired social role or emotional functioning and noncompliance.

Psychosocial variables and the therapeutic patient-provider relationship, as previously noted, are among the most significant affecting compliance. Dynamic assessment of the patient and his or her family's past and present coping styles is essential. The areas of premorbid weakness will be exaggerated, and the areas of strength tested. Counseling, individual or family, should be directed toward identifying and activating social support networks, identifying and diminishing environmental stresses, enhancing positive communication skills, crystalizing sources of fear or anxiety, clarifying misconceptions, and providing information. The key element is the provision of an environment in which the patient and family feel free to discuss these areas, form new attitudes, and test modifications of their coping style. The environmental strategies identified in Table 3 are all applicable and the reader can undoubtedly add significantly to this preliminary list.

Investigators have found that counseling efforts are most effective when they are incorporated in the patient's overall management or rehabilitation program (Dudley et al., 1980). Research further suggests that counseling efforts are less threatening when they are focused on the impact that the disease has on the patient and/or family's ability to cope rather than the effect of their premorbid coping styles on the disease (Post and Collins, 1981-82; Dudley et al., 1980b; Pattison et al., 1971).

The physical measures of breathing retraining, positioning, relaxation, energy conservation, work simplification, and desensitization techniques are effective because of the relative immediate relief and positive feedback they provide. Patient and family teaching as described earlier is a strategy to increase their knowledge, sense of control, and active participation in the health care team.

IV. Summary and Conclusion

The nursing care of patients with COPD is complex, demanding, and at times can be overwhelming and frustrating. The care is complex in part because the social, psychological, and physiological aberrations are multiple and varied among persons with the same diagnosis. While COPD affects primarily the lungs, the secondary effect on other body systems can be equally incapacitating. The care can be frustrating because COPD is a chronic progressive disease that, despite the patient's or nurse's best efforts, results in disability and death. The goal of nursing care is to assist the patient in maintaining the highest level of self-care function allowed by his biopsychosocial reserves.

References

Alkalay, I., Kaplan, A. S., Sharma, R., and Kimbel, P. (1980). Chronic obstructive pulmonary disease: rehabilitation program with continuation on an outpatient basis. *J. Am. Geriatric Soc.* **28**:88-92.

Angle, D. P., Baum, G. L., Chester, E. H., and Wendt, M. (1973). Multidiscipline treatment of chronic pulmonary insufficiency: Part I. Psychologic aspects of rehabilitation. *Psychosom. Med.* **35**:41-49.

ATS News (Summer, 1981). Standards for nursing care of patients with COPD. pp. 31-37.

Baekland, F., and Lundwall, L. (1975). Dropping out of treatment: a clinical review. *Psychol. Bull.* **82**:738-783.

Barstow, R. E. (1975). Coping with emphysema. *Nursing Clin. North Am.* **19**:137-145.

Barstow, R. E. (1979). Coping with emphysema: a field study. *Respir. Care* **24**:913-920.

Becker, M. H. (1976). Sociobehavioral determinants of compliance. In *Compliance with Therapeutic Regimens.* Edited by D. L. Sackett and R. B. Haynes. Baltimore, Johns Hopkins University Press, pp. 40-50.

Bergofsky, E. H. (1973). Rehabilitation medicine and prospects for prevention of disability from chronic obstructive lung disease. *Prev. Med.* **2**: 43-56.

Bille, D. A. (1977). The role of body images in patient compliance and education. *Heart Lung* **6**:143-148.

Blackwell, B. (1973). Drug therapy: patient compliance. *N. Engl. J. Med.* **289**:249-253.

Bonnevie, O. (1977). Causes of death in duodenal and gastric ulcers. *Gastroenterology* **73**:1000-1004.

Burrows, B., and Earle, R. H. (1969). Course and prognosis of chronic obstructive lung disease. *N. Engl. J. Med.* **280**:397-404.

Caplan, C., and Killilea, M. (1976). *Support Systems and Mutual Help.* New York, Grune & Stratton.

Caplan, R., Robinson, E., French, J., Caldwell, J., and Shinn, M. (1976). *Adhering to Medical Regimens.* Ann Arbor, MI, Ann Arbor Institute for Social Research, University of Michigan.

Charney, E. (1972). Patient-doctor communication: implications for the clinician. *Pediatr. Clin. North Am.* **19**:263-279.

Chetty, K. G., Brown, S. E., and Light R. N. (1983). Improved exercise tolerance of the polycythemic lung patient following phlebotomy. *Am. J. Med.* **74**:415-420.

Cohen, B. H., Bios, W. B., Chase, G. A., Diamond, E. L., Graves, C. G., Levy, D. A., Menkes, H., Meyer, M. B., Permutt, S., and Tockman, M. S. (1980). Is ABH nonsecretor status a risk factor for obstructive lung disease? *Am. J. Epidemiol.* **111**:285-291.

Collins, B. E., and Hoyt, M. F. (1972). Personal responsibility for consequences: an integration and extension of the forced compliance literature. *J. Exp. Soc. Psychol.* **8**:558-592.

Daughton, D. M., Fix, A. J., Kass, I., Patil, K. D., and Bell, C. W. (1979). Physiological-intellectual components of rehabilitation success in patients with chronic obstructive pulmonary disease. *J. Chron. Dis.* **32**: 405-409.

Davido, J. (1981). Pulmonary rehabilitation. *Nursing Clin. North Am.* **16**: 275-283.

Davis, M. S., and Eichhorn, R. L. (1963). Compliance with medical regimens: a panel study. *J. Health Hum. Behav.* **4**:240-249.

DiMatteo, M. R. (1979). A social-psychological analysis of physician-patient rapport: toward a science of the art of medicine. *J. Soc. Issues* **35**: 12-33.

Dirks, J. F., Fross, K. H., and Evans, N. W. (1977). Panic-fear in asthma: generalized personality trait vs. specific situational state. *J. Asthma Res.* **15**:171-178.

Dirks, J. F., Horton, D. J., Kinsman, R. A., Fross, K. H., and Jones, J. G. (1978a). Patient and physician characteristics influencing medical decisions in asthma. *J. Asthma Res.* **15**:171-178.

Dirks, J. F., and Kinsman, R. A. (1978). Clinical prediction of medical rehospitalization: psychological assessment with the battery of asthma illness behavior. *J. Personality Assess.* **45**:608-613.

Dirks, J. F., Kinsman, R. A., Jones, N. F., and Fross, K. H. (1978b). New developments in the panic-fear research in asthma: validity and stability of the MMPI fear-panic scale. *Br. J. Med. Psychol.* **57**:119-126.

Dirks, J., Fross, K., and Paley, A. (1978). Panic-fear in asthma—State trait relationship and rehospitalization. *J. Chronic Dis.* **31**:605-609.

Donabedian, A., and Rosenfeld, L. S. (1964). Follow up study on chronically ill patients discharged from the hospital. *J. Chron. Dis.* **17**:847-862.

Dudley, D. L. (1981). Coping with COPD: therapeutic options. *Geriatrics* **36**:69-74.

Dudley, D. L., Glaser, E. M., Jorgenson, B. N., and Adhozan, D. L. (1980a). Psychosocial and psychological concomitants to rehabilitation in chronic obstructive pulmonary disease, Part I. *Chest* **77**:413-419.

Dudley, D. L., Glaser, E. M., Jorgenson, B. N., and Logan, D. L. (1980b). Psychosocial concomitants to rehabilitation in chronic obstructive pulmonary disease, Part 2. *Chest* **77**:544-551.

Dudley, D. L., and Pitts-Poarch, A. R. (1980). Psychophysiologic aspects of respiratory control. *Clin. Chest Med.* **1**:131-143.

Dyksterhuis, J. E. (1972). Vocational rehabilitation of chronic obstructive pulmonary disease patients. *Rehab. Lit.* **33**:136-147.

Finnerty, F. A., Jr., Mattie, E. C., and Finnerty, F. A. III (1973). Hypertension in the Inner City. I. Analysis of clinical dropouts. *Circulation* **47**: 73-75.

Fix, A. J., Daughton, D., Kass, I., Bell, C. W., and Golden, C. J. (1980). Emotional intellectual and physiological predictors of vocational outcome of pulmonary rehabilitation patients. *Psychol. Rep.* **46**:379-382.

Fix, A. J., Daughton, D., Kass, I., Patil, K. D., Kass, M., and Polenz, D. (1978). Personality traits affecting vocational rehabilitation success in patients with chronic obstructive pulmonary disease. *Psychol. Rep.* **43**:939-944.

Fletcher, E. C., and Martin, R. J. (1982). Sexual dysfunction and erectile impotence in chronic obstructive pulmonary disease. *Chest* **81**:413-421.

Flick, M. R., and Block, A. J. (1979). Nocturnal vs. diurnal cardiac arrhythmias in patients with chronic obstructive pulmonary disease. *Chest* **75**: 8-11.

Friedman, H. S., and DiMatteo, M. R. (1979). Health care as an interpersonal process. *J. Soc. Issues* **35**:1-11.

Gates, S., and Colburn, D. (1976). Lowering appointment failures in a neighborhood health center. *Med. Care* **14**:263-267.

Gillum, R. F., and Barsky, A. J. (1974). Diagnosis and management of patient noncompliance. *J.A.M.A.* **228**:1563-1567.

Grant, I., Heaton, R. K., McSweeny, A. J., Adams, K., and Timms, R. M. (1980). Brain dysfunction in COPD. *Chest* **77**:308-309.

Hallburg, J. (1976). Teaching of aged adults. *J. Gerontol. Nursing* **2**:13-19.

Hass, A., and Cardon, H. (1969). Rehabilitation in chronic obstructive pulmonary disease. *Med. Clin. North Am.* **53**:593-606.

Haynes, R. B. (1976). A critical review of the determinants of patient compliance with therapeutic regimens. In *Compliance with Therapeutic Regimens.* Edited by D. L. Sackett and R. B. Haynes. Baltimore, Johns Hopkins University Press, pp. 26-39.

Hulka, B. S., Cassel, J. C., Kupper, L. L., and Burdette, J. A. (1976). Communication, compliance and concordance between physicians and patients with prescribed medications. *Am. J. Public Health* **66**:847-853.

Joseph, L. (1980). Self-care and the nursing process. *Nursing Clin. North Am.* **15**:131-142.

Kasel, S. V. (1975). Issues in patient adherence to health care regimens. *J. Hum. Stress* **1**:5-8.

Kass, I., Dyksterhuis, J., Rubin, R., and Patel, K. (1975). Correlation of psychophysiologic variables with vocational rehabilitation outcomes in patients with chronic obstructive pulmonary disease. *Chest* **67**:433-440.

Kent, D. C., and Smith, J. K. (1977). Psychological implications of pulmonary disease. *Clin. Notes Respir. Dis.* **1**:3-11.

Kinsman, R. A., Dirks, J. F., and Dahlem, N. W. (1980). Noncompliance to prescribe-as-needed (PRN) medication use in asthma: usage patterns and patient characteristics. *J. Psychosom. Res.* **24**:97-107.

Kirscht, J. P., and Rosenstock, I. M. (1979). Patient problems in following recommendations of health experts. In *Health Psychology*. Edited by G. C. Stone, F. Cohen, and N. E. Adler and Associates. San Francisco, Jossey-Bass, pp. 189-215.

Kleiger, R. E., and Senior, R. M. (1974). Longterm electrocardiographic monitoring of ambulatory patients with chronic airway obstruction. *Chest* **65**:483-487.

Langman, M. J., and Cooke, A. R. (1976). Gastric and duodenal ulcer and their associated diseases. *Lancet* **1**:680-683.

Lazarus, R. S. (1960). *Psychological Stress and the Coping Process*. New York, McGraw-Hill.

Lertzman, M. M., and Cherniak, R. M. (1976). Rehabilitation of patients with chronic obstructive pulmonary disease. *Am. Rev. Respir. Dis.* **114**:1145-1165.

Lippman, M., and Fein, A. (1981). Pulmonary embolism in patients with chronic obstructive pulmonary disease. *Chest* **79**:39-42.

Lustig, F. M., Hass, A., and Castillo, R. (1972). Clinical and rehabilitation regime in patients with COPD. *Arch. Phys. Med. Rehab.* **53**:315-322.

Marston, M. (1970). Compliance with medical regimens: a review of the literature. *Nursing Res.* **19**:312-323.

Mazzulo, J. M., Lasagna, L., and Griner, P. F. (1974). Variations in interpretation of prescription instruction. *J.A.M.A.* **227**:929-931.

McAlister, A. L., Farquhar, J. W., Thoreson, C. E., and Maccoby, N. (1976). Behavioral science applied to cardiovascular health: progress and research need in the modification of risk-taking habits in adult populations. *Health Ed. Monographs* **4**:45-74.

McSweeny, A. J., Heaton, R. K., Grant, I., Cugell, D., Solliday, N., and

Timms, R. (1980). Chronic obstructive pulmonary disease: socio-emotional adjustment and life quality. *Chest* **77**:309-310

McSweeny, A. J., Grant, I., Heaton, R. K., Adams, K., Timms, R. (1982). Life quality of patients with chronic obstructive pulmonary disease. *Arch. Intern. Med.* **142**:473-478.

Monson, R. R. (1970). Duodenal ulcer as a second disease. *Gastroenterology* **59**:712-716.

Moser, K. M. (1977). Pulmonary embolism: state of the art. *Am. Rev. Respir. Dis.* **115**:829-850.

Neeley, E., and Patrick, M. L. (1968). Problems of aged persons taking medications at home. *Nursing Res.* **17**:52-55.

Orem, D. (1980). *Nursing Concepts of Practice,* 2nd edition. New York, McGraw-Hill, pp. 87-116.

Patel, A. K., Skatrud, J. B., and Thomsen, J. H. (1981). Cardiac arrhythmias due to oral aminophylline in patients with chronic obstructive pulmonary disease. *Chest* **80**:661-665.

Pattison, M. E., Rhodes, R. J., and Dudley, D. L. (1971). Response to group treatment in patients with severe chronic obstructive pulmonary lung disease. *Int. J. Group Psychother.* **21**:214-225.

Pearlin, L., and Schooler, C. (1978). The structure of coping. *J. Health Soc. Behav.* **19**:2-21.

Petty, T. L. (1970). Ambulatory care for emphysema and chronic bronchitis. *Chest* **58**:441-448.

Petty, T. L. (1974). Does treatment for severe emphysema and chronic bronchitis really help? (A response). *Chest* **65**:124-126.

Petty, T. L. (1976). Pulmonary rehabilitation. *J. Maine Med. Assoc.* **67**:199-205.

Petty, T. L., and Cherniak, R. M. (1981). Comprehensive care of COPD. *Clin. Notes Respir. Dis.* Winter:3-12.

Petty, T. L., MacIlroy, E. R., Swigert, M. A., and Brink, G. A. (1970). Chronic airway obstruction and gainful employment. *Arch. Environ. Health* **21**:71-78.

Post, L., and Collins, C. (1981-82). The poorly coping COPD patient: a psychotherapeutic perspective. *Int. J. Psychiatry Med.* **11**:173-183.

Prescott, S. M., Richards, K. L., Tikoff, G., Armstrong, J. D., and Shigeoka, J. W. (1981). Venous thromboembolism in decompensated chronic obstructive pulmonary disease. *Am. Rev. Respir. Dis.* **123**:32-36.

Rodin, J., and Janis, I. L. (1979). The social power of health care practitioners as agents of change. *J. Soc. Issues* **35**:60-81.

Rogers, C. R. (1968). The characteristics of a helping relationship. In *Interpersonal Dynamics: Essays and Readings in Human Interaction,* 3rd edition. Edited by W. G. Bennis, E. H. Schein, D. E. Berle, and F. I. Steel. Homewood, IL, Dorsey Press, pp. 309-325.

Roser, R., and Geiz, A. (1981). Psychological approaches to breathlessness and its treatment. *J. Psychosom. Res.* **25**:439-447.

Rutter, B. (1979). The prognostic significance of psychological factors in the management of chronic bronchitis. *Psychol. Med.* **9**:63-70.

Rutter, B. (1976). Measurement of psychological factors in chronic illness. *Rheumatol. Rehab.* **15**:174-178.

Sackett, D. L., Haynes, R. B., Gibson, E. S., Taylor, D. W., Roberts, R. W., and Johnson, A. L. (1977). Hypertension control, compliance and science. *Am. Heart J.* **94**:666-667.

Seligman, M. E. P. (1975). *Helplessness.* San Francisco, W. H. Freeman & Company Publishers.

Senior, R. M., Lefrak, S. S., and Kleiger, R. E. (1979). The heart in chronic obstructive pulmonary disease. Editorial. *Chest* **75**:1-2.

Sleisenger, M. H., and Fordtran, J. S. (1983). *Gastrointestinal Diseases,* 3rd ed. Philadelphia, W. B. Saunders, p. 644.

Soll, A. H., and Isenberg, J. I. (1983). Duodenal ulcer disease. In *Gastrointestinal Disease,* 3rd edition. Edited by M. H. Sleisenger and J. S. Fordtron. Philadelphia, Saunders, pp. 644-645.

Stanford, D. (1977). All about sex after middle age. *Am. J. Nursing* **77**: 608-611.

Staudenmayer, H., Kinsman, R. A., Dirks, J. F., Sheldon, L. S., and Wangaard, C. (1979). Medical outcomes in asthmatic patients: effects of airways hyperreactivity and symptom-focused anxiety. *Psychosom. Med.* **41**: 109-117.

Stockdale-Woolley, R. (1983). Sexual dysfunction and COPD: problems and management. *Nurse Practitioner* **8**:16-20.

Stone, G. (1979). Compliance and the role of the expert. *J. Soc. Issues* **35**: 34-59.

Tagliacozzo, D. M., Luskin, D. B., Lashoff, J. C., and Inman, K. (1974). Nurse intervention and patient behavior. *Am. J. Public Health* **64**: 596-603.

Wallston, K. A., Maides, S., and Wallston, B. (1976). Health related information seeking as a function of health related locus of control and health value. *J. Res. Personal.* **10**:215-222.

Wynne, J. W., and Block, A. J. (1973). Ambulatory care and rehabilitation in COPD. *Postgrad. Med.* **54**:173-178.

11

Behavioral Science Aspects of COPD: Current Status and Future Directions

SYDNEY R. PARKER

National Heart, Lung, and Blood Institute
National Institutes of Health
Bethesda, Maryland

I. Introduction

Chronic obstructive pulmonary disease (COPD) is a condition that has been largely ignored by the behavioral science community. Although it is an important and increasing cause of morbidity and mortality in the United States, it has not received the attention of behavioral scientists warranted by its public health importance. Morbidity from COPD, which includes emphysema and chronic bronchitis, affects nearly 10 million persons in the United States alone and results in annual health care costs exceeding $6.5 billion. It is the fifth leading cause of death in this country. If current trends continue, it may be the fourth or even third leading cause of death by the year 2000. (National Heart, Lung, and Blood Institute, 1984a). In fact, the death rate has risen over 15% from 1912 to 1982 (National Heart, Lung, and Blood Institute, 1984b).

The only aspect of COPD that has generated much behavioral science research is smoking cessation. Smoking is the overwhelming risk factor for the development of COPD; nonsmokers rarely develop the condition. Other factors in the development and manifestation of COPD have not been systematically addressed by behavioral science research for two important reasons. First, risk factors besides smoking for the development of COPD are not clearly established, and suspected risk factors would be difficult to modify. The only other risk factor clearly linked to decline in lung function is the presence of a genetically linked deficiency in $alpha_1$ antitrypsin. Other risk factors that may play a part in abnormal decline include genetically determined secretion of ABH antigen, airways hyperreactivity, familial factors (whether genetic or family aggregation of body habits, atopic status, history of childhood respiratory infections, exposure to occupational irritants), and socioeconomic status (USDHHS, 1984). Although a few of these factors may be modifiable, the specific behaviors that must be changed to reduce them have not been clearly spelled out. Even if the suspected risk factors may be modified, there is no empirical evidence that a reduction in the risk factors can prevent the development of COPD. Thus application of behavioral science techniques cannot be expected to alter the course of COPD significantly once it is established. Progressive pulmonary function decline in the disease is irreversible, and no treatment can be expected to result in a cure.

However, many facets of the disease lend themselves to the application of behavioral science technology and may result in a greater understanding of the disease and its effects, a decrease in symptoms, or an improvement in the quality of life for these patients. The following section in this chapter will review the current literature on the behavioral aspects of lung disease and will make recommendations for future research. The area of smoking research is only briefly mentioned since it is covered more completely elsewhere in this volume (see Chapter 12). However, smoking cessation studies will be reviewed that have been conducted on individuals with COPD or those identified as having specific pulmonary risk factors. Other topics reviewed in this chapter, such as quality of life and neuropsychological status, are also covered more completely in this volume, but herein is presented a summary of the many aspects of COPD that can be described and investigated by behavioral methods. I hope that this review will stimulate more behavioral scientists to apply their methods to lung disease and will encourage the pulmonary community to explore the use of behavioral science research to enhance the treatment of patients with this condition.

II. Impact of the Disease

A. Psychosocial Functioning

Psychosocial issues are an important factor in the total picture of the COPD patient and may exacerbate existing symptoms and decrease compliance with treatment. Dudley (1980; Dudley et al., 1968) was among the first to describe thoroughly the psychological state of the patient and make suggestions to the physician for dealing with the patient's negative feelings. He described the COPD patient as frequently anxious and depressed, with low self-esteem. For patients with few psychological assets such as a vital interest in life, financial resources, and social support, the disease can be devastating. Agle and Baum (1977) noted that male COPD patients exhibit frequent sadness, tearfulness, sense of worthlessness, lack of motivation, loss of sexual activity, excessive body preoccupation, alcoholism, and paranoia. Although exercise is recommended for these patients, they may show a phobic avoidance of activity, for fear of dyspnea. It is possible that the COPD patient experiences an increase in symptoms when he or she experiences extreme states of both action, such as anxiety, anger, or euphoria, and extreme states of inaction such as apathy, depression, and deep relaxation (Dudley, 1980; Dudley et al., 1968).

Impairment of the psychosocial functioning and quality of life of the patient with advanced COPD has been thoroughly described by McSweeny and his colleagues (1980, 1982) with data from the Nocturnal Oxygen Therapy Trial (1980). In this trial, which compared the effects of continuous (24 hr) with nocturnal (12 hr) low-flow oxygen therapy, COPD patients were compared with a group of healthy controls on four dimensions of life quality: emotional function, social role function, daily living activities, and ability to engage in enjoyable hobbies and recreational pasttimes. The COPD patients were impaired in almost all respects. According to the Minnesota Multiphasic Personality Inventory, 42% of the patients were depressed, versus 9% of controls. They were dissatisfied with life and were preoccupied with somatic concerns. The patients were not unusually paranoid or hostile, although some showed evidence of hysteria, hyponchondriasis, and manipulative character disorder. The mood of the COPD patients was tense, depressed, and confused. Recreational activities, home management, sleep, and rest were affected, and the patients were socially withdrawn and somewhat obstreperous. In addition, quality of life was significantly related to severity of disease. This finding is consistent with an observation by Kimbel et al. (1971) that patients with more severe disease have more somatic concerns, depression, and conversion tendencies, all of which decrease their quality of life.

Patients with less severe disease are also impaired in quality of life indices. In a sample of 100 mildly hypoxemic patients in the Intermittent Positive Pressure Breathing Trial (1983), it was found that this group was less physically limited than the NOTT patients, but showed about equal impairment in psychosocial functioning and dysphoric mood, indicating that the degree of psychosocial limitation is not determined directly by the degree of pulmonary disease, once COPD is present (Prigatano et al., 1983).

The potential depth of depression and decreased quality of life are suggested by the number of suicides in one of the NOTT Clinical Centers (Sawyer et al., 1983). Although the numbers are small, of 43 patients in one center, 3 committed suicide, 1 succeeding in a second attempt. In one of the cases, the patient was extremely debilitated and depressed, with chronic neck and back pain, osteoarthritis, arteriosclerosis with angina, gastric ulcer, status postcholecystectomy and oopherectomy. This case presents an example of the frequently occurring presence of concomitant conditions that can exacerbate the effects of COPD.

Dyspnea, or breathlessness, is a major symptom of COPD. Although the sensation of dyspnea may serve a protective function in limiting the strain on respiratory muscles approaching the limits of their force-generating capacity, the symptom itself is an important cause of suffering and disability. However, no treatment for relief of dyspnea has been investigated by physiologists and the current emphasis of research is on the function and performance of respiratory muscles (Altose et al., 1985). Although emotional factors are believed to influence the experience of dyspnea, their role is unclear, as is the relationship between respiratory sensation and behavioral control of breathing.

From previous research, an understanding of the psychological functioning of the COPD patient has evolved. However, many questions are yet unanswered regarding the natural behavioral history of patients with COPD. For example, what are the changes in behavior, quality of life, and lifestyle over time in these patients? Are there environmental and psychosocial mediators of the psychological effects of COPD over time? As recommended in the Report of the Workshop on Lung Disease and Behavior (NHLBI, 1983b), research is needed to assess the variables associated with the decline in psychological state and functioning, which often occurs in stages, in contrast with pulmonary function, which declines gradually. Studies are also needed to investigate the clinical observation that some COPD patients remain active, despite their condition, while others with the same level of pulmonary function are more disabled. Very little is known about the effects of psychosocial stress on the immune system in COPD patients, exacerbations of the disease, and the patient's perception of dyspnea. Finally, psychophysiological studies of the relationship between respiratory sensation and the behavioral control of breathing may be useful in developing approaches to the management of dyspnea.

B. Neuropsychological Functioning

Neuropsychological test performance is impaired in COPD patients, and the dysfunction seems to be roughly correlated with hypoxemia (Grant et al., 1982). In two large clinical trials, the neuropsychological functioning of COPD patients was carefully assessed in relation to all the physiological parameters examined. These studies are reviewed elsewhere in this volume, but a summary will be presented here. The Nocturnal Oxygen Therapy Trial (1980) compared the effects of receiving 12 or 24 hr oxygen on 203 moderately to severely impaired COPD patients. Study patients were aged 35 or older, with a ratio of forced expiratory volume in 1 sec to forced vital capacity (FEV_1/FVC) less than 70% after the inhalation of $beta_2$ agonists with a metered dose inhaler, total lung capacity greater than 80% of normal, and partial pressure of arterial oxygen (PaO_2) greater than 60 mmHg. The mean level of PaO_2 in the population was 51 mmHg, with a mean FEV_1 of 0.74 liters. Neuropsychological assessment by the Halstead-Reitan Test Battery (Grant et al., 1982) and other measures was completed on 74 of the patients and 74 controls matched for age, sex, race, and neighborhood of residence. Results showed that study patients performed significantly worse on virtually all neuropsychologic tests, with 77% of all the COPD patients showing some defects. Moderate to severe impairment, suggestive of cerebral dysfunction, was indicated in 43% of the patients, as compared with 14% of controls. Higher cognitive functioning, that is, abstracting ability and complex perceptual-motor integration, was nore severely affected in the patients, and one-half showed decrements in motor speed, strength, and coordination. The COPD patients were significantly more impaired in their ability to acquire and retain new information, form new concepts and think flexibly, perform complex perceptual motor maneuvers, and engage in simple perceptual discrimination. They were also impaired in motor dexterity, strength, quickness, and grip strength. Patients performed worse than controls in every area of function. However, the authors found no association between neuropsychological defects and any of the pulmonary function or hemodynamic indices. The only physiological measures showing even modest associations were PaO_2, arterial oxygen saturation (SaO_2), oxygen transport, work capacity, and hemoglobin level. These would support the notion that cerebral dysfunction in COPD could be due to insufficient oxygen to the brain. Additional studies by Grant and his colleagues (1986) support this notion.

Patients in a less impaired, ambulatory COPD population were also found to have neuropsychological impairment (Prigatano et al., 1983). In the intermittent Positive Pressure Breathing Trial (1983), home IPPB treatment was compared to treatment with compressor-powered nebulizer as methods for inhaling aerosolized medication. Baseline neuropsychological measurements, including the Halstead-Reiten Neuropsychological Test Battery, were made on 100 of the 985 study patients, and 25 healthy matched controls. Patients in the IPPB group all were between 30 and 74 years, with prebronchodilator FEV_1 of less than 60% of predicted, and the PaO_2 of the patient group was 66 mmHg. Results showed mild neuropsychological impairment in the COPD patients, with overall indices of neurological dysfunction correlated with resisting PaO_2. Patients were impaired in categorization skills, perceptual-motor learning, language functioning, memory, visual reproduction, and paired associate learning. Also impaired were speed of finger tapping, speech-sounds perception, rhythm perception, and basic sensory-perceptual abilities. When the COPD patients were compared to the matched controls, these findings were generally confirmed. When effects of age and education were partialed out, a modest but reliable correlation was found between overall measures of neuropsychological impairment and resting PaO_2. The authors suggested that the level of blood oxygenation plays some role in the degree of neuropsychological impairment of these patients. Depression and motivation could not account for these impairments, since depression accounted for the only 1 or 2% of the variance, and the patients performed adequately on the exercise test, given their individual level of age and education.

Some of the neuropsychological impairment seen in COPD patients may be reversible by long-term low-flow oxygen (Krop et al., 1973). After 4 weeks of oxygen therapy, significant improvement has been observed in some aspects of neuropsychological performance and emotional functioning.

COPD patients are impaired in abstract reasoning, memory, perceptual ability, and speed of performance. The realization of these deficits must be a factor in the increased anxiety and depression often seen in COPD patients. Job requirements, interpersonal relations, and daily activities are more difficult and are additional reminders of the losses of functioning evident in patients with this chronic disease.

Additional research is needed on the effects of decreased neuropsychological functioning on the course of COPD. The extent to which any of these deficits may be reversible with treatment should be studied further. Other topics for future research were enumerated in the Report of the Workshop on Lung Disease and Behavior (NHLBI 1983b) including research on the relationship of emotional status, particularly depression, to neuropsychological functioning. Additional work is needed on the interaction of normal aging, neuropsychological functioning, and COPD. A short screening battery for identifying potential neuropsychological deficiencies in COPD patients also would be useful. Finally, investigation is needed into the influence of neuro- psychological or other psychological factors on adherence to therapeutic regimens.

C. Sexual Functioning

Not surprisingly, sexual functioning is an area affected by COPD. Although there are no definitive data on the presence of sexual dysfunction in COPD, especially among women, male COPD patients have been reported to com- plain frequently when asked of a decrease in sexual interest and ability (Fletcher and Martin, 1982; Kravetz, 1982; Agle and Baum, 1977), although Kass et al. (1972) have attributed sexual dysfunction in COPD patients to marital and psychic conflicts rather than to disease status. Angle and Baum (1977) found that shortness of breath was blamed for the decrease in sexual activity, but there was no direct relationship between physiological impair- ment and degree of interference with sexual performance.

It is likely that, in at least some patients, sexual dysfunction is related to worsening lung function. Fletcher and Martin (1982) studied 20 men aged 46-60 with COPD and found that 7 had completely ceased sexual activity, and the rest were functioning at 16% of premorbid sexual activity levels. It is important to note, however, that the sample was not randomly chosen since some of the subjects were referred because of sexual complaints. Over all, the mean level of activity for the group was 25% of premorbid levels. Nocturnal penile tumescence monitoring showed that six of the men had organogenic erectile impotence. The decrease in sexual activity was also re- lated to worsening lung function, as measured by pulmonary function tests, measurement of blood gases, and exercise tests. Other concomitant condi- tions such as neurovascular function impairment, diabetes, or hormonal dys- function, could not account for the sexual dysfunction.

Anxiety and depression, which often accompany COPD, may play a role in the decreased libido of the COPD patient. For a man who has lost his job, earning power, and his traditional masculine role because of his ill- ness, sexual functioning may represent one of the few remaining roles, and therefore become greater in importance than in the past. Threats to this area of function may exacerbate existing anxieties. Fletcher and Martin (1982) reported that 7 of their 20 subjects showed elevated scores on the hypochondriasis, depression, and hysteria scales of the Minnesota Multiphasic Personality Inventory, indicating abnormally high anxiety and concern over bodily function. The fear of rejection is also an important psychological variable undermining sexual functioning (Kravetz, 1982).

Treatment of the sexual dysfunction of the COPD patient has been limited. Fletcher and Martin (1982) treated some of the dysfunctional COPD patients with corticosteroids, home oxygen, and counseling, reporting that 9 of the 20 patients improved in libido and activity. Kravetz (1982) has outlined specific advice for the physician to give to the patient, and has developed educational materials to go with this advice. The physician should give the patient (1) permission to talk about this sensitive topic, (2) information concerning his condition, and (3) specific suggestions as to ways to make sexual activity more comfortable, such as inhaling a bronchodilator, resting prior to activity, and using positions that require less effort for the patient.

D. Nutrition

Malnutrition may play a role in exacerbating the effects of COPD. There is some evidence of an association between malnutrition and COPD, since a significant proportion of patients experience weight loss, (Oppenbrier et al., 1983; Hunter et al., 1981). Although low weight seems to correlate with poor prognosis (Vandenberg et al., 1967), the reasons for this are not clear. It may be that low weight is simply a marker for severely impaired lung function, which is the primary risk factor for increased morbidity and mortality. Although the reasons for weight reduction in COPD patients may not be understood at this time, it is likely that studies of the patterns of eating behavior in COPD patients will be forthcoming, and interventions may be attempted to increase and maintain certain levels of caloric intake. Behavioral science methods may play an important part in the analysis of eating behavior in these patients and in the possible development of interventions to encourage weight gain in malnourished patients.

III. Management and Rehabilitation

A. Comprehensive Management

Comprehensive management for the COPD patient has been well delineated (Lertzman and Cherniak, 1976; Hodgkin, 1979; Petty, this volume), although measures for the treatment of this condition are not curative. Comprehensive care is comprised of many specific components. These can be separated into those for which the physician is primarily responsible, and those for which the patient is primarily responsible, although the roles for performing these responsibilities are greatly interdependent. The physician's responsibilities include the prescribing of appropriate medications, perhaps including bronchodilators, influenza immunizations, immunotherapy, aggressive treatment of exacerbations and infections, and the provision of low-flow oxygen therapy if appropriate. The physician is also responsible for educating the patient and his or her family regarding care of the COPD condition and addressing psychosocial issues such as patient depression.

Successful management of the disease, however, depends ultimately upon the patient adhering to the physician's recommendations and assuming responsibility for taking many specific actions to control the condition. These specific behaviors are often complicated, perhaps involving extensive changes in life style as well as adhering to the prescribed medication regimen. Respiratory therapy may require the inhalation of a bronchodilator several times a day, and the devices used to deliver aerosols in this procedure must be thoroughly disinfected to prevent growth of bacteria. Patients should avoid smoking and other inhaled irritants, infection, and excessively hot or cold environments. Adequate hydration is necessary, as is proper nutrition to prevent excessive weight loss.

There are several additional behaviors that patients must learn and use regularly in order to participate fully in the management of the condition (Hodgkin, 1979). Learning relaxation may help in relieving anxiety and decreasing compensatory muscle contractions. Biofeedback may be used in this process, although its efficacy in the COPD patient has not been demonstrated. Breathing retraining is useful in the control of dyspnea in that it slows down respiration, increases alveolar ventilation, and decreases the energy cost of breathing through the use of the diaphragm. Chest percussion and postural drainage are useful, as is a regular exercise program. Vocational rehabilitation may be necessary if the patient can no longer perform the tasks required for his job. Finally, weight reduction may be indicated if the patient is obese, since the work of breathing is increased, cough effectiveness is decreased, and spontaneous physical activity is less likely.

B. Rehabilitation

In rehabilitating COPD patients, "the aim of therapy is to prevent progression of the underlying disease and to overcome, insofar as possible, the functional disturbances that are present, thereby lessening symptoms" (Lertzman and

Cherniak, 1976). Rehabilitation programs are useful in encouraging positive changes in functioning, since the psychological condition is improved, adjustment is better, patients are less likely to be hospitalized, and quality of life is improved, although physiological functioning may not be improved. Although there is some disagreement concerning effectiveness (Alkalay, 1977), pulmonary rehabilitation is an established method of care for advanced stages of COPD. The question of survival has not been answered, but there is a suggestion that rehabilitation can improve survival (Petty, 1980).

In one of the earlier reports, Haas and Cardon (1969) monitored 252 male patients for 5 years following a respiratory rehabilitation program. They found that the rate of deterioration in pulmonary function in program participants was no different from the rate in patients not in the program. However, a greater number of program participants were gainfully employed and able to care for themselves, fewer required nursing home care, and mortality due to respiratory failure was less than in patients who did not participate in the program. Improvement in patients' activity level was also found by Fishman and Petty (1971) in an evaluation of a rehabilitation program for 182 patients. The program involved individual and group instruction about the disease and respiratory hygiene, breathing retraining, physiological conditioning, medication, and oxygen for some patients. After 1 year, a subsample of 30 patients demonstrated improved maximum voluntary ventilation and tolerance for walking, and decreased affective distress. Moreover, the pulmonary function of the patients did not decrease over the year, as might be expected. A 10-year follow-up of the entire 182 patients (Sahn et al., 1980) revealed that only 28 (17%) were still living. Although no control group was available for comparison, the authors indicate that these patients showed an improved survival rate compared to other studies being carried out at the time.

Obley and Preiser (1974) reported more striking results in an evaluation of 59 patients followed up for 9 months after a rehabilitation program. The program included training in proper breathing, airway hygiene, respiratory efficiency, exercise, and routine medical management as well as training in life style and diet, hydration, social involvement, environmental control, prevention of infection, and avoidance of stress. The specific interventions in the program are not described. After 9 months, 97% of the participants reported functional improvement, 7 patients (11%) showed increased in pulmonary function of 30% or more, increased daily walking, reduction in the taking of steroids, and decreased hospital admissions. Increases in walking and some functional improvement in patients were also found by White et al. (1979) following a five-session program. Data from both of these studies must be qualified, however, since neither study was controlled. Moreover, Obley and Preiser included no measurement of reversibility of the airflow limitation, and patients with asthma may have been included in this group.

In controlled studies, exercise tolerance generally has been found to increase while pulmonary function does not change. Chester et al. (1977) report a study of 21 COPD patients and 8 controls, in which the trained patients improved in amount of work performed on a treadmill after a 4-week exercise program. No improvement was found in cardiopulmonary function, and the authors speculate that the increase in walking tolerance may be due to increased efficiency in walking and increased motivation. Perhaps the patient also becomes desensitized to the sensation of dyspnea while exercising under controlled and supportive circumstances. Similarly, Mohsenifar et al. (1983) found small but significant reductions in exercise heart rate and blood lactate levels following an exercise and breathing retraining program, while no significant changes in pulmonary function were observed.

In the above described rehabilitation programs, the psychosocial aspects of the program were either not mentioned or described briefly. Several additional authors have specifically mentioned the need for psychological intervention, viewing this intervention as a form of psychotherapy. In addition to advocating a careful evaluation of the patients' psychological status, Miller (1971) recommended that the patient read a book on relaxation. Another early study used an experimental design to examine the effect of a psychological intervention in comparison to the physical rehabilitation intervention. Lustig and co-workers (1972) assigned 45 COPD patients to one of three groups: pulmonary rehabilitation (including exercise, relaxation, breathing training, and postural drainage), psychotherapy, or no treatment. Results indicate that the pulmonary rehabilitation program resulted in an increase in vocational activities, the psychotherapy group improved somewhat in attitude but not in work, and both groups improved psychologically. The authors conclude that all-inclusive programs are needed to assist in COPD rehabilitation. Hughes and Davison (1983), in a review of exercise conditioning in COPD, conclude that the effort to rehabilitate the patient must be comprehensive, and must include the psychological component. It should include (1) the administration of oxygen to prolong survival, increase endurance, and decrease the sensation of dyspnea; (2) administration of drugs such as theophylline and beta$_2$ bronchodilators; (3) intervention with psychological defenses; (4) encouragement of adequate nutrition; and (5) respiratory muscle exercises. The authors consider the psychological aspect of rehabilitation vital to a successful program, but note that it is a poorly understood component.

They question whether "psychotherapy" will prove to be an effective addition to exercise reconditioning and speculate that exercise itself may improve the psychological attitude of patients, perhaps even more than traditional psychotherapy.

In all the aforementioned studies, the rehabilitation program is seen as the treatment, and the effect is later measured by the patient's subsequent ability to walk a certain amount, or to fulfill more activities of daily living, to be hospitalized less, or live longer. However, recent work in behavioral medicine has begun to study the process that intervenes between a medical intervention and the subsequent outcome. Education of the patient may be a part of this process, and patient education regarding COPD has been shown to be successful in increasing knowledge (Black and Mitchell, 1977). However, patient education must recognize another intervening variable: the behavior of the patient, including compliance with medication, following exercise prescription, as well as practicing and using new breathing techniques. All of these play an important part in the effectiveness of the program.

Compliance with treatment is an issue that has received increasing attention in the past decade. It has become increasingly clear that the discrepancy between the therapeutic regimen prescribed by the physician and the actual behavior of the patient relative to his or her health is large. In general, physicians are not aware of the magnitude of their patients' noncompliance and are not good predictors of their patient's behavior. A comprehensive review of 537 original studies (Sackett and Snow, 1981) of compliance has revealed that, although short-term regimens may be followed at a fairly high rate, there may be rapid declines in compliance after the first 10 days of therapy. Rates of compliance with a wide variety of medication for different illnesses tend to converge at approximately 50%. When overuse, underuse, and scheduling errors are combined, the total average error may be as high as 58% (Hulka, 1981).

Various classes of drugs are associated with differing compliance rates, with cardiac and antidiabetic drugs achieving the greatest compliance rates: 89% and 78%, respectively. Antituberculosis drugs show lower rates of about 42%, while studies of adult asthmatics have shown distressingly low levels of compliance. One study of 157 adult asthmatics indicated that 68% had no bronchodilator medication at home, and 24% used an inhaler ineffectively (Avery et al., 1980). Another study of 100 adult patients reported at least 54% noncompliance, with patients underusing and overusing medications, as well as doing both cyclically (Kleiger and Dirks, 1979).

Behavioral science researchers have investigated predictors of compliance in many different diseases (Haynes, 1981). Drawing from this research, it may be predicted that COPD patients will not be good compliers with therapy for several reasons. First COPD is a chronic disease, and adherence to medication generally decreases with time. Second, COPD patients are generally older patients, and may have several other ailments requiring medication. In general, the more prescriptions a patient has, the lower the compliance. Third, hypoxemia in these patients may cause memory deficits that may further complicate the problem of compliance. Fourth, the dyspnea experienced by the COPD patient is a constant symptom, and it has been observed that increasing symptoms may be associated with a decrease in compliance. On the other hand, the degree of the patient's disability may influence compliance in a positive direction, so disabled COPD patients may have more incentive to comply.

Although reliable estimates of compliance of COPD patients are not available, one study has documented the noncompliance of ambulatory COPD patients to a prescribed aerosolized medication. In the intermittent positive pressure breathing (IPPB) trial, patients were instructed to use their machines, either IPPB or compressor-powered nebulizer (CN), to inhale an aerosolized bronchodilator for at least 30 min a day. The patients were followed up with monthly home visits and quarterly clinic visits. Even with such an intensive follow-up, only half of the 985 patients used their machines for more than 25 min a day. Approximately one-fifth of them averaged less than 10 min per day. Patients were equally noncompliant between the IPPB and the CN groups (IPPB Trial Group, 1983).

Several behavioral strategies for improving compliance have been suggested and evaluated in recent years. These include simple reminders around the home, contingency contracting to perform a certain behavior, using a graduated regimen of implementation, self-monitoring, reinforcing compliance behavior, tailoring the intervention to individual needs, and maintaining long-term behavior change through self-reinforcement and social support (Dunbar et al., 1981). These methods have not been used systematically in studies of pulmonary rehabilitation. In fact, only a few studies of rehabilitation in COPD have focused on the patient's compliance behavior as an outcome variable or used behavioral techniques to increase compliance.

Ashikaga and co-wrokers (1980) measured patients' reports of attitudes and behaviors prior to and 4 months after a pulmonary education workshop for COPD patients. After six sessions dealing with medication, nutrition, effective coughing, breathing retraining, relaxation, exercise endurance, respiratory anatomy and physiology, they compared the experimental group with a wait-list control group. The experimental group showed greater knowledge and understanding of COPD, were more ready to take action to help themselves, were more compliant with therapy, and showed increased positive affect. Oddly enough, the control group at 4 months was more optimistic about their chances of improvement as time went by, showed less negative affect, and lower perception of themselves as socially disabled. This unexpected change in perceptions of the control group may be the result of unrealistically high expectations of the benefit of the upcoming program, while in the experimental group a realistic approach to the disease was encouraged. This COPD rehabilitation study is important in that it is the first report that specifically takes into account the patient's knowledge attitudes, and behavior with observed compliance or physical functioning. The inclusion of these patient variables added an important dimension to the rehabilitation literature.

The emphasis on patient behavior in COPD rehabilitation has finally reached the stage of controlled experimentation and observable behavior in recent work using behavioral methods to enhance treatment (Atkins and Kaplan, 1984). Three methods of encouraging exercise in COPD patients were compared. In the behavior modification group, patients were instructed in the use of environmental, situational, and social determinants of behavior and used these to cue and reward themselves for exercising. The cognitive modification group used cognitive restructuring to create and maintain motivation, based on the premise that cognitive change is necessary for long-term behavior change. In this group, patients were instructed to alter their internal dialogues: what they say to themselves in stressful situations. A third group combined behavior modification with cognitive restructuring. Two control groups were included, one received an equivalent amount of attention from the experimenters but no treatment, while the other was a no treatment control. Results indicate that treatment groups walked more than the control groups. The cognitive-behavior modification group walked significantly more than either the cognitive or the behavior modification group alone. No change was seen in the patients' pulmonary function, as measured by FEV_1, blood pressure, or oxygen saturation, which is consistent with other rehabilitation program results. The findings also agree with prevailing notions that exercise tolerance is increased following an exercise program. The combined cognitive-behavior modification group increased 149% in exercise tolerance.

Results of this work have demonstrated that behavioral methods can be useful in increasing compliance to one component of a pulmonary rehabilitation program. Additional research is needed to document the level and patterns of compliance in the COPD population. In addition, research on the process of pulmonary rehabilitation needs to be undertaken, as noted in the Report of the Workshop on Lung Disease and Behavior (NHLBI, 1983b). Randomized controlled evaluations of pulmonary rehabilitation programs are needed as are evaluations of the individual program components generally accepted as useful in rehabilitation. Behavioral research may contribute to increasing compliance with these components as exercise, was increased in the Atkins and Kaplan (1984) study. Methods for increasing medication compliance, use of postural draining, and diaphragmatic breathing would be useful. The role of social support in both families and patient support group needs to be defined; if specific types of social support are found to enhance the process, ways of increasing this adjunct to therapy may be developed. The usefulness of teaching patients skills for coping with the depression and limitaions of activity needs to be investigated. Objective methods are also needed for assessing individual patient compliance behaviors, and ways of encouraging and monitoring long-term behavior change would be useful. Specific smoking-cessation programs for the COPD patient need to be developed, since a surprisingly high proportion of patients continue to smoke. Finally, attention has recently been focused on the underweight nutritional status of many COPD patients. Behavioral science researchers concerned with eating behavior may usefully apply their approaches to the study of eating behavior in COPD.

C. Biofeedback

Biofeedback has been recommended as a possible adjunct to pulmonary rehabilitation (Hodgkin, 1979). It may provide some relief from bronchoconstriction in the COPD patients who have some reversible airway obstruction and may help relieve dyspnea through a reduction in general muscle tension and oxygen consumption. Bronchoconstriction may be influenced by biofeedback in COPD patients, since facial muscle relaxation has been shown to be related to peak expiratory flow rate in controlled trials with asthmatic children (Kotses et al., 1976).

Little biofeedback research has been conducted with COPD patients. In a limited study, muscle tension and anxiety were reduced in a small group of patients given two training sessions 1 week apart (Jones, 1980). No other physiological effects were seen in this short period of time. In a more intensive study of four COPD patients, biofeedback was shown to reduce frontalis muscle tension in three. Improvement was maintained after 6 weeks (Warnock et al., 1980). Although the effect of this biofeedback training was not separated out from the general effects of the pulmonary rehabilitation program, the authors conclude that this treatment is a valuable addition to the program, especially since the patient becomes more actively involved in his or her treatment rather than taking a passive role. More research testing the efficacy of the use of biofeedback as an adjunct to pulmonary rehabilitation is needed, with a long-term follow-up of both psychological and physiological effects.

D. Smoking

Cigarette smoking is the major cause of COPD in the United States, and 80-90% of the COPD in this country can be attributed to cigarette smoking (USDHHS, 1984). In several epidemiologic studies, smoking is the only significant predictor of COPD. In fact, the rate of decline in pulmonary function with increasing age is greater for smokers than for nonsmokers. However, after cessation of smoking, the rate of decline gradually reverts to a more normal rate, although the function that has already been lost is not generally regained. By the time a patient is diagnosed with COPD, a significant amount of lung function has been lost (Fletcher et al., 1976).

If a patient diagnosed with COPD continues to smoke, cessation is recommended in the self-care or rehabilitation regimen. However, rarely do reports of rehabilitation programs discuss smoking cessation advice given to the patient. One must hope and assume that if the practioner or program director were aware of the patient's continued smoking, appropriate advice was given for the patient to quit. Unfortunately, its lack of visibility in rehabilitation reports is probably evidence of a lack of organized attention to this important topic. Perhaps clinicians have given up hope that a COPD patient might quit smoking. Nevertheless, any self-care program should discourage smoking COPD patients from their habits.

The diagnosis of COPD motivates some individuals to quit smoking, but many continue to smoke in spite of this disease. A review of quit rates among pulmonary patients following their physicians' advice indicates quit rates between 15 and 51%, although none of the studies include a no-advice group (USDHHS, 1984). Burns (1969), in a study of 120 COPD patients (94 smokers) coming to the respiratory clinic, found that 47% had given up smoking since the diagnosis was made, 21% reduced their level of intake, and 32% continued to smoke. Daughton et al. (1980) similarly found that 67% of COPD patients had already quit, but 33% were still smoking when they were coming in to the rehabilitation program. Subsequently, 31% of those smokers quit during the program. The IPPB clinical trial likewise found that 40% of its COPD patients were still smoking at baseline. During the study, about 20% of these quit (IPPB Trial Group, 1983).

A smoking cessation program specifically targeted for patients with cardiopulmonary disease has recently been reported by Hall and co-workers (1983) in a small number of patients (11 cardiac and 24 pulmonary patients). The smokers in this initial study received either a health motivation intervention or an aversive smoking intervention. Although the motivation group was 26% abstinent at 26 weeks, compared to 6% for the aversive smoking group, the differences were not significant, due to a differential drop-out rate in the aversive smoking group. Although this study does not give much information on the treatment of choice, it appears that the aversive smoking procedure was so aversive that patients dropped out at an abnormally high rate, indicating that this procedure has a minimal usefulness when applied to COPD patient populations. More research on the process of smoking cessation in COPD patients and the effectiveness of both self-help and formal cessation programs in this population is needed. The usefulness of nicotine gum as an adjunct to instructions in quitting needs to be investigated, since many COPD patients are heavy smokers and may be heavily nicotine-dependent.

E. Early Detection

Pulmonary function gradually declines with age in normal adults (Fletcher et al., 1976; Fletcher and Peto, 1977). Some smokers experience a rate of decline similar to this normal rate. However, other smokers show an abnormally rapid rate of decline, which will progress to the development of COPD and ultimately death is not slowed down by smoking cessation. By the time patients experience breathlessness of a severity that causes them to consult a doctor, the airflow obstruction has reduced FEV_1 to less than 1 liter, or less than half of normal airflow. From that point, the condition usually progresses relentlessly over 5 or more years, with further losses in FEV_1, more disability, and eventually death caused by respiratory failure. Smokers who eventually die of COPD have usually already experienced appreciable loss of pulmonary function in their 40s. Smokers who already show below-normal pulmonary function by early middle age are at greater risk of death from airflow obstruction unless they quit immediately. The FEV_1 and the ratio of FEV_1 to FVC are standard measures for detecting this airflow obstruction and should be used more widely, especially for middle-aged smokers and others exposed to environmental and occupational hazards.

More sensitive tests of early airways disease are also available, but their prediction of later airways disease is not known (Becklake and Permutt, 1979). A method for personalizing risk of developing COPD, called the Tecumseh Index of Risk, has been developed based on a data from the Tecumseh epidemiologic study (Higgins et al., 1982; Higgins and Keller, 1983). By using the individual's age, sex, FEV_1, current smoking habits, and height, one can predict a person's risk of developing COPD in the next ten years. For example, a 51-year-old man who smokes two packs a day and has a FEV_1 of 85% would have about a 1:4 chance of developing airway obstruction in the next 15 years if he continues to smoke. If he quits, he reduces his risk to almost 1:10. Although the Tecumseh Index of Risk has not been tested as a motivating factor in cessation, it may be used in conjunction with routine spirometry and to enhance the effectiveness of smoking counseling at this time. It is generally assumed that smoking cessation for those with abnormally low pulmonary function will be beneficial. No controlled trial has yet been conducted to examine the effects of smoking cessation in those with mild airflow obstruction. However, it is likely that such an intervention would prevent further rapid decline in pulmonary function and thereby prevent the development of COPD.

One trial has been conducted with patients determined to be at risk for cardiopulmonary disorders, based on known cardiac and pulmonary risk factors (Rose and Hamilton, 1978). In this study 1445 high-risk male smokers aged 40-59 were identified. All subjects were given complete medical examinations. Half were given a 15 min counseling session with a physician regarding the hazards of smoking, with advice to quit, and for the other half results of the medical examination were sent to their general practitioners. Results showed that at 1 year, 51% of the intervention group versus 10% of the control group were not smoking. By 3 years, 36% and 14%, respectively, were not smoking. However, these results were not validated with biochemical tests for smoking. Yet rate of decline in the intervention group was 14% slower than in the control group, dyspnea was reduced, even when the respiratory function was the same between the groups, and morning phlegm was reduced by half in the intervention group. Although this study was not specifically targeted to those with reduced pulmonary function, it does indicate that subjects at risk for chronic diseases can be convinced to stop smoking, resulting in a decrease in the rate of decline in pulmonary function. Results of the Multiple Risk Factor Intervention Trial (MRFIT) also show that those individuals at risk for heart disease can be convinced to stop, as evidenced by the 43% quit rate at the end of 1 year in the intervention group, as opposed to a quit rate of 14% in the control group (MRFIT Group, 1982). This increased to 46% and 29%, respectively, at the end of 6 years. Research is needed to determine the effects of such a preventive intervention in those at risk specifically for respiratory diseases. If early intervention is found to be effective in preventing rapid decline in lung function, results of this study have the potential for encouraging widespread national efforts to prevent COPD.

IV. Behavioral Medicine and COPD

In this chapter, recommendations have been made for the application of behavioral science techniques to the study and treatment of COPD. These applications will contribute to the growing body of knowledge of health and behavior known as behavioral medicine. As recently as 1977, behavioral medicine was given its name as a specialized field of research (Schwarts and Weiss, 1977):

> Behavioral medicine is the field concerned with the development of behavioral science knowledge and techniques relevant to the understanding of physical health and illness and the application of this knowledge and these techniques to prevention, diagnosis, treatment, and rehabilitation. Psychosis, neurosis, and substance abuse are included only insofar as they contribute to physical disorders as endpoint.

Since 1977, the field has grown tremendously, with most work conducted in heart disease and cancer. Three things need to happen in order for the study of COPD, and lung disease in general, to receive the benefit of attention by behavioral medicine researchers. First, networks of communication must be established among an array of disciplines not previously well connected, which is a requirement for the development of behavioral medicine in general (Agras, 1982). Behavioral, social, and biomedical scientists must interact with pulmonary medicine researchers to investigate the emerging pathways from basic research to clinical applications. Ways of increasing contact between scientists working in different areas and of transferring information between them need to be developed.

Second, joint research efforts must be developed to study the links between lung disease and behavior. Such joint ventures are not without difficulty. Through its program of Demonstration and Education research (NHLBI 1983a), the National Heart, Lung, and Blood Institute has attempted to stimulate multidisciplinary interventions to prevent and treat diseases of interest to the Institute. However, it has been observed that medical specialists are unaware of the possibilities of behavioral contributions to the prevention and treatment of heart, lung, or blood disease, and behavioral scientists may have simplistic conceptions of the physical processes under study. In addition, investigators in one field have difficulty in judging the expertise and competence of their co-workers in another field. This may result in the choice of a competent collaborator who does not have the expertise necessary, or the choice of a convenient, but inexperienced coinvestigator. This misjudging of qualifications occurs in both directions, with pulmonary researchers and behavioral scientists alike feeling frustrated when peer-reviewed grant applications are not successful. Although these observations have been made concerning the development of interventions, more basic multidisciplinary research may suffer from similar problems.

The third requirement for the development of behavioral medicine related to lung disease is the need for multidisciplinary training programs to encourage young scientists to study the causes, treatment, management, and prevention of lung disease from a number of perspectives. To date, there are no behavioral medicine training programs related to lung disease. The development of such programs will provide a cadre of scientists trained to think broadly about the phenomenon of lung disease. When multidisciplinary teams of researchers apply their techniques to investigating the prevention, early detection, and management of COPD, the quality of life of a significant number of adults may be enhanced.

References

Agle, D. P., and Baum, G. L. (1977). Psychological aspects of chronic obstructive pulmonary disease. *Med. Clin. North Am.* **61**(4):749-757.

Agras, W. S. (1982). Behavioral medicine in the 1980's. *J. Consult. Clin. Psychol.* **50**(6):797-803.

Alkalay, I. (1977). Rehabilitation in chronic obstructive pulmonary disease: myth or reality. *Ann. Allergy* **38**(5):371.

Altose, M., Cherniak, N., and Fishman, A. (1985). Respiratory sensations and dyspnea. *J. Appl. Psychol.* **58**(4):1051-1054.

Ashikaga, T., Vacek, P. M., and Lewis, S. O. (1980). Evaluation of a community based education program for individuals with chronic obstructive pulmonary disease. *J. Rehab.* **280**(6225):1229.

Atkins, C. J., and Kaplan, R. M. (1984). Behavioral programs for exercise compliance in chronic obstructive pulmonary disease. *J. Consult. Clin. Psychol.* **52**:591-603.

Avery, C. H., March, J., and Brook, R. H. (1980). An assessment of the adequacy of self-care by adult asthmatics. *J. Community Health* **5**:167-180.

Becklake, M., and Permutt, S. (1979). Evaluation of tests of lung function for "screening" for early detection of chronic obstructive lung disease. In *The Lung in the Transition Between Health and Disease.* Edited by P. Macklem and S. Permutt. New York, Marcel Dekker.

Black, L. F., and Mitchell, M. M. (1977). Evaluation of a patient education program for chronic obstructive pulmonary disease. *Mayo Clin. Proc.* **52**(2):106-111.

Burns, B. H. (1969). Chronic chest disease, personality, and success in quitting smoking. *Br. J. Prev. Soc. Med.* **23**:23-27.

Chester, E. H., Belman, M. J., Bahler, R. C., Baum, G. L., Shez, G., and Busch, P. (1977). The effect of physical training on cardiopulmonary disease: Multidisciplinary treatment of chronic pulmonary insufficiency. *Chest* **72**(6):695-702.

Daughton, D. M., Fix, A. J., Kass, I., and Patil, K. D. (1980). Smoking cessation among patients with chronic obstructive pulmonary disease. *Addic. Behav.* **5**(2):125-128.

Dudley, D. L. (1980). Psychosocial concomitants to rehabilitation in chronic obstructive pulmonary disease. *Chest* **77**(3):413-420.

Dudley, D., Martin, C. J., and Holmes, T. H. (1968). Dyspnea: psychologic and physiologic observations. *J. Psychosom. Res.* **11**:325-339.

Dunbar, J. M., Marshall, G. D., and Hovell, M. F. (1981). Behavior strategies for improving compliance. In *Compliance in Health Care.* Edited by R. B. Haynes, D. W. Taylor, and D. L. Sackett. Baltimore, Johns Hopkins University Press, pp. 174-190.

Fletcher, C. M., and Peto, R. (1977). The natural history of chronic airflow obstruction. *Br. Med. J.* **1**:1645-1648.

Fletcher, C. M., Peto, R., Tinker, C., and Speizer, F. E. (1976). *The Natural History of Chronic Bronchitis and Emphysema, an Eight-Year Study of Early Chronic Obstructive Lung Disease in Working Men in London.* New York, Oxford, Oxford University Press.

Fletcher, E. C., and Martin, R. J. (1982). Sexual dysfunction and erectile impotence in chronic obstructive pulmonary disease. *Chest* **81**:413-421.

Fishman, D. B., and Petty, T. L. (1971). Physical, symptomatic and psychological improvement in patients receiving comprehensive care for chronic airway obstruction. *J. Chron. Dis.* **24**:775-785.

Grant, I., Heaton, R. K., McSweeny, A. J., Adams, K. M., and Timms, R. M. (1982). Neuropsychologic findings in hypoxemic chronic obstructive pulmonary disease. *Arch. Intern. Med.* **142**:1470-1476.

Grant, I., Prigatano, G. P., Heaton, R. K., McSweeny, A. J., Wright, E. C., and Adams, K. M. (1987). Progressive neuropsychological impairment in relation to hypoxemia in chronic obstructive pulmonary disease. *Arch. Gen. Psychiatry,* in press.

Haas, A., and Cardon, H. (1969). Rehabilitation in chronic obstructive pulmonary disease: a 5-year study of 252 male patients. *Med. Clin. North Am.* **53**:593.

Hall, S., Bachman, J., Henderson, J., Barstow, R., and Jones, R. T. (1983).

Smoking cessation in patients with cardiopulmonary disease: an initial study. *Addic. Behav.* 8:33-42.

Haynes, R. B., (1981). Determinants of compliance. The disease and mechanics of treatment. In *Compliance and Health Care.* Edited by R. B. Haynes, D. W. Taylor, and D. L. Sackett. Baltimore, Johns Hopkins University Press, pp. 49-62.

Higgins, M. W., Keller, J. B., Becker, M., Landis, J. R., Rotman, H., Weg, J. G., and Higgins, I. (1982). An index of risk for obstructive airways disease. *Am. Rev. Respir. Dis.* **125**:144-151.

Higgins, M. W., and Keller, J. B. (1983). Estimating your patient's risk of COPD. How to target your preventive efforts at high risk patients. *J. Respir. Dis.* **4**:97-108.

Hodgkin, J. E. (1979). *Chronic Obstructive Pulmonary Disease: Current concepts in Diagnosis and Comprehensive Care.* Park Ridge, IL, American College of Chest Physicians, pp. 35-83.

Hughes, R. L., and Davison, R. (1983). Limitations of exercise reconditioning in C.O.L.D. *Chest* **2**:241-249.

Hulka, B. S. (1981). Patient-clinician interactions and compliance. In *Compliance and Health Care.* Edited by R. B. Haynes, D. W. Taylor, and D. L. Sackett. Baltimore, John Hopkins University Press, pp. 63-77.

Hunter, A. M. B., Carey, M. A., and Larsh, H. W. (1981). The nutritional status of patients with chronic obstructive pulmonary disease. *Am. Rev. Respir. Dis.* **124**:381.

Intermittent Positive Pressure Breathing Trial Group. (1983). Therapy of chronic obstructive pulmonary disease; a clinical trial. *Ann. Intern. Med.* **99**:612-620.

Jones, J. N. (1980). Selected physiologic and psychologic responses of chronic obstructive pulmonary disease patients to relaxation. *Dissertation Abstr. Int.* **41**(6-B):2121-2122.

Kass, I., Indegraff, K., and Muffly, R. B. (1972). Sex in chronic obstructive pulmonary disease. *Med. Aspects Human Sexuality* **6**:33-42.

Kimbel, P., Kaplan, A. S., Alkalay, I., and Lester, D. (1971). An in hospital program for rehabilitation of patients with chronic obstructive pulmonary disease. *Chest* **60**(2):6-10 (Suppl).

Kleiger, J. H., and Dirks, J. F. (1979). Medication compliance in chronic asthmatic patients. *J. Asthma Res.* **16**:193-196.

Kotses, H., Glaus, K. D., Crawford, P. L., Edwards, J. E., and Scherr, M. (1976). Operant reduction of frontalis EMG activity in the treatment of asthma in children. *J. Psychosom. Res.* **20**:453-459.

Kravetz, H. M. (1982). Sexual counseling for the COPD patient. *Clin. Challenge Cardiopulmon. Med.* 4:1-6.

Krop, H. D., Block, A. J., and Cohen, E. (1973). Neuropsychologic effects of continuous oxygen therapy in chronic obstructive pulmonary disease. *Chest* **64**:317.

Lertzman, M. M., and Cherniak, R. N. (1976). State-of-the-art rehabilitation of patients with chronic obstructive pulmonary disease. *Am. Rev. Respir. Dis.* **114**:1145-1165.

Lustig, F., Haas, A., and Castillo, R. (1972). Clinical and rehabilitation program in patients with chronic obstructive pulmonary disease. *Arch. Phys. Med. Rehab.* **53**:315-322.

McSweeny, A. J., Heaton, R. K., Grant, I. G., Cugell, D., Solliday, N., Petty, T., and Timms, R. (1980). Chronic obstructive pulmonary disease: socioemotional adjustment and life quality. *Chest* **77**(2):309-311 (Suppl.).

McSweeny, A. J., Grant, I., Heaton, R. K., Adams, K., and Timms, R. (1982). Life quality of patients with chronic obstructive pulmonary disease. *Arch. Intern. Med.* **142**:473-479.

Miller, W. (1971). Useful methods of therapy. *Chest* **60**(2):2-5 (Suppl.).

Mohsenifar, Z., Horak, D., Brown, H. V., and Koerner, S. K. (1983). Sensitive indices of improvement in a pulmonary rehabilitation program. *Chest* 2:189-192.

Multiple Risk Factor Intervention Trial Group (1980). Multiple risk factor intervention trial: risk factor changes and mortality results. *J.A.M.A.* **248**:1465-1477.

National Heart, Lung, and Blood Institute (1977). *Respiratory Diseases: Task Force on Prevention, Education, and Control.* Department of Health, Education and Welfare Publication No. (NIH) 77-1248. Washington, D.C., U.S. Government Printing Office.

National Heart, Lung, and Blood Institute (1983a). *Guidelines for Demonstration and Education Research,* 1983. Bethesda, MD, U.S. Department of Health and Human Services, Public Health Service, National Institutes of Health.

National Heart, Lung, and Blood Institute (1983b). *Report of Workshop on Lung Disease and Behavior.* Bethesda, MD, U.S. Department of Health and Human Services, Public Health Service, National Institutes of Health, National Heart, Lung, and Blood Institute, Division of Lung Diseases.

National Heart, Lung, and Blood Institute (1984a). *National Heart, Lung, and Blood Institute Fact Book for Fiscal 1984.* Bethesda, MD, U.S.

Department of Health and Human Services, Public Health Service, National Institutes of Health.

National Heart, Lung, and Blood Institute (1984b). *Tenth Report f the Director, National Heart, Lung, and Blood Institute. Ten Year Review and Five Year Plan, Vol. 3 Lung Diseases.* Bethesda, MD, U.S. Department of Health and Human Services, Public Health Service, National Institutes of Health Publication.

Nocturnal Oxygen Therapy Trial Group (1980). Continuous or nocturnal oxygen therapy in hypoxemic chronic obstructive lung disease: a clinical trial: risk factor changes and mortality results. *Arch. Intern. Med.* **93**: 391-398.

Obley, F. A., and Preiser, F. M. (1974). Comprehensive outpatient respiratory care: a program conducted in a suburban private practice. *J. Am. Gerontol. Soc.* **22**(11):521-524.

Oppenbrier, D. R., Irwin, M. M., Rogers, R. M., Gottlieb, G. P., Dauber, J. H., Van Thiel, D. H., and Pennock, B. E. (1983). Nutritional status and lung function in patients with emphysema and chronic bronchitis. *Chest* **83**: 17-22.

Petty, T. L. (1980). Pulmonary rehabilitation. *Am. Rev. Respir. Dis.* **122**(5): 159-161.

Prigatano, G. D., Parson, O., Wright, E., Levin, D. C., and Hawryluk, G. (1983). Neuropsychological test performance in mildly hypoxemic patients with chronic obstructive pulmonary disease. *J. Consull. Clin. Psychol.* **51**(1): 108-116.

Rose, G., and Hamilton, P. J. S. (1978). A randomized controlled trial of the effect on middle aged men of advice to stop smoking. *J. Epidemiol. Community Health* **32**:275-281.

Sackett, D. L., and Snow, J. (1981). The magnitude of compliance and noncompliance. In *Compliance in Health Care.* Edited by R. B. Haynes, D. W. Taylor, and D. L. Sackett. Baltimore, Johns Hopkins University Press, pp. 11-21.

Sahn, S. S., Nett, L. M., and Petty, T. L. (1980). Ten-year follow up of a comprehensive rehabilitation program for severe COPD. *Chest* **77**(2):311-314.

Sawyer, J. D., Adams, K. M., Conway, W. L., Reeves, J., and Kvale, P. (1983). Survival in cases of chronic obstructive pulmonary disease. *J. Psychiatr. Treat. Eval.* **5**:281-283.

Schwartz, G. E., and Weiss, S. M. (1977). *Proceedings of the Yale Conference on Behavioral Medicine.* U.S. Department of Health, Education, and Welfare Publication No. (NIH) 78-1424. Washington, D.C., U.S. Government Printing Office.

United States Department of Health and Human Services (1984). *Chronic Obstructive Lung Disease. The Health Consequences of Smoking. A Report of the Surgeon General.* DHHS Publication No. 84-2677. Washington, D.C., U.S. Department of Health and Human Services, Public Health Service, Office of the Assistant Secretary for Health, Office of Smoking and Health.

Vandenberg, E., van de Woestigne, and Gyselen, A. (1967). Weight changes in the terminal stages of chronic obstructive pulmonary disease. *Am. Rev. Respir. Dis.* **95**:556-566.

Warnock, J. K., Standard, B., and Mintz, S. I. (1980). Health promotion and maintenance for patients with chronic obstructive pulmonary disease: a review. *J. Chron. Dis.* **33**(1):5-12.

White, B., Andrew, J., Morgan, J., and Downes-Voge, P. (1979). Pulmonary rehabilitation in an ambulatory group practice setting. *Med. Clin. North Am.* **63**(2):379-390.

AUTHOR INDEX

Italic numbers give the page on which the complete reference is listed.

A

Adams, K., 246, 248, *275, 277*
Adams, K. M., 32, *36*, 40, 41,
45, 46, 47, 48, 50, 52, 54,
55, 56, 60, 61, 63, 66, 67,
68, 69, 70, 72, 73, 74, *84*,
100, *102*, 105, 106, 108, 114,
115, 116, 117, *120,* 123, *159,*
281, 282, 283, *299, 301, 302*
Adhozan, D. L., 247, 248, *274*
Adkins, D., 167, *181*
Agle, D. P., 66, 67, *82*
Agras, W. S., 297, *298*
Aickin, M., 186, *234*
Albert, M. L., 40, *55*
Alkalay, I., *273*, 281, 288, *298,
300*
Allen, B. P., 155, *157*
Allison, J. A., 128, *156*
Altose, M., 282, *298*
Anderson, J. P., 137, *156*
Anderson, S. D., 128, *156*

Andrew, J., 288, *303*
Angle, D. P., *273*, 281, 285, *298*
Anthonisen, N. R., 127, *156*
Anthony, W. Z., 41, *55*, 108, *120*
Arand, D. L., 28, *34, 37*
Archer, R. K., 127, 151, *160*
Archibald, C., 127, 150, 151, 153,
159, 160
Armstrong, J. D., 242, *277*
Asher, H. B., 74, *82*
Ashikaga, T., 291, *298*
Astin, T. W., 123, *156*
Atkins, C. J., 125, 126, 148, 152,
156, 158, 161, 292, 293, *298*
Avery, C. H., 290, *298*

B

Bachman, J., 295, *299, 300*
Baekland, F., 250, *273*
Bahler, R. C., 289, *299*
Baile, W. F., Jr., 166, *178*